Instant Clinical Diagnosis in Ophthalmology
Anterior Segment Diseases

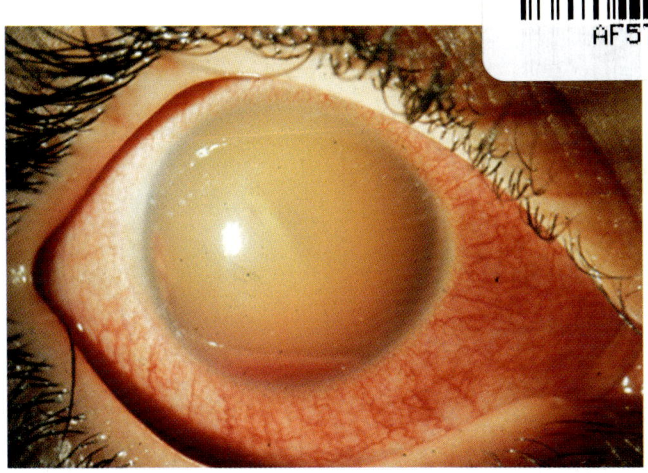

Instant Clinical Diagnosis in Ophthalmology

Anterior Segment Diseases

Series Editors

Ashok Garg
MS PhD FIAO (Bel) FRSM FAIMS ADM FICA
International and National Gold Medalist
Chairman and Medical Director
Garg Eye Institute and Research Centre
235-Model Town, Dabra Chowk
Hisar-125 005 (India)

Emanuel Rosen
MD
Medical Director
Rosen Eye Associates
Harbour City, Salford Quays
M50 3 BH
UK

Editors

Arturo Perez Arteaga
MD
Medical Director
Centro Oftalmologico Tlalnepantla
Dr Perez-Arteaga Vallarta No. 42
Tlalnepantla, Centro Estado de Mexico
54000, Mexico

Ashok Sharma
MD
Medical Director
Dr Ashok Sharma's Corneal
Centre, SCO 833-834 (2nd floor)
Sector 22-A
Chandigarh, India

Foreword

Boris Malyugin

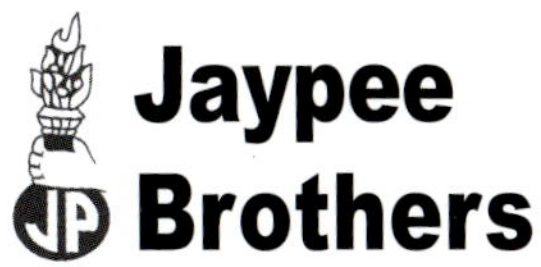

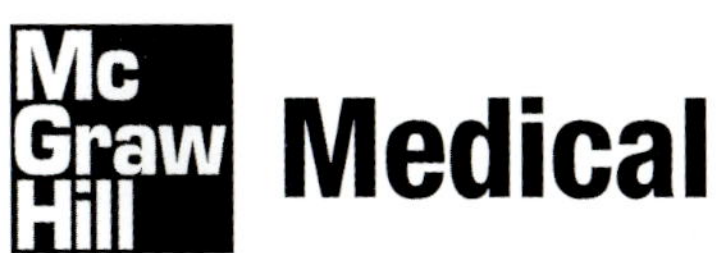

First published in India in 2009 by

Jaypee Brothers Medical Publishers (P) Ltd.

Corporate Office

4838/24 Ansari Road, Daryaganj, **New Delhi** - 110002, India, +91-11-43574357

Registered Office

B-3 EMCA House, 23/23B Ansari Road, Daryaganj, **New Delhi** 110 002, India
Phones: +91-11-23272143, +91-11-23272703, +91-11-23282021,
+91-11-23245672, Rel: +91-11-32558559 Fax: +91-11-23276490, +91-11-23245683
e-mail: jaypee@jaypeebrothers.com, Website: www.jaypeebrothers.com

First published in USA by The McGraw-Hill Companies, 2 Penn Plaza, New York, NY 10121. Exclusively worldwide distributor except South Asia (India, Nepal, Sri Lanka, Bhutan, Pakistan, Bangladesh, Malaysia).

ISBN-13: 978-0-07-166726-5
ISBN-10: 0-07-166726-1

Dedicated to

- My Respected Param Pujya Guru Sant Gurmeet Ram Rahim Singh Ji for his Blessings and Motivation
- My Respected Parents, Teachers, My Wife Dr Aruna Garg, Son Abhishek and Daughter Anshul for their Constant Support and Patience during all these days of Hard Work
- My Dear Friend Dr Amar Agarwal, a Renowned International Ophthalmologist for his Constant Support, Guidance and Expertise

— Ashok Garg

The Memory of My Step Daughter Nicola Ross who Enjoyed Benefits from Refractive Surgery was Cut Short by a Tragic Fatal Illness

— Emanuel Rosen

I dedicate my work to all the people in the world with ophthalmic diseases, with the best wish that we can improve with this kind of material our quality of care. I also dedicate this opus to Prof Ashok Garg, because he has trusted in my work many times

— Arturo Perez Arteaga

I thank my wife Sushma, my sons Rajan and Raghav who graciously allowed me to contribute to this project

— Ashok Sharma

Contributors

Abhiyan Kumar MD
Consultant, Refractive Surgery
Dr. Pattnaik's Laser Eye Institute
New Delhi
India

Anita Panda MD
Professor and Head
Department of Cornea Services
Dr RP Centre for Ophthalmic Sciences
AIIMS
Ansari Nagar
New Delhi 110 029
India

Arif Adenwala MS DNB FRCS ICO
Consultant Ophthalmologist
P. Box No. 457
Zulekha Hospital
Sharjah (UAE)

Arturo Perez Arteaga MD
Medical Director
Centro Oftalmologico Tlalnepantla
Dr Perez-Arteaga Vallarta No. 42
Tlalnepantla, Centro
Estado de Mexico
54000, Mexico

Ashok Garg MS PhD FRSM
Chairman and Medical Director
Garg Eye Institute and Research Centre
235-Model Town
Dabra Chowk
Hisar 125 005
India

Ashok Sharma MD
Director
Dr Ashok Sharma's Corneal Centre
SCO 833-834 (2nd Floor)
Sector 22-A
Chandigarh 160 022
India

Belquiz A Nassaralla MD PhD
Goiania Eye Institute
Department of Cornea and Refractive
Surgery, Goiania
GO
Brazil

David Meyer MB ChB MMed FCoph
Professor and Head
Department of Ophthalmology
Faculty of Health Sciences
University of Stellenbosch
South Africa

Earl R Crouch MD
Eastern Virginia Medical School
880, Kemphsville Road
Suite 2500, Norflock, Virginia 23502
USA

Eric Crouch MD
Assistant Professor of Pediatric
Ophthalmology
Eastern Virginia Medical School
880, Kemphsville Road
Suite 2500, Norflock
Virginia 23502
USA

Eric D Donnenfeld MD FACS
Ophthalmic Consultants of Long Island
Suit 402
2000 North Village Ave
Rockville Centre
NY 11570
USA

Emanuel Rosen MD
Medical Director
Rosen Eye Associates
Harbour City
Salford Quays
M50 - 3 BH
UK

Flavio A Marigo MD
Consultant Ophthalmologist
New York Ophthalmic Oncology
Centre, 5th Floor, 115-East, 61st Street
New York, NY
USA

Geeta Behera MD
Department of Cornea Services
Dr RP Centre for Ophthalmic Sciences
AIIMS
Ansari Nagar
New Delhi 110 029
India

Hala M Elhilaly MD
Profesor of Ophthalmology
Department of Ophthalmology
Cairo University, Cairo
Egypt

Henry D Perry MD FACS
Chief of Corneal Services
Nassau University Medical Center
East Meadow, New York
2000 North Village Ave
Rockville Centre
NY 11570
USA

Hoda M Mostafa MD
Lecturer of Ophthalmology
Department of Ophthalmology
Cairo University
Cairo
Egypt

Joao J Nassaralla MD PhD
Rua L nº 53 # 12º andar, Setro Oeste
Goiania, Goias
Brazil, ZC : 74.120-050

John D Sheppard MD MMSc
Associate Professor of Ophthalmology
Microbiology and Immunology
Clinical Director, Thomas R Lee
Centre for Ocular Pharmacology
Eastern Virginia Medical School
Norfolk, Virginia 23501
USA

Mahesh Dalvi MS
Consultant
Pediatric Ophthalmology
Tejomay Eye Hospital
Kohlapur
Maharashtra
India

Paul T Finger MD
Consultant Ophthalmologist
New York Ophthalmic Oncology
Centre, 5th Floor, 115-East, 61st Street
New York-NY
USA

Rania EI Essawy MD
Department of Ophthalmology
Cairo University
Cairo
Egypt

Sandeep Kumar MD
Associate Professor
Subharati Medical College, Meerut
India

Shibal Bhartiya MD
Pool Officer
Dr RP Centre for Ophthalmic Sciences
AIIMS, Ansari Nagar
New Delhi 110 029
India

Foreword

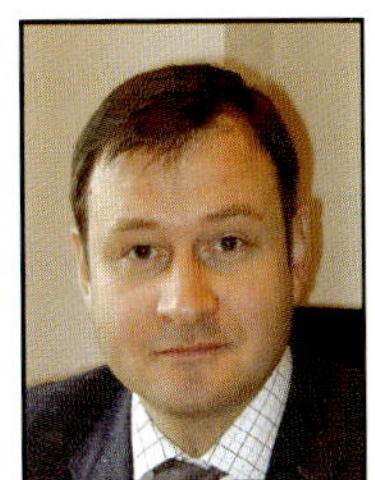

Nowadays we face the dramatic changes in many diagnostic and treatment modalities of the eye anterior segment diseases. New technologies utilizing high frequency ultrasound, wave front analysis, optical coherence tomography and other sophisticated equipment became routine and indispensable tools.

But their availability has not eliminated the need of classical principles of diagnostics and management of ocular pathology and even underscored the role of physician in establishing the correct diagnosis. In many cases the latter can save precious time and allows prescribing the correct and timely treatment.

This book is new, comprehensive and clinically relevant with in-depth focus on anterior segment diseases. Among the latter the authors concentrated on the vital areas of the eye surface abnormalities including pathology of tear film, diseases of conjunctiva, eyelids, cornea and sclera, developmental abnormalities and tumors.

The majority of the book chapters follow the template including: introduction; clinical signs and symptoms; investigations; differential diagnosis; general principles of treatment and prognosis.

This advanced book has a primary goal on presenting the updated guidelines that I consider extremely valuable for the ophthalmologists.

In realization of this ambitious project the works of the editors Dr A Garg and Dr E Rosen and Section Authors have been essential in achieving the goal for it, namely "establishing the instant and correct clinical diagnosis".

Boris Malyugin
MD PhD
Department of Cataract and Implant Surgery, Chief
Deputy Director General
S. Fyodorov Eye Microsurgery Complex State Institution
127486, Beskudnikovsky blvd 59 A
Moscow, Russia.
Tel: +7 (495) 488-8511
Tel/Fax: +7 (495) 905-8051
E-mail: boris.malyugin@gmail.com

Preface

The modern day busy and fast life ophthalmologists are glued to their clinical and surgical practice and have little time to read large volume books. The need of hour is to have pocket size ready recokner enriched with complete and up-to-date information of the diseases in a most comprehensive manner. At present very few Quality Ready Reference books are available at an International level.

After detail research and need of ophthalmologists we have developed a series of 10 Volume Ready Reference Books termed as Instant Clinical Diagnosis in Ophthalmology. This series covers Oculoplastic and Reconstructive Surgery, Retina, Lens, Glaucoma, Refractive Surgery, Pediatric Ophthalmology, Strabismus, Anterior Segment Diseases, Cornea and Neuro-ophthalmology. Present series has been designed to provide up-to-date information of concerned disease in a comprehensive and a lucid manner along with high quality clinical photographs in an easy to read format. International Masters of concerned subject have contributed chapters in this series covering pathophysiology, clinical signs and symptoms, investigations, differential diagnosis, treatment and prognosis in a simplified manner.

Present volume deals with all types of anterior segment diseases specially congenital and developmental anomalies, tear film disorders specially dry eye, various conjunctival and corneal diseases (infectious, inflammatory, neoplastic, degenerative and trauma), sclera and episclera, iris and ciliary body and finally keratoplasty in a comprehensive manner. Anterior segment diseases are clinically very significant specially corneal diseases which are one of the major causes of irreversible blindness worldwide. Proper and intime diagnosis of corneal diseases is very crucial. This volume shall help the ophthalmologists achieve this goal.

We are highly thankful to our publisher M/s Jaypee Brothers Medical Publishers Pvt. Ltd. specially Sh. Jitendar P Vij (CEO), Mr. Tarun Duneja (Director, Publishing) and all staff members for their dedication and hard efforts put in the preparation of High Quality Series of Instant Clinical Books.

We hope this 10 volume set of ready reference pocket size books shall provide complete and useful clinical information to ophthalmologists all around the world and shall help them accurately and precisely diagnose, treat and manage their clinical case confidently to the satisfaction and expectations of their valued patients. We also hope this ready reckoner shall serve as useful companion on to every clinician desk.

Editors

Contents

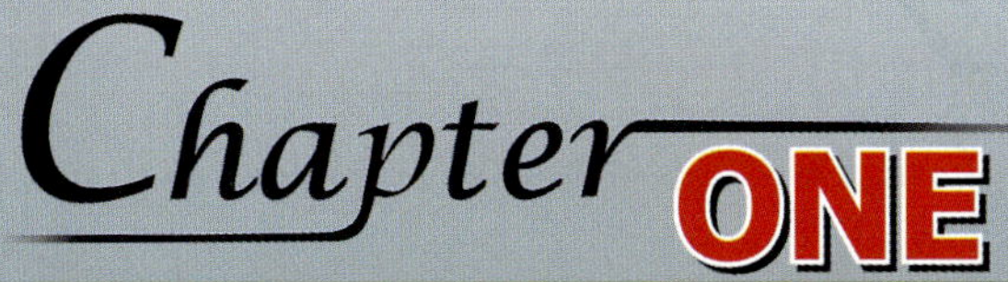

Congenital Anomalies of the Anterior Segment

Hala M Elhilaly
Rania El Essawy
Hoda M Mostafa (Egypt)

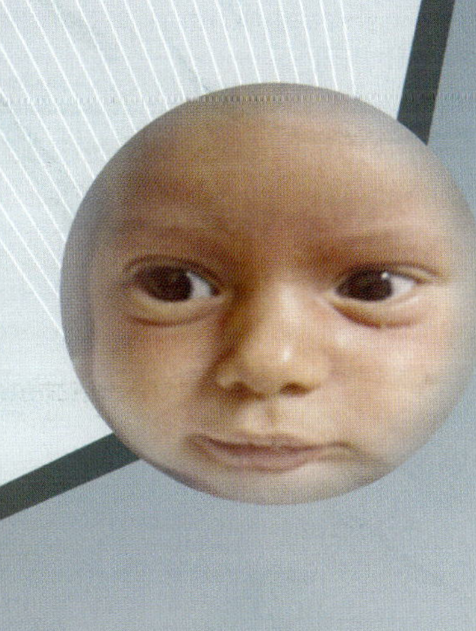

ANOPHTHALMOS/MICROPHTHALMOS

Anophthalmos and Microphthalmos are major congenital structural ocular malformations that occur as a result of insults to the developing eye during the first 8 weeks of gestation. It could be isolated or associated with other congenital anomalies.

Prevalence

The ***prevalence*** of both Anophthalmos and Microphthalmos is estimated to lie between 1 and 3.5 per 10,000 with no predilection to sex or race, however, an increased incidence has been noticed in low socioeconomic societies, and consanguinity is a known predisposing factor.

Anophthalmos is the congenital absence of the globe. True Anophthalmos may be difficult to differentiate both clinically and radiologically from extreme Microphthalmos (clinical Anophthalmos) where a very small globe can only be detected by serial histological sections of the orbital contents.

Mann Classified Anophthalmos into Three Distinct Types

Primary Anophthalmos: caused by failure of development of the optic vesicle from the forebrain before 2 mm stage of embryonic life. It is usually bilateral and sporadic.

Secondary Anophthalmos: an extremely rare and lethal anomaly due to complete suppression or grossly anomalous development of the entire anterior neural tube: the forebrain and its derivatives, the optic vesicles.

Consecutive or degenerative Anophthalmos: occurs when the optic vesicle forms but subsequently degenerates due to insults during the second stage of development: 4-8 weeks of embryonic life.

Anophthalmos is most commonly bilateral, sometimes occurring on one side and Microphthalmos on the opposite side. The orbit and eyelids are formed but small (micro-orbitism and micro-blepharism), the eyelids are shortened in all directions, often with a dystrophic levator muscle, the fornices are shallow, the extraocular muscles are present but may be maldeveloped.

Infants with true bilateral anophthalmia show an absence of the optic nerves and optic chiasma with maldeveloped optic foramina. Lack of properly established connections from the developing eyes to the optic pathways results in hypoplasia or absence of the related white matter tracts and lateral geniculate ganglia. Dysgenesis or absence of the corpus callosum may also be seen suggesting an anomalous formation of the lamina terminalis which is a precursor of the forebrain and the corpus callosum.

Microphthalmos is a condition in which the affected eye is smaller than 15 mm in greatest diameter at birth (normally 16-19 mm), less than 19 mm at 1 year or 22 mm in adulthood.

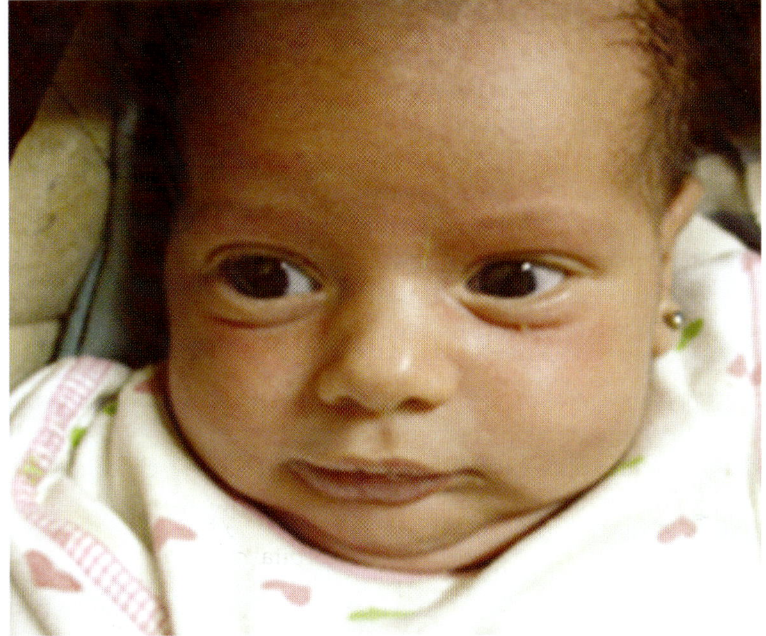

Fig. 1: Left microphthalmos

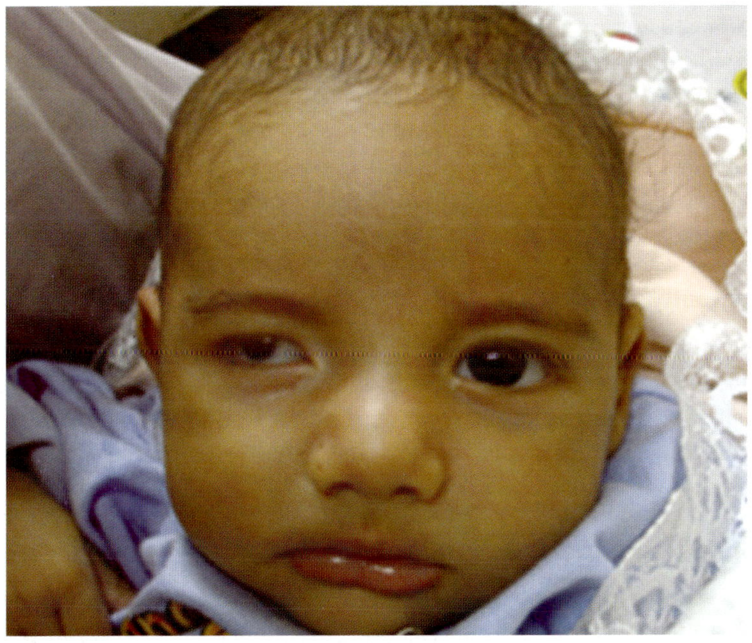

Fig. 2: Right microphthalmos

Microphthalmos occurs between 7 and 14 mm stages of embryonic development when the primary optic vesicle already has invaginated but the fetal cleft (embryonic neuroectodermal fissure) has not closed. It is due to intrauterine involution of the optic vesicle and interference with the normal fusion of that fissure. Three types of microphthalmia are recognized:

Simple Microphthalmos (nanophthalmos) is a very rare form. The eye is small, but normal, with no other gross abnormalities; however the relative lens/eye volume is high making it susceptible to acute and chronic angle closure glaucoma. Also there is hypermetropia, thick sclera and a tendency towards postoperative or even spontaneous uveal effusion and secondary choroidal or retinal detachment.

Microphthalmos associated with other ocular anomalies or more generalized systemic malformations as in congenital Rubella and Trisomy 13. The eye is reduced in size with a microcornea often an iris, ciliary body, choroidal or optic nerve coloboma, and may be corneal opacities, posterior synechiae, cataract or retinal detachment.

Microphthalmos with a cyst (Colobomatous Microphthalmos) where the sclera is thin and ectatic appearing as a cyst of variable size that may grow to become bigger than and obscuring the microphthalmic globe itself. The microphthalmic eye is usually displaced upwards behind the upper lid by a cyst located inferiorly and presenting as a bulge in the lower eyelid. Rarely the cyst is located posteriorly causing proptosis.

Duke Elder described three categories of cysts associated with Microphthalmos: a relatively normal eye with a small cyst not apparent clinically; an obvious cyst associated with a grossly deformed eye; a large cyst which has pushed the globe backwards so, that it is no longer visible clinically. The condition is usually unilateral but frequently the other eye shows the evidence of a coloboma.

Histologically

Histologically there is an eversion of the retina through the unclosed fissure to form a lining of rudimentary neuroectodermal tissue covered with a fibrous outer coat of variable thickness which may be continuous with the sclera but the choroid is absent. The cavity of the cyst is usually in direct continuity with the vitreous cavity and is filled with a clear fluid.

Differential Diagnosis

Differential diagnosis is from *congenital cystic eyeball* where there is failure of invagination of the primary optic vesicle occurring between 2 and 7 mm stage of embryonic development. The orbit shows a cystic structure of a bluish color due to contained fluid and uveal pigment. In some instances, invagination occurs but is incomplete leading to a condition known as *congenital non-attachment of the retina.*

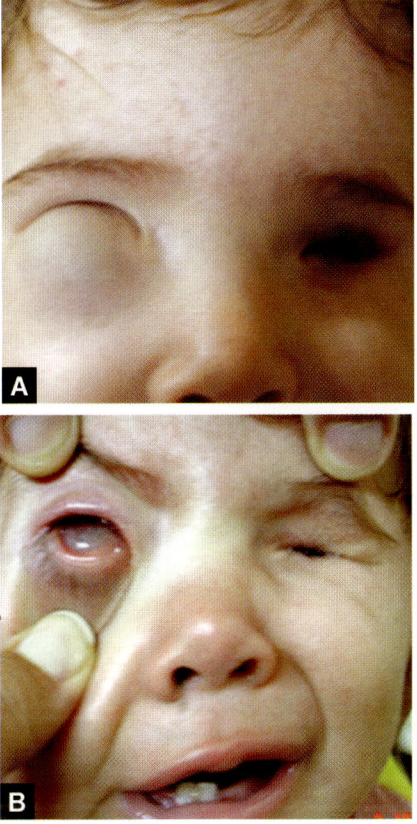

Figs 3A and B: Right microphthalmos with cyst and left clinical anophthalmos

Etiology

Anophthalmos/Microphthalmos may be due to genetic or non-genetic factors that cause the disease to occur in isolation or as a part of a syndrome. All patterns of inheritance are observed: autosomal dominant, autosomal recessive, X-linked dominant and recessive or sporadic. Chromosomal aberrations commonly in the form of trisomy (Trisomy 13, 18 and 22) and deletions may account for 16% of all cases of anophthalmia and microphthalmia. *Non-genetic factors* include maternal exposure to infections as Rubella, Toxoplasma and Cytomegalovirus, influenza and fever. A number of potential environmental teratogens have been proposed including: alcohol, drugs such as thalidomide, retinoids, warfarin, and carbamazepine, vitamin A deficiency, hyperthermia and exposure to X-rays or agricultural pesticides; the evidence in their support however is only preliminary and the condition may result from a variety of different exposures alone or in combination. It is also probable that a background of genetic susceptibility is required.

Ocular and Systemic Associations

The condition may be associated with microcornea, sclerocornea, Peter's anomaly, cataract, persistent fetal vasculature (posterior hyperplastic primary vitreous), iris coloboma, aniridia, choroidal, retinal or optic nerve colobomata. *Systemic Associations* differ according to the syndrome (see table), there may be syndactyly or polydactyly; ear anomalies; nasal anomalies such as a thin pinched nose; orodental anomalies such as thin lips, high arched palate, macrostomia, micrognathia, bifid tongue or delayed eruption of teeth; hypoplastic or ambiguous external genitalia. Also Cardiac anomalies, esophageal atresia and skin defects in the form of hypo or hyperpigmentation. Both cranial and intracranial anomalies may be seen as: microcephaly, hydrocephaly, hemifacial atrophy, facial clefting, hypogenesis of corpus callosum and cerebellar hypoplasia.

CT scan and MRI are of value in:

1. Demonstration of anophthalmia or microphthalmia by showing an absent or a small globe
2. Assessment of associated craniofacial anomalies, and
3. Detection of associated intracranial anomalies.

Management

The management is a challenge especially in cases of anophthalmia and severe microphthalmia. Treatment could be long and complicated with multiple orbital, conjunctival and eyelid reconstruction surgeries required throughout the child's life, and even then results may be disappointing because a perfectly normal-looking orbit will not be achieved. Psychological support for both the parents and the child is necessary.

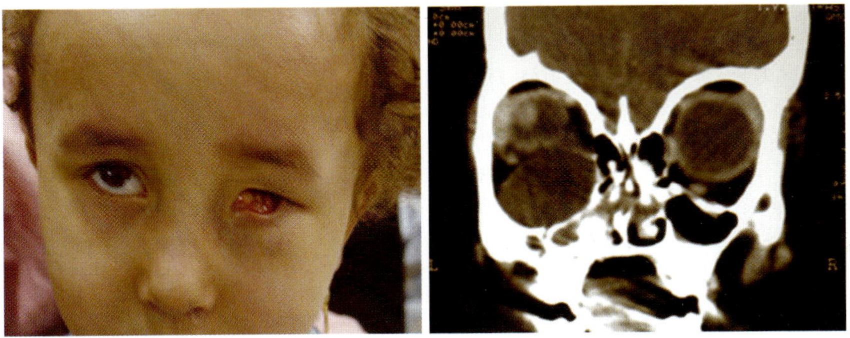

Fig. 4: Left microphthalmia with a cyst and its CT scan appearance

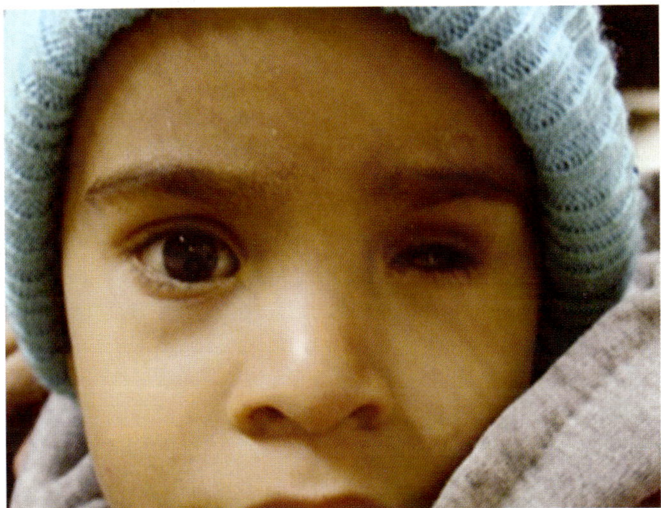

Fig. 5: Left anophthalmia with an artificial eye and a right iris coloboma

Examination and management of other ocular anomalies wherever possible such as associated cataract, exclusion of other system malformations by the pediatrician and genetic counselling when required are all appropriate measures.

The *timing* of surgery differs according to the severity of the condition: early interference is only required in cases of large orbital cysts protruding through the palpebral fissure and in anophthalmia where the results are much better if treatment is initiated in the first year. Recent studies have confirmed that enucleation in childhood compromises orbital growth, cases with small or medium sized cysts with an associated ocular remnant help stimulate orbital expansion better than any artificial orbital implant so, although parents are often keen to have the microphthalmic eye or the cyst removed to improve cosmoses, elective enucleation is better postponed to school age.

Syndrome	*Ocular associations*	*Systemic associations*
Trisomy 13 (Patau's syndrome)	Iris or ciliary body colobomata, cataract, persistent fetal vasculature, corneal dysgenesis, retinal dysplasia	Mental retardation, low set ears, cleft palate, cleft lip, polydactyly, cryptorchidism
Trisomy 18 (Edward's syndrome	Narrow palpebral aperture, ptosis, epicanthus, hypo- or hypertelorism, proptosis, nystagmus, rarely corneal opacities, colobomata, cataract	Mental retardation, low set ears, micrognathia, prominent occipit, narrow pelvis and maybe hip subluxation, flexed overlapping fingers, cardiac and renal anomalies
Lenz microphthalmia syndrome		Mental retardation, malformed ears, skeletal anomalies, urogenital anomalies
Fryns anophthalmia-plus syndrome		Nasal deformity, choanal atresia, bifid uvula, facial cleft
Anophthalmia-esophageal-genital syndrome		Esophageal atresia, cryptorchidism
Fetal rubella syndrome	Corneal opacity, cataract, glaucoma, chorioretinitis,	Deafness, cardiac anomalies
Fetal alcohol syndrome	Short palpebral fissures, ptosis	Microcephaly, cardiac anomalies
CHARGE syndrome	Colobomata most commonly retinal	Cardiac anomalies, choanal atresia, ear anomalies, deafness, genital anomalies
Aicardi syndrome	Chorioretinal lacunae	Infantile spasms, agenesis of corpus callosum
Focal dermal hypoplasia (Golz syndrome)		Skin anomalies, skeletal anomalies, dental anomalies
Microphthalmia and linear skin defect syndrome (MLS)	Sclerocornea, chorioretinal abnormalities	Skin anomalies, agenesis of corpus callosum, hydrocephalus, infantile seizures, mental retardation, cardiac anomalies
Goldenhar syndrome	Epibulbar dermoids, accessory auricular appendages,	Vertebral anomalies
Hallermann-Streiff syndrome	Microcornea, cataract	Mandibular hypoplasia, parrot-beak nose, bird-like facies

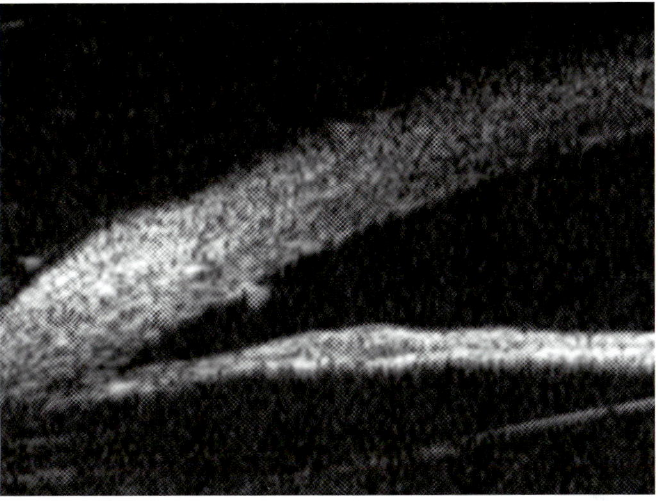

Fig. 6: Posterior embryotoxon may not be easily detected clinically, but with the high resolution of UBM, its detection may be easier (*UBM image courtesy of Z El Sanabary, MD, Cairo University)*

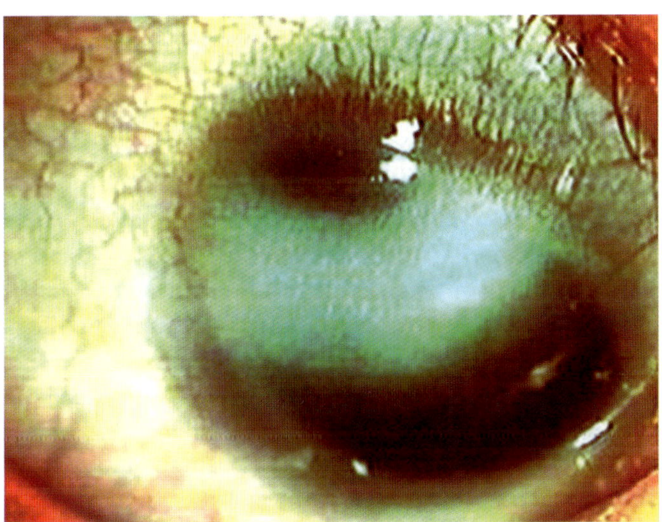

Fig. 7: Color image of a patient with Peter's anomaly

Management of Anophthalmos

Orbital Surgery

Orbital expansion can be achieved by:

1. Progressively increasing the size of a *Solid Conformer*
2. An *Inflatable Silicone Expander* reconstituted with saline through a tube placed at the lateral orbital rim.
3. *Osmotic Tissue Expander* which is a recently introduced self-inflating Hydrogel or HEMMA expander. Once expansion of the orbit and fornices permits, fitting of an ocular prosthesis improves the appearance. More volume enhancement can be achieved by orbital implants when feasible.

In cases of late referral with severe micro-orbitism or insufficient orbital volume, a *three dimensional orbital bone expansion* surgery for the bony orbit with or without bone grafts to augment the deficient contours is needed.

Eyelid Surgery

Fitting of the prosthesis is often limited by the palpebral fissure and eyelid shortening. The palpebral fissure may be widened by a lateral and/or a medial canthotomy or canthoplasty. Additional lengthening of eyelids can be accomplished by a combination of skin, mucosal or cartilage grafts, but this is best postponed until maximum expansion has been achieved by conformer therapy as early treatment may lead to cicatricial tissue formation.

Management of Microphthalmos

Patients with poor orbital volume can achieve very good cosmetic results if treated with conformers as early as possible, microphthalmic eyes with some residual vision can be treated with clear conformers that do not obscure the visual axis, cosmetic scleral shells with optical correction have also been recently introduced. Cysts may be aspirated but this is frequently followed by fluid re-accumulation, in this case surgical excision and orbital implantation is indicated. Silicone, acrylic, hydroxyappatite and other implants may be used but the Dermis fat graft has the advantage of being autogenous and with the ability to enlarge as the child grows.

Anterior Segment Dysgenesis

Anterior segment dysgenesis (ASD) constitutes a spectrum of developmental disorders involving the cornea, angle, iris and lens. It most likely represents an abnormal embryonic development of the cranial neural ectoderm. Many theories on the pathogenesis of ASD have been proposed. A developmental arrest, late in gestation, of certain anterior segment structures derived from neural crest cells is the most likely mechanism. First, abnormal retention of the primordial endothelial layer on the surface of the iris and anterior clamber angle, with

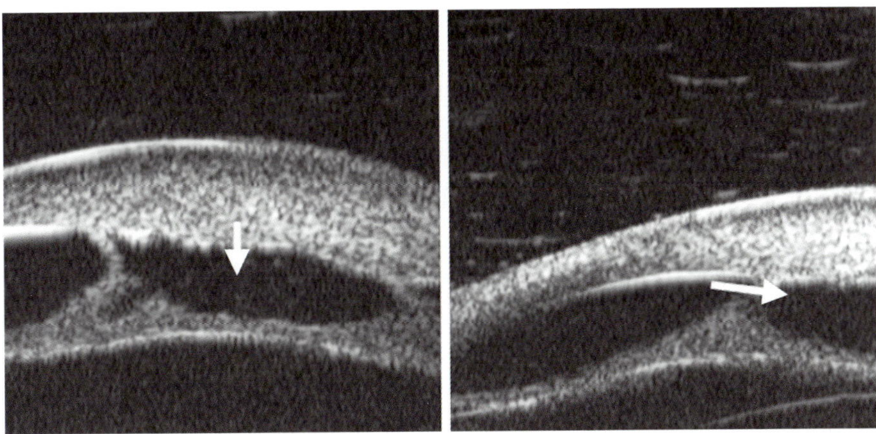

Fig. 8: Typical Peter's anomaly with defective central Descemet's membrane (down arrow) and iridocorneal synechiae at the edges of the defect (right arrow) (*UBM image courtesy of Z El Sanabary, MD, Cairo University)*

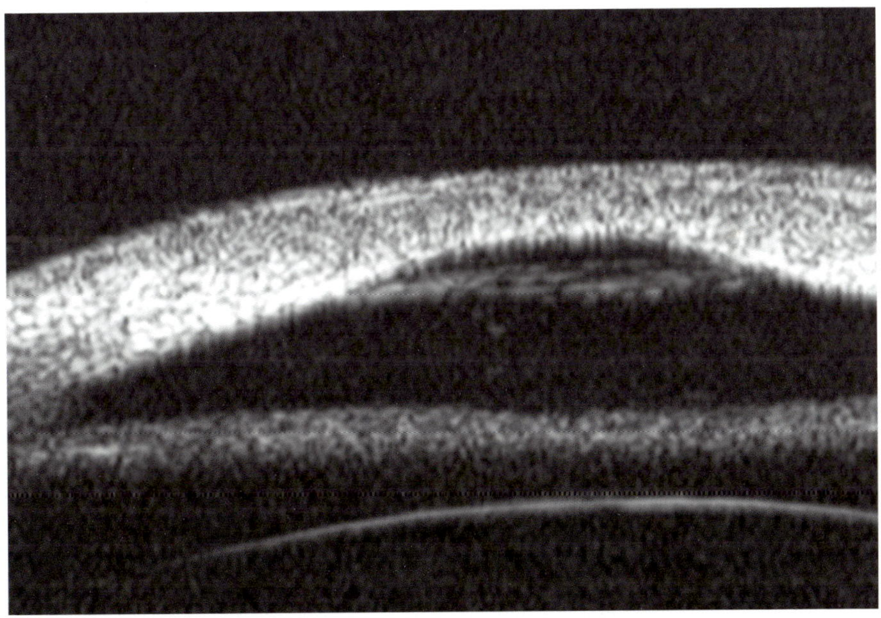

Fig. 9: Variant of Peter's anomaly with poorly developed DM (*UBM image courtesy of Z El Sanabary, MD, Cairo University)*

subsequent contraction, is believed to account for the iris changes and the tissue strands in the anterior clamber angle. Furthermore, deposition of basement membrane by these cells is felt to result in a prominent Schwalbe's line. Secondly, a developmental arrest in the posterior recession of the iris root during the third trimester, results in a high insertion into the posterior aspect of the trabecular meshwork. Lastly, incomplete development of the trabecular meshwork and Schlemm's canal represents further evidence of developmental arrest occurring during the third trimester.

Posterior Embryotoxon

Posterior embryotoxon is a prominent, anteriorly displaced Schwalbe's line. It can be found in up to 15% of normal eyes without any clinical significance or may represent a form fruste of anterior segment dysgenesis .

On slit-lamp examination, it appears as a whitish, irregular arcuate ridge located 0.5 to 2 mm central to the limbus. The majority of posterior embryotoxon is seen temporally and limited to a few clock hours, but in some patients it can be seen for 360 degrees.

Alagille syndrome or arteriohepatic dysplasia is an autosomal dominant condition involving jaundice caused by a developmental scarcity of intrahepatic bile ducts. It has characteristic cardiovascular, skeletal, facial and ocular features. A prominent Schwalbe line occurs in 90% of cases of Alagille's syndrome and is identified as an important marker. Early recognition of the syndrome is helpful in establishing the proper diagnosis to avoid unnecessary abdominal surgery and institute vitamin therapy.

Axenfeld-Rieger Syndrome

The presence of posterior embryotoxon in association with numerous iris processes is known as Axenfeld's anomaly. If there is iris hypoplasia in addition to Axenfeld's anomaly, then the condition is referred to as Rieger's anomaly. If systemic features are present it is referred to as Rieger's syndrome. Many eponyms exist for Axenfeld-Rieger syndrome (ARS) including anterior cleavage syndrome and anterior segment mesodermal dysgenesis disorders.

The historical classification of ARS based on phenotypes has been challenged with the advent of the Human Genome Project and more of the molecular biology mechanisms underlying development are being unravelled. It has now become apparent that ARS shares genotypic and phenotypic overlap with other anterior segment dysgenesis such as iridogoniodysgenesis anomaly, iridogoniodysgenesis syndrome, iris hypoplasia and familial glaucoma iridogoniodysplasia. It has been proposed that all these overlapping groups of conditions should be classified under the umbrella term of ARS to eliminate the confusing sub-classification and to facilitate communication between clinicians.

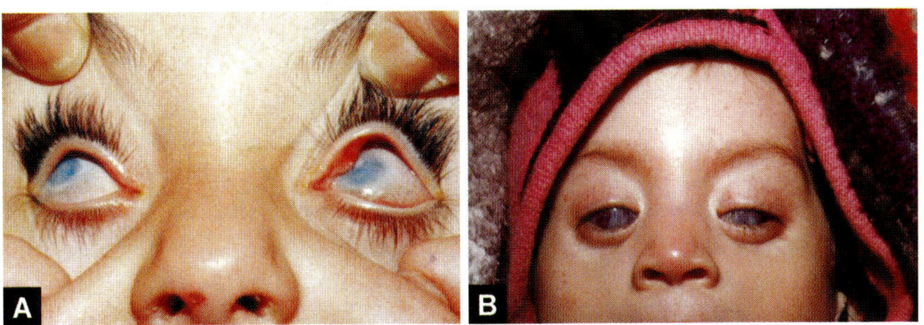

Figs 10A and B: Showing bilateral corneal opacification consistent with sclerocornea

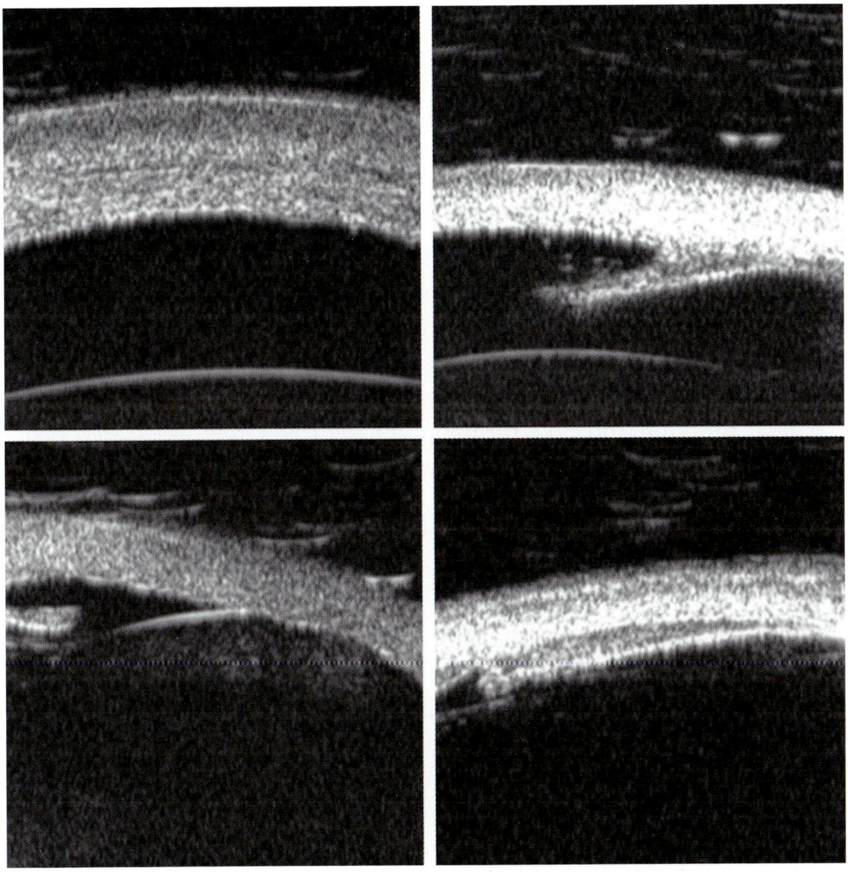

Fig. 11: Sclerocornea with different lenticulo-corneal relationships
(UBM image courtesy of Z El Sanabary,MD, Cairo University)

Axenfeld-Rieger syndrome is inherited in an autosomal dominant pattern. Three chromosomal loci (4q 25, 6p 25, 13q 14) have recently been demonstrated to link to ARS and related phenotypes. The PITX2 gene, on chromosome 4q 25, and the FOXC1 gene, on chromosome 6p 25, have been implicated. These are genes coding for paired-like homeodomain and forkhead/winged-helix transcription-factor families. Mutation in DNA binding domain of these genes can cause a wide variety of phenotypes that share features with ARS. Mutation resulting in increased PITX2 activity has been found to correlate with more severe ARS ocular phenotype. A plyomorphism in the GJA1 gene has been recently identified in association with ARS and raises the possibility of its participation as a modifier gene.

In ARS, gonioscopic examination reveals that the anterior chamber angle is open and the trabecular meshwork is visible, but the scleral spur is obscured by the more anterior insertion of the peripheral iris into the posterior portion of the trabecular meshwork.

In Rieger's anomaly, iris pathology can range from mild stromal thinning (iris hypoplasia) to marked atrophy with hole formation, corectopia and ectropion uvea. When corectopia is present, the pupil is displaced towards a prominent peripheral iridocorneal adhesion; the atrophy and hole formation occurs in the quadrant away from the direction of the pupil.

Abnormalities of the anterior chamber angle do not appear to progress after birth except for occasional thickening of iris strands. Abnormalities of the central iris are usually stable, but have been observed to progress during the first years of life. These changes consist of distortion or displacement of the pupil and occasional thinning and hole formation of the iris. Other associated ocular anomalies include sclerocornea, persistent pupillary membrane, microphthalmus and typical iris coloboma.

Glaucoma develops in 50 to 60% of patients with ARS. It may manifest itself during infancy but more commonly appears in childhood or young adulthood. Glaucoma is felt to occur more often in patients with centric iridic changes and in those with more pronounced anterior peripheral iris insertion into the trabecular meshwork.

Rieger's syndrome is associated with many systemic anomalies, in particular, those involving developmental defects of the teeth and facial bones. Dental defects may include a reduction in crown size (microdontia), a decreased but evenly spaced number of teeth (hypodontia), and a focal absence of teeth (oligodontia or anodontia). Facial anomalies may include maxillary hypoplasia with flattening of the midface and a receding upper lip and prominent lower lip. Hypertelorism, telecanthus, and broad flat nose have also been described.

Other non-ocular associations of ARS include congenital lip abnormalities, hydrocephalus, empty sella syndrome, middle ear deafness, kidney abnormalities, hypospadias, umbilical skin folds and heart defects. There is considerable variation in non-ocular features, even among family members with ARS.

All associated ocular and systemic anomalies appear to arise from the maldevelopment of the neural crest cells. Patients with ARS should be examined for the presence of anomalies in the tissues of neural crest origin.

Management of glaucoma in patients with Axenfeld-Rieger syndrome is difficult. Medications, particularly aqueous humor suppressants may be effective, although many patients will require surgery. Goniotomy is reported to be effective in some younger patients, but this procedure can be complicated by extensive iris processes and should probably be avoided in patients with large areas of contact between the iris and cornea. Trabeculotomy, too has a high risk for substantial bleeding, endothelial cell damage, and inflammation in eyes with thick iridocorneal adhesions. Some authors believe that filtering surgery with anti-metabolites is the best surgical procedure for these patients. Eyes that fail trabeculectomy may require an aqueous shunt, or ultimately diode cyclophotocoagulation.

Peters Anomaly

Peter's anomaly is a congenital, mostly bilateral condition in which a central corneal opacity is present with corresponding defects in the posterior corneal stroma, Descemet's membrane and endothelium. The condition is usually sporadic, although autosomal recessive and autosomal dominant transmission both have been reported. Approximately, 50% of patients will have associated glaucoma. Some cases can have the peripheral anterior chamber angle abnormalities of Axenfeld-Rieger syndrome since they are both defects of neural crest cell origin which may lead to diagnostic confusion.

Peter's anomaly is often classified into three groups: (i) posterior corneal defect with leucoma alone; (ii) posterior corneal defect with leucoma and adherent iris strands and (iii) posterior corneal defect with leucoma, adherent iris strands, and keratolenticular contact or cataract.

The corneal opacity in Peter's anomaly is usually central, oval and well-defined, but it may sectorial and have diffuse margins. The affected cornea is rarely vascularized and the peripheral cornea is usually clear although scleralization of the limbus may occur in Peter's anomaly type II, the lens either lies in juxtaposition to the corneal surface or is in normal position with an intact surface but cataract is present. In contrast to the first two forms of Peter's anomaly, the last variant may occur in eyes with microphthalmia, persistent hyperplastic primary vitreous (PHPV) and retinal dysplasia.

Peter's plus syndrome is a multiple malformation syndrome characterized by a combination of Peter's anomaly of the eye and other extraocular defects, including short-limb dwarfism, a thin upper lip, hypoplastic columella, and a round face. Hypothyroidism, multiple midline defects such as cleft lip and palate, cardiac anomalies, an atretic cranial meningocele as well as malformations of the ear have also been reported.

Histopathology

Histopathology in Peter's anomaly shows an abnormal, immature or absent Descemet's membrane and attenuated, endothelial cells in the area of the corneal opacity, in addition to thinning or even complete absence of Bowman's membrane. It has been suggested that there is failure of the normal differentiation of the mesoderm into normal endothelium and trabecular meshwork.

Differential Diagnosis

Differential diagnosis of Peters anomaly includes causes of corneal opacities that may be seen in children. These include sclerocornea, where the entire cornea is opacified, aniridia, trauma associated with forceps delivery during birth, congenital glaucoma, mucopolysacharidoses, congenital hereditary endothelial dystrophy (CHED) and a perforated corneal ulcer.

Ultrasound Biomicroscopy

Ultrasound biomicroscopy (UBM) has proved to be useful in confirming the diagnosis of Peter's anomaly. It also acts as a preoperative guide in cases undergoing penetrating keratoplasty by detecting keratolenticular and iridocorneal adhesions.

Management of Peter's anomaly primarily relies on controlling glaucoma, when present and preventing amblyopia. Detection of glaucoma is complicated by the corneal opacity, which affects the accuracy of tonometry and obscures the clinician's view of the anterior chamber angle and optic nerve head. Although some cases may respond to medical management, many cases ultimately may require filtering surgery. Multiple procedures and adjunctive medical therapy are often required to achieve and maintain adequate IOP control. Visual results are poor due to uncontrolled glaucoma, amblyopia, and other anterior and posterior segment anomalies that may accompany Peter's anomaly. Patients undergoing keratoplasty after adequate pressure control are reported to have long-term graft clarity in 36% of cases.

Sclerocornea

Sclerocornea is one of the common causes of corneal clouding or opacification in the newborn. It presents at birth by non-progressive, non-inflammatory opacification of the peripheral and to a lesser degree the central cornea with vascularisation. Despite its characteristic presentation it should be differentiated from other pathologies such as congenital glaucoma, trauma, infectious diseases, dystrophies, metabolic causes and other forms of ocular dysgenesis.

The sclera and choroid develop from mesenchymal tissue of neural crest origin. Sclerocornea results from mesenchymal dysgenesis leading to anomalous development of this portion of the anterior segment. It has been suggested that the wave of mesenchymal tissue that normally forms the corneal stroma fails to form the clear cornea and forms tissue resembling sclera instead. This wave of tissue remains as homogenous sheets throughout the 7th–10th week of gestation until the limbal anlage develops. Failure of the limbal anlage to develop or its central displacement may be responsible for various forms of sclerocornea.

Most cases are sporadic however inheritance patterns have been demonstrated. Autosomal dominant patterns as well as autosomal recessive traits have been reported. Cases with an autosomal dominant pattern are invariably less severe.

Sclerocornea is usually bilateral and affects male and female newborns equally. Sclerocornea presents in a newborn with opacification of the peripheral cornea with vasculariziation. Although the axial portion of the cornea may also be involved to a varying degree, the peripheral opacification is usually denser. The limbus is indistinct and blends with the surrounding sclera. Some cases may present with involvement of only a small arc at the periphery. Where relatively clear cornea is present it is invariably flatter than normal. Accurate visualization of the anterior segment is often hindered by the opaque cornea. It should be noted that in cases of total sclerocornea the relative clarity of the central cornea as compared to the periphery can be important in differentiating sclerocornea from Peter's anomaly.

Histologically

Histologically there is thickened collagen fibers in the superficial stroma of the cornea as compared to the posterior stroma. This is a pattern similar to that seen in the sclera. Recent evidence however suggests that sulphation patterns of interfibrillar keratan sulphate proteoglycan within the tissue matrix may resemble cornea rather than sclera as previously postulated.

Ultrasound Biomicroscopy

Ultrasound Biomicroscopy (UBM) has proven to be a vital tool in assessing the nature and extent of structural defects as well as confirming the presence of associated anterior segment anomalies in cases of sclerocornea thus aiding in the surgical decision making process.

Differential Diagnosis

Differential diagnosis of sclerocornea is that of causes of a cloudy cornea in a newborn, this includes infantile glaucoma, forceps injury, congenital hereditary endothelial dystrophy, congenital rubella, and congenital syphilis. Other conditions presenting with corneal opacities such as Peter's anomaly, congenital hereditary stromal dystrophy, mucopolysaccharidosis, mucolipidosis and cystinosis may also be confused with sclerocornea.

Laterality, intraocular pressure and associated findings will usually aid in determining the pathology underlying the corneal opacification. However, although many of these entities may seem quite different, the various degrees of affection in sclerocornea may sometimes make an accurate diagnosis difficult. UBM is a useful tool in such cases.

Ocular associations may commonly be encountered in cases of sclerocornea. microphthalmia, iris anomalies, anterior chamber irregularities have been documented in cases of sclerocornea. UBM has dramatically improved the clinician's ability to diagnose associated ocular anomalies which may not be readily diagnosed by routine anterior segment examination.

Systemic associations may be encountered in cases of sclerocornea such as skeletal anomalies, various cerebellar, cranial and cardiac anomalies.

Sclerocornea may also present as part of the a documented syndrome such as the MIDAS **(microphthalmia-dermal aplasia-sclerocornea)** syndrome. This syndrome is synonymous with the microphthalmia with linear skin defects (MLS) syndrome. This syndrome includes linear areas of erythematous skin dysplasia involving the chin, neck, and head, occurring in association with microphthalmia, corneal opacities, and orbital cysts. Additional findings may include agenesis of corpus callosum, sclerocornea, chorioretinal abnormalities, hydrocephalus, seizures, mental retardation, and nail dystrophy. Some features of the phenotype of this syndrome overlap those of Aicardi and Goltz syndromes.

As with the majority of congenital corneal opacities the ultimate aim in the absence of extensive associated ocular anomalies is to clear the visual axis by performing a penetrating keratoplasty. Associated conditions such as anterior segment anomalies and glaucoma must also be addressed. The timing of this intervention is a debatable issue however in most cases a single or sometimes multiple keratoplasties are indicated to prevent deprivation amblyopia.

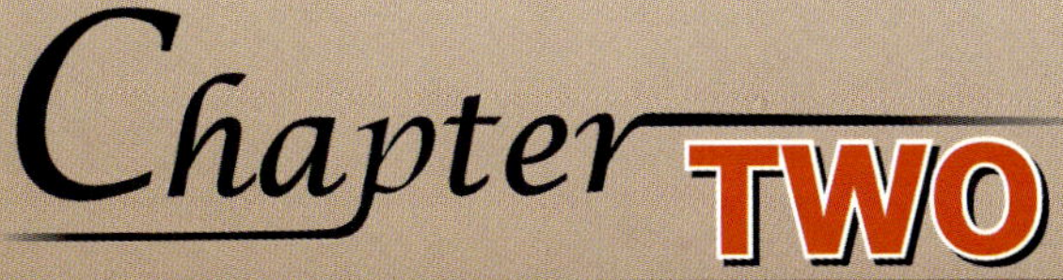

Developmental Abnormalities

Arturo Perez Arteaga (Mexico)

- Axenfeld Rieger Syndrome
- Peters Anomaly
- Aniridia

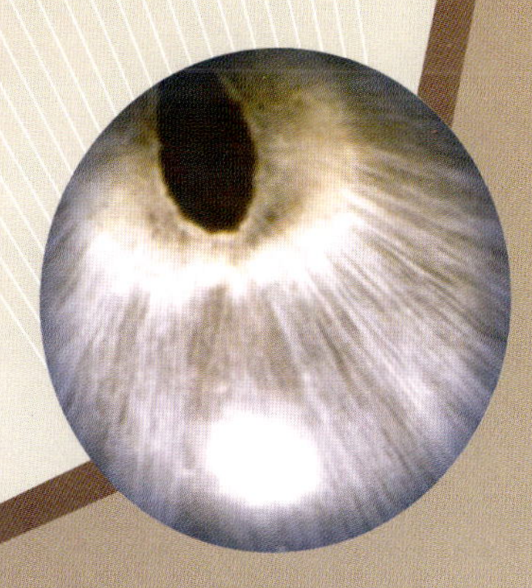

AXENFELD RIEGER SYNDROME

Introduction

Rieger syndrome is an autosomal dominant disorder of morphogenesis that leads to abnormal development of the anterior segment of the eye, and results in blindness primarily from glaucoma in almost 50% of cases. Systemic anomalies associated are dental hypoplasia, failure of involution of periumbilical skin, and maxillary hypoplasia. Historically, this condition was classified under the broader heading of anterior chamber cleavage syndromes that includes Axenfeld's anomaly, Axenfeld's syndrome, Rieger's anomaly, and Rieger's syndrome. Current theory now holds that these conditions are probably a continuum of a single developmental disorder, hence the name Axenfeld-Rieger syndrome.

Clinical Signs and Symptoms

Patients displaying Axenfeld-Rieger syndrome are generally asymptomatic. The condition is diagnosed based upon findings from routine biomicroscopic and gonioscopic evaluation; many times the ophthalmologist is a consultant. The clinical feature of this anterior segment disorder is posterior embryotoxon (a prominent, anteriorly displaced Schwalbe's line) and one or more of the following findings: iris strands adherent to Schwalbe's line, iris hypoplasia, focal iris atrophy with hole formation, corectopia, and ectropion uveae. Glaucoma may develop in approximately 50 percent of patients with A-R syndrome, but is more common in those with central iris changes and pronounced anterior iris insertion. Systemic manifestations of A-R syndrome may include developmental defects of the teeth and facial bones, pituitary anomalies, cardiac disease, oculocutaneous albinism, and redundant periumbilical skin. A-R syndrome is always bilateral but many times asymmetric.

Investigations

There has been much speculation as to the embryonic pathogenesis of A-R syndrome but there's an amply confirmation about its autosomal dominant inheritance. The current and most widely held theory suggests a developmental arrest of specific anterior segment tissues derived from neural crest cells, which apparently occurs late in gestation. It is not understood why such a developmental arrest occurs, but the result is the retention of a primordial endothelial cell layer on portions of the iris and angle structures. Contraction of these endothelial "membranes" leads to the associated abnormalities in form and function of the anterior segment structures. Presumably, this same developmental arrest can affect other organ systems, resulting in orofacial and other anomalies sometimes encountered in A-R syndrome.

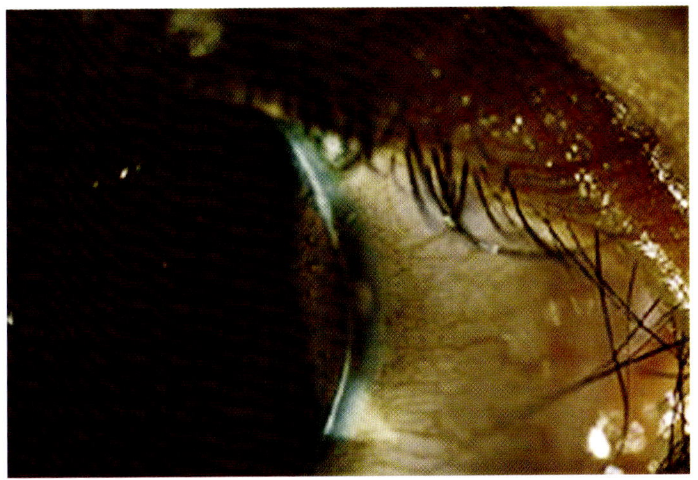

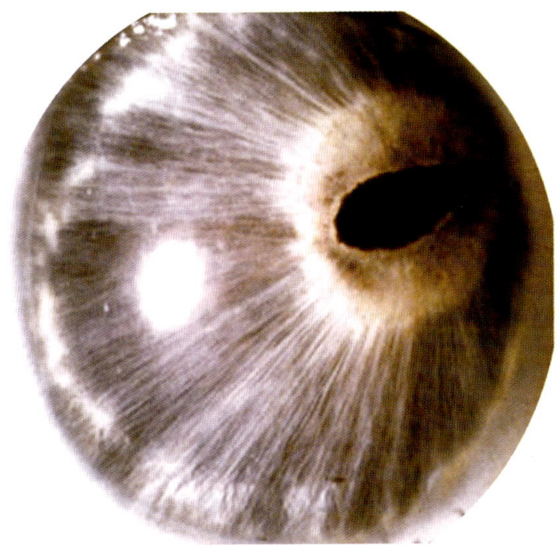

Figs 1 and 2: Axenfeld Rieger syndrome

Differential Diagnosis

Axenfeld-Rieger syndrome is described as a rare, congenital ocular disorder. Still, some authors have found many patients with manifestations of A-R syndrome, some of which are not characteristic. In general, A-R syndrome is more academically interesting than it is clinically challenging. Glaucoma must be a concern in every patient presenting with this disorder. In fact, when glaucoma does occur, it can be quite severe. In addition, patients with A-R syndrome should undergo both a comprehensive medical and dental evaluation to rule out non-ocular manifestations.

Treatment

A-R syndrome, a congenital disorder, generally requires little therapeutic intervention. In those instances where iris atrophy results in pseudopolycoria, patients may be fitted with opaque, cosmetic contact lenses to improve their appearance and decrease optical aberrations; also interventions for corectopia can be performed. The greatest concern in patients with A-R syndrome is the development of secondary glaucoma; patients must be monitored throughout life for elevations in intraocular pressure and optic nerve head changes. Glaucoma therapy follows the same regimen as for primary open angle glaucoma; typical therapy begins with topical -blockers (e.g. Betoptic-S) or topical carbonic anhydrase inhibitors (e.g. Azopt). Unfortunately, many of these glaucoma cases become recalcitrant, and glaucoma surgical intervention is often necessary but not frequently successful.

Prognosis

Blindness from glaucoma affects approximately 50% of individuals. Because of the known inheritance pattern and variable expression, recommend ocular evaluation for all family members when you detect A-R syndrome.

Peters Anomaly

Introduction

Peters anomaly was first described in 1906 by Dr Alfred Peters. The anomaly affects the eyes of people of both genders and from all ethnic groups. Peters anomaly is a developmental error occurring during pregnancy (10-16 weeks). It consists of a central corneal leukoma, absence of the posterior corneal stroma and descemet membrane, and a variable degree of iris and lenticular attachments to the central aspect of the posterior cornea (anterior sinechia). It occurs as an isolated ocular abnormality or in association with other ocular defects like cataract and microcornea.

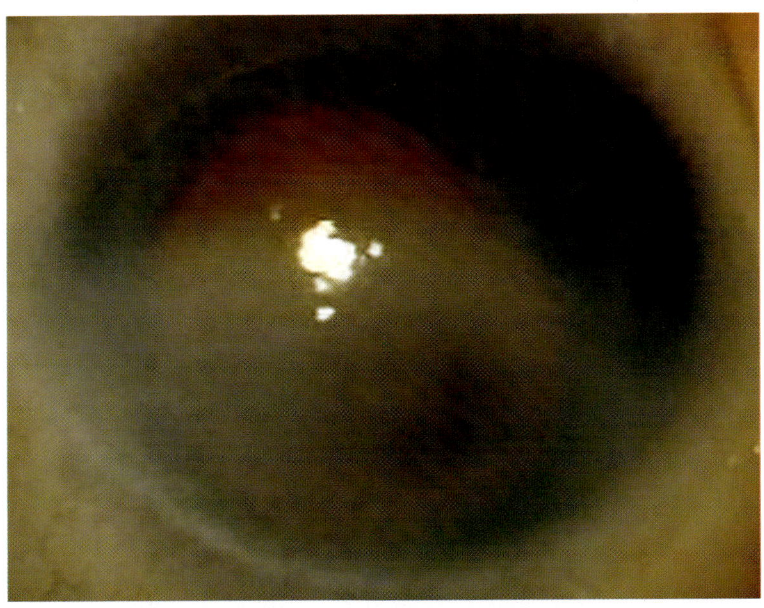

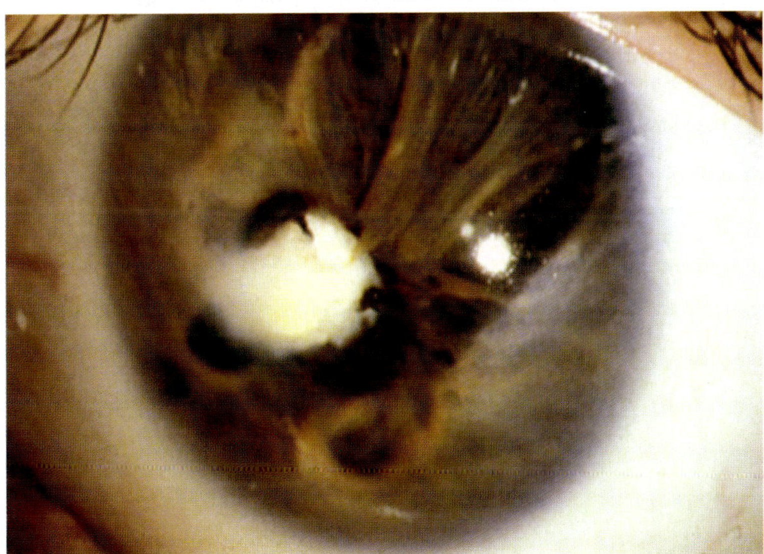

Figs 3 and 4: Peters anomaly

Clinical Signs and Symptoms

Corneal opacity is always present; it can be central, paracentral, or complete. Usually, no vascularization of this opacity occurs; this data is helpful in distinguish it from other causes of congenital corneal opacity. Some investigators have classified Peters anomaly in two groups:

- Type 1: Only 80% of the cases are bilateral. There is not a complete corneal opacity; there is only a central or paracentral annular opacity. The surrounding peripheral cornea may be clear or edematous because of glaucoma. The opacity is caused by a defect in the underlying corneal endothelium and the Descemet membrane.
- Type 2: Almost all cases are bilateral. The corneal opacity is denser and can be either central or eccentric. The lens is usually cataractous. The posterior stroma, the Descemet membrane, and the endothelium are defective.
- Other ocular abnormalities are microcornea, cornea plana, sclerocornea aniridia, and glaucoma due to dysgenesis of the angle. Glaucoma occurs in up to 90% of cases. Colobomas of the iris and choroid and optic nerve hypoplasia or atrophy also can occur.

Systemic associations in Peters anomaly include developmental delay, congenital heart disease, structural defects of the neurologic system, spinal defects, genitourinary abnormalities, external ear abnormalities, hearing loss, cleft lip and palate, and short stature.

Investigations

Peters anomaly can be caused by mutations in the PAX6 gene, the PITX2 gene, the CYP1B1 gene, or the FOXC1 gene. In a family with dominantly inherited anterior segment malformations with variable expression, including typical Peters anomaly the investigators identified a mutation in the PAX6 gene.

Differential Diagnosis

Intrauterine keratitis, mucopolysaccharidoses, congenital hereditary endothelial dystrophy, corneal dermoids, congenital hereditary endothelial dystrophy and posterior polymorphous dystrophy.

Treatment

The systemic treatments include a thorough physical examination by a pediatrician and genetic counseling. The ocular treatment includes in first line, glaucoma treatment, because is the main cause of visual loss in these cases. Surgery might be indicated according the particular case: if a clear peripheral cornea exist, a peripheral optical iridectomy can be useful for glaucoma prevention and improve of vision; if bilateral visually corneal opacity exist, the penetrating keratoplasty is recommended in order to prevent amblyopia; the earlier is performed, the better.

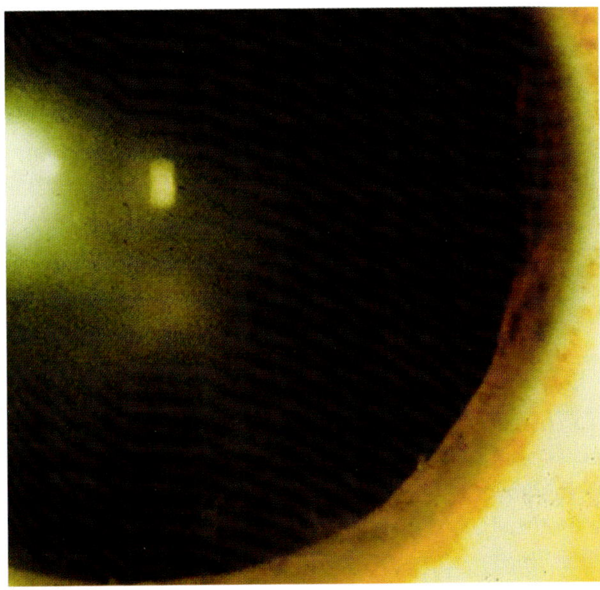

Fig. 5: Aniridia

Prognosis

- The visual prognosis is guarded. The earlier the keratoplasty is performed, the better the chances of preventing deprivation amblyopia. The visual acuity in patients after keratoplasty is reported to be 20/80 or worse. Also, in most series, the chances that patients maintain a clear graft were 30-50% at 10 years. Patients with glaucoma and cataract had a worse prognosis.
- The prognosis for life depends on other systemic anomalies.

Aniridia

Introduction

Aniridia is a congenital, hereditary, bilateral, extreme form of iris hypoplasia that may be associated with other ocular defects. Because of this iris hypoplasia the iris appears absent on superficial clinical examination. Gonioscopy shows the presence of the iris root. It is not a malformation confined to the anterior segment; it is really a panocular disorder with macular and optic nerve hypoplasia, cataract, and corneal changes, anomalies that lead to decreased vision. Glaucoma is a secondary problem and the leading cause of visual loss. Because a poor macular development exist, low vision aids are very helpful. Lifelong regular follow-up care is necessary.

Clinical Signs and Symptoms

In contrast with other developmental abnormalities, sometimes the diagnosis of aniridia is delayed. The patient presents with absence of iris, nystagmus, strabismus and reduced vision. The ocular examination may reveal nystagmus, strabismus, photophobia, corneal pannus, epithelial ulcers, aniridic keratopathy, arcus juvenilis and microcornea. There is a complete absence of iris at oblique illumination, atypical coloboma of pupil and the root of the iris can be visible at gonioscopy where also can be seen the trabecular meshwork partially or completely covered by the iris stump. The crystalline lens can be transparent or opaque with a subluxation and even a complete luxation. The ocular fundus might reveal optic nerve hipoplasia, macular reflex dull and glaucomatous disk. The IOP can be normal or increased, according the associated glaucoma and the vision is poor.

Investigations

Aniridia occurs because an autosomal dominant disorder, as an identifiable chromosome deletion of the short arm of chromosome 11, including band p13 and also as a sporadic case. The exact defect in iris morphogenesis giving rise to aniridia is unknown. Because the iris pigment epithelium, the iris musculature, the retina, and the optic nerve are derived from neuroectoderm, there may be a

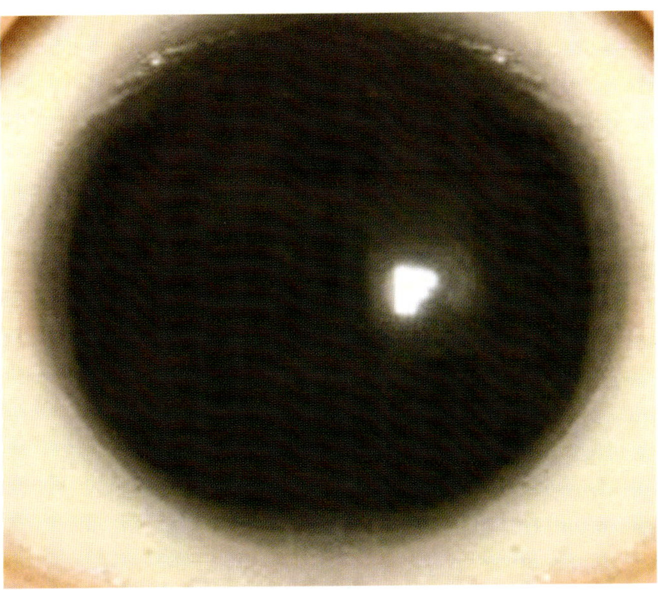

Fig. 6: Aniridia

common embryologic origin for these anomalies. As an isolated ocular malformation, aniridia is an autosomal dominant disorder, which is caused by a mutation in the PAX6 (paired box gene family) gene.

Differential Diagnosis

Rieger syndrome with iridocorneal dysgenesis, congenital coloboma of the iris, hereditary iris hypoplasia, traumatic iris injury, surgical iris coloboma and bilateral congenital mydriasis.

Treatment

Prophylaxis is directed toward the prevention of glaucoma, which includes medical treatment with miotics and surgical separation of the iris from the trabecular meshwork in selected cases. The medical treatment is directed toward control of intraocular pressure, which includes the topical use of miotics, beta-blockers, sympathomimetics, carbonic anhydrase inhibitors and prostaglandin analogues. The chances of failure with local antiglaucoma treatment are high. For visual rehabilitation and to reduce the amplitude and frequency of nystagmus as much as possible, is very important the treatment of photophobia and nystagmus with tinted or iris contact lenses, tinted spectacle lenses and even tinted intraocular lenses (IOLs). Also a careful refraction and complete correction are mandatory. Supports groups worldwide, can play a major role in the acceptation and rehabilitation of the disease.

Prognosis

Prognosis varies from patient to patient. A sustained elevation in the intraocular pressure may damage vision permanently. Cataract may require surgery and progressive corneal opacification may need corneal grafting.

Chapter THREE

Conjunctival Disorders

Arturo Perez Arteaga (Mexico)

- Infectious Diseases
- Inflammatory Diseases
- Neoplastic Disorders
- Degenerations

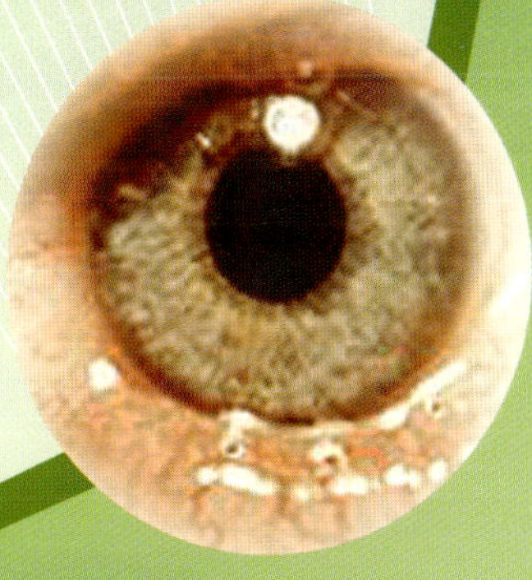

Infectious Diseases

Trachoma

Introduction

Trachoma is the leading infectious cause of blindness worldwide. In Western countries, few people know about the disease, but in the poorest countries in Africa, prevalence among children can reach 40 percent. The World Health Organization (WHO) estimates that 8 million people worldwide have been visually impaired by trachoma. The bacterium that causes trachoma spreads through direct contact with the eye, nose or throat secretions of infected people. It's very contagious and almost always affects both eyes. Untreated trachoma can lead to blindness.

Clinical Signs and Symptoms

The World Health Organization has identified a grading system with five stages in the development of trachoma. They are as follows:

Follicular Inflammation

The infection is just beginning. Five or more follicles — small bumps that contain lymphocytes are visible on the conjunctiva of the superior tarsus.

Intense Inflammation

In this stage, the eye is now highly infectious and becomes irritated, with a thickening or swelling of the upper eyelid.

Eyelid Scarring

Repeated infections lead to scarring of the inner eyelid; the scars often appear as white lines in the tarsus. The eyelid may become distorted and entropion may become.

Trichiasis Stage

The scarred inner lining of the eyelid continues to deform, causing the lashes to turn in so that they rub on and scratch the transparent outer surface of the cornea. Only about 1 percent of people with trachoma develop this painful condition.

Corneal Clouding

The cornea becomes affected by an inflammation that is most commonly seen under the upper lid. Continual inflammation compounded by scratching from

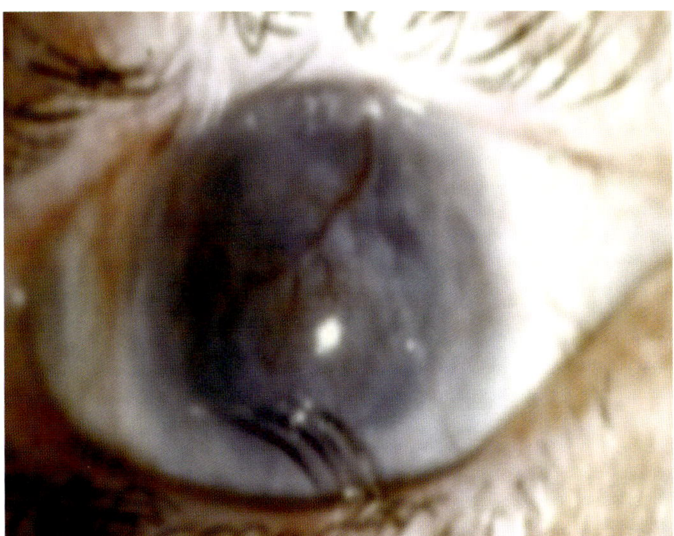

Fig. 1: Trachoma

the turned lashes leads to clouding of the cornea. Secondary infection can lead to development of ulcers on the cornea and eventually partial or complete blindness.

Investigations

The cause of trachoma is certain subtypes of chlamydia trachomatis, a bacterium that can also cause the sexually transmitted disease, chlamydia. Trachoma spreads through contact with discharge from the eyes or nose of an infected person. Hands, clothing, towels and insects can all be routes for transmission. In the developing countries, flies are a major means of transmission.

Differential Diagnosis

Some other inflammatory conditions of the cornea and conjunctiva, like Cicatricial Pemphigoid and Stevens-Johnson.

Treatment

Medications

In the early stages of trachoma, treatment with antibiotics alone may be enough to eliminate the infection. The two drugs currently in use include a tetracycline eye ointment and oral azithromycin (Zithromax). Although azithromycin appears to be more effective than tetracycline, azithromycin is more expensive. In poor communities, the drug used often depends on which one is available and affordable.

Surgery

Treatment of later stages of trachoma — including painful eyelid deformities — may require surgery. An eyelid rotation surgery (bilamellar tarsal rotation) can sometimes be indicated to avoid corneal damage. The procedure limits the progression of corneal scarring and can improve eyesight. Generally, this procedure can be performed on an outpatient basis. The procedure takes less than 15 minutes and has a good long-term success rate.

Prognosis

Untreated trachoma can lead to blindness. Trachoma is preventable and, if treated early, the prognosis for people with trachoma is excellent. If the cornea has become clouded enough to seriously impair vision, corneal transplantation is an option that offers some hope of improved vision; frequently, however, the results are not good, because the chronic inflammatory process at the cornea.

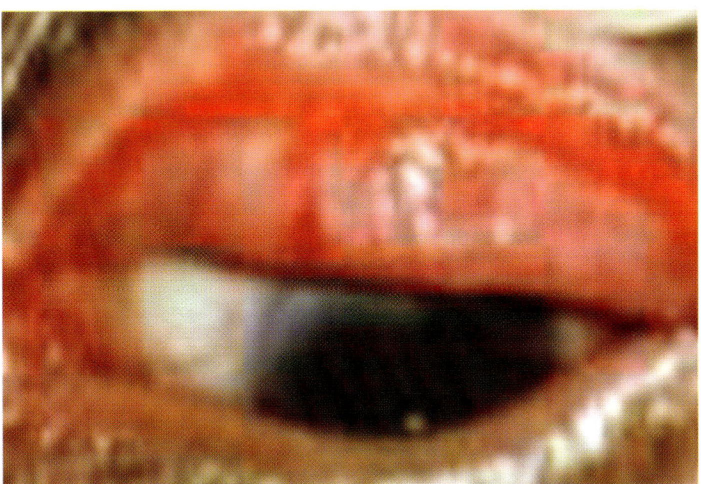

Fig. 2: Trachoma

Bacterial Conjunctivitis

Introduction

Bacterial conjunctivitis is a microbial infection involving the mucous membrane of the surface of the eye. This condition, which is usually a benign self-limited illness, sometimes can be serious or signify a severe underlying systemic disease. Occasionally, significant ocular and systemic morbidity may result.

Investigations

The surface tissues of the eye and the periocular tissues are colonized by normal flora such as *streptococci*, *staphylococci*, and *corynebacterium* strains. Alterations in the host defense or in the species of bacteria can lead to clinical infection. An alteration in the flora can occur by external contamination, by spread from adjacent sites, or via a blood-borne pathway. The primary defense against infection is the epithelial layer covering the conjunctiva. Disruption of this barrier can lead to infection. Secondary defenses include hematologic immune mechanisms carried by the conjunctival vasculature; tear film immunoglobulins and lysozyme; and the rinsing action of lacrimation and blinking.

Clinical Signs and Symptoms

- Conjunctival injection may be present segmentally or diffusely. The palpebral conjunctival pattern may hold clues as to the etiology.
- Using slit lamp biomicroscopy, the inflammation of the conjunctiva can be characterized as being follicular or papillary.
  - A follicular pattern has blood vessels circumferentially around the base of the tiny elevated lesions. This pattern is characteristic of viral or chlamydia conjunctivitis.
  - A papillary pattern has vessels coming up the center of the tiny elevated lesion and is characteristic of bacterial or allergic conjunctivitis.
- The discharge in bacterial conjunctivitis is typically more purulent than the watery discharge of viral conjunctivitis. Thus, there is more "mattering" of the lid margins and associated difficulty in prying the lids open following sleep.
- In uncomplicated bacterial conjunctivitis, slit lamp examination reveals a quiet anterior chamber that has not visible cells. The vitreous is also unaffected.
- A preauricular lymph node is unusual in bacterial conjunctivitis but is found in severe conjunctivitis caused by *N. gonorrhoeae*. It is associated with viral ocular syndromes, typically herpes simplex keratitis and epidemic keratoconjunctivitis.
- Eyelid edema is often present, but it is mild in most cases of bacterial conjunctivitis. Severe lid edema in the presence of copious purulent discharge raises the suspicion *N. gonorrhoeae* infection.

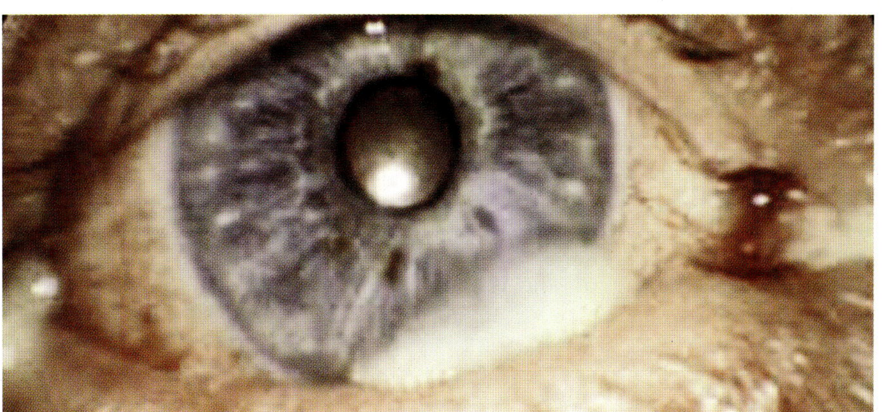

Fig. 3: Bacterial conjunctivitis

- Visual acuity is preserved in bacterial conjunctivitis, except for the expected mild blur secondary to the discharge and debris in the tear film.
- The pupil reacts normally in bacterial conjunctivitis.
- Dilation and tortuosity of the major vessel injection suggests a cavernous sinus-carotid artery fistula rather than conjunctivitis.

Differential Diagnosis

Because the differential diagnosis should me made with some other types of conjunctivitis, some studies can be very helpful; conjunctival scrapings and cultures most often are used in laboratory studies.

- Cultures can be completed for viral, chlamydial, and bacterial agents.
- If testing for *N. gonorrhoeae*, specific procedures should be followed.
- Fungal culture would be unusual.
- Conjunctival scrapings can be performed with topical anesthetic and gentle use of a platinum spatula or similar blunt metallic object.
- Gram stain is useful to identify bacterial characteristics.
- Giemsa stain is helpful to screen for intracellular inclusion bodies of *chlamydia*.
- Additionally, the nature of the inflammatory reaction is reflected in the cellular response. Lymphocytes predominate in viral infections, neutrophils in bacterial infections, and eosinophils in allergic reactions.

Treatment

The mainstay of medical treatment of bacterial conjunctivitis is topical antibiotic therapy. Systemic antibiotics are indicated only for *N. gonorrhoeae* (a single dose of intramuscular ceftriaxone 125 mg followed by oral doxycycline 100 mg twice daily for 7 days) and chlamydial infections (doxycycline 100 mg orally twice daily for 7 days). Practice patterns for prescribing topical antibiotics vary from doctor to doctor. Most practitioners prescribe a broad-spectrum agent on an empirical basis without culture for a routine, mild-to-moderate case of bacterial conjunctivitis. Always be aware of the differential diagnosis, and instruct patients to seek follow-up care if the expected improvement does not occur or if vision becomes affected. Sodium sulfacetamide, gentamicin, tobramycin, neomycin, trimethoprim and polymyxin B combination, ciprofloxacin, ofloxacin, gatifloxacin, and erythromycin are representatives of commonly used first-line agents. Eye drops have the advantage of not interfering with vision. Ointments have the advantage of prolonged contact with the ocular surface and an accompanying soothing effect.

Prognosis

Frequently good.

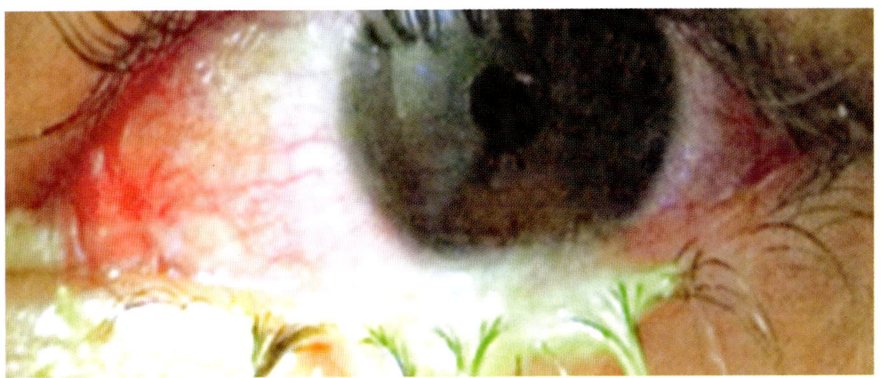

Fig. 4: Bacterial conjunctivitis

Adenoviral Keratoconjunctivitis

Introduction

Viruses are a common cause of conjunctivitis in patients of all ages. A variety of viruses can be responsible for conjunctival infection; however, adenovirus is by far the most common cause, and herpes simplex virus (HSV) is the most problematic. Less common causes include varicella-zoster virus (VZV), picornavirus (enterovirus 70, Coxsackie A24), poxvirus (molluscum contagiosum, vaccinia), and human immunodeficiency virus (HIV). Viral conjunctivitis, although usually benign and self-limited, unfortunately tends to follow a longer course than acute bacterial conjunctivitis, lasting for approximately 2-4 weeks. Viral infection is characterized commonly by an acute follicular conjunctival reaction and preauricular adenopathy.

Clinical Signs and Symptoms

Patients with adenoviral conjunctivitis may give a history of recent exposure to an individual with red eye at home, school, or work, or they may have a history of recent symptoms of an upper respiratory tract infection, also a common source of infection. The eye infection may be unilateral or bilateral. The main complains are ocular itching, foreign body sensation, tearing, redness, and photophobia. Typical signs of adenoviral conjunctivitis include preauricular adenopathy, epiphora, hyperemia, chemosis, subconjunctival hemorrhage, follicular conjunctival reaction, and occasionally a pseudomembranous or cicatricial conjunctival reaction. The cornea often demonstrates a punctate epitheliopathy. The eyelids often are edematous and ecchymotic. In severe cases, there can be a corneal epithelial defect. It typically begins in one eye and progresses to the fellow eye over a few days. The second eye is usually less significantly involved. In contrast acute hemorrhagic conjunctivitis starts unilaterally but rapidly involves the fellow eye within 1 or 2 days. Signs on examination include a swollen, edematous eyelid, and pronounced hemorrhage beneath the bulbar conjunctiva.

Investigations

Adenoviral conjunctivitis is the most common cause of viral conjunctivitis. Particular subtypes of adenoviral conjunctivitis include epidemic keratoconjunctivitis (pink eye) and pharyngoconjunctival fever. Transmission occurs through contact with infected upper respiratory droplets, fomites, and contaminated swimming pools. When conjunctivitis occurs in a patient with AIDS, it tends to follow a more severe and prolonged course. In general, patients with AIDS may develop a transient nonspecific conjunctivitis, characterized by irritation, hyperemia, and tearing, that requires no specific treatment.

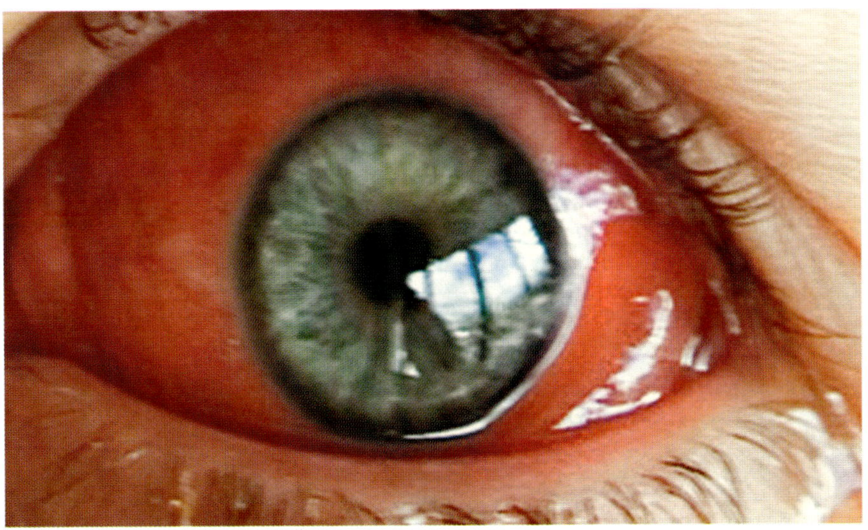

Fig. 5: Adenoviral conjunctivitis

Differential Diagnosis

Generally, a diagnosis of viral conjunctivitis is made on the clinical features alone. Such findings include the classic follicular conjunctivitis, and preauricular adenopathy associated with adenoviral infection. Differential diagnosis is with HSV keratoconjunctivitis, VZV keratoconjunctivitis, ocular chlamydial infections, vernal keratoconjunctivitis, blepharoconjunctivitis, contact lens keratoconjunctivitis, foreign body and epithelial keratitis.

Treatment

Treatment of adenoviral conjunctivitis is supportive. No evidence exists that demonstrates efficacy of antiviral agents. Patients should be instructed to use cold compresses and lubricants, such as artificial tears, for symptoms relief. Topical steroids may be used for pseudomembranes or when subepithelial infiltrates impair vision, although subepithelial infiltrates may recur after discontinuing the steroids. Extreme caution should be taken when using corticosteroids, as they may worsen an underlying infection. Complications include the following: punctate keratitis with subepithelial infiltrates, bacterial superinfection, corneal ulceration with keratoconjunctivitis, and chronic infection, in particular in patients with impaired immune system.

Prognosis

Most cases of viral conjunctivitis are acute, benign, and self-limited. The infection usually resolves spontaneously within 2-4 weeks. Subepithelial infiltrates may last for several months, and, if in the visual axis, they may cause decreased vision or glare.

Chlamydial Conjunctivitis

Introduction

Bacterial conjunctivitis is common worldwide. Community sequelae can be devastating in areas affected by blinding infections of newborns as well as in areas heavily affected by *chlamydia trachomatis.* The practitioner must be vigilant in considering sexually transmitted diseases caused by *chlamydia* in sexually active age groups and in newborns that may have been exposed during birth. Tactful and confidential history taking are a necessary skill, in particular in countries where legal issues are important regarding this topic.

Clinical Signs and Symptoms

Chlamydial infection in the newborn can lead to pneumonia and/or otitis media. Morbidity in terms of discomfort, ocular discharge, and redness are common in benign cases and often lead to absence from work and school.

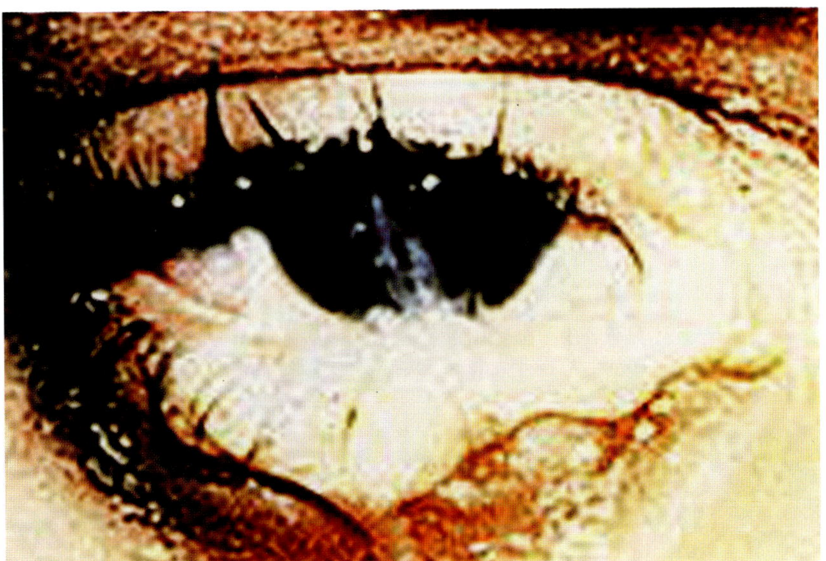

Fig. 6: Chlamydial conjunctivitis

Morbidity can be associated with misdiagnosis. Since many eye diseases cause the redness, it is beneficial to have a solid approach to diagnosis. Patients at a sexually active age should be considered for venereal diseases. If the conjunctivitis is associated with copious purulence, severe injection, and chemosis, then a discussion of possible exposure to *N. gonorrhoeae* must take place. Bacterial cultures, including Thayer-Martin and chocolate agar, and a Gram stain must be taken. A history of sexual partners must be obtained if the cultures/stain verifies this condition so that they also can be treated. The practitioner must be aware that laws require reporting incidences of this disease to the appropriate board of health. This history is mandatory to be obtained when chlamydial conjunctivitis is suspected.

Investigations

Chlamydia is transmitted via the birth canal of an infected mother, and neonates exposed to *chlamydia* at birth may develop conjunctivitis 5-13 days later. *C. trachomatis* immunotypes A-C, which are endemic in Africa, causes a chronic conjunctivitis. *Chlamydia trachomatis* is an obligate, intracellular bacterium with 15 immunotypes, as follows: A-C cause trachoma (chronic conjunctivitis); D-K, genital tract infections; and L1-L3, lymphogranuloma venereum (associated with genital ulcer disease). *chlamydia* is the most commonly reported bacterial sexually transmitted disease in the United States and is one of the most important causes of infertility in women.

Differential Diagnosis

Laboratory test are very helpful to avoid a misdiagnosis. The most reliable are cell culture, direct fluorescent antibody, nucleic acid amplification techniques, enzyme immunoassay and giemsa stain, that is very helpful to screen for intracellular inclusion bodies of *chlamydia*. Other forms of conjunctivitis must be excluded, in particular some sexually transmitted conjunctivitis, like *N. gonorrhoeae.*

Treatment

Chlamydial infection of the newborn requires systemic treatment of the neonate, the mother, and at-risk contacts. The neonate may be treated with erythromycin orally in liquid form 50 mg/kg/day in 4 divided doses for 2 weeks. The mother and at-risk contacts may be treated with doxycycline 100 mg orally twice daily for 7 days.

Prognosis

Only cases with extremely pathogenic bacteria, such as *Chlamydia trachomatis* or *N. gonorrhoeae,* are expected to develop complications in these kinds of conjuntivitis.

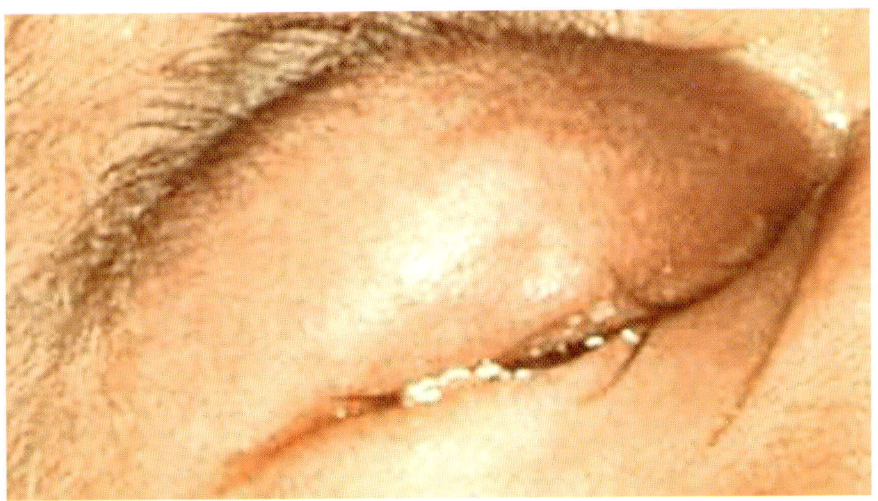

Fig. 7: Chlamydial conjunctivitis

Inflammatory Diseases

Allergic Conjunctivitis

Introduction

The conjunctiva may exhibit a wide variety of immunologic responses that may result in conjunctival and even corneal inflammation. In the Gell and Coombs classification system for various immunologic hypersensitivity reactions, 5 classes of reactions are recognized, and so, allergic conjunctivitis can be divided into 5 major subcategories. Seasonal allergic conjunctivitis (SAC) and perineal allergic conjunctivitis (PAC) are commonly grouped together. Vernal keratoconjunctivitis (VKC), atopic conjunctivitis (AKC), and giant papillary conjunctivitis (GPC) constitute the remaining subtypes of allergic conjunctivitis.

Clinical Signs and Symptoms

Diagnosis of allergic conjunctivitis generally is made by taking a thorough history and by careful clinical observation. Important features of history include a personal or family history of atopic disease, such as allergic rhinitis, bronchial asthma, and even atopic dermatitis. Perhaps the most important feature in the clinical history is the symptom of itching; without itching, the diagnosis of allergic conjunctivitis is suspect. Classic signs of allergic conjunctivitis include injection of conjunctival vessels as well as varying degrees of chemosis and eyelid edema. The conjunctiva often has a milky appearance due to obscuration of superficial blood vessels by edema within the conjunctival tissue of the conjunctiva. Edema is generally believed to be the direct result of increased vascular permeability caused by release of histamine from conjunctival mast cells.

Investigations

Since conjunctiva is a mucosal surface similar to the nasal mucosa, the same allergens that trigger allergic rhinitis may be involved in the pathogenesis of allergic conjunctivitis. Common airborne antigens, including pollen, grass, and weeds, may provoke the symptoms of acute allergic conjunctivitis, such as ocular itching, redness, burning, and tearing. The main distinction between SAC and PAC, as implied by the name, is the timing of symptoms during the year. VKC is a chronic bilateral inflammation of the conjunctiva commonly associated with a personal and/or family history of atopy. More than 90% of patients with VKC exhibit one or more atopic conditions, such as asthma, eczema, or seasonal allergic rhinitis.

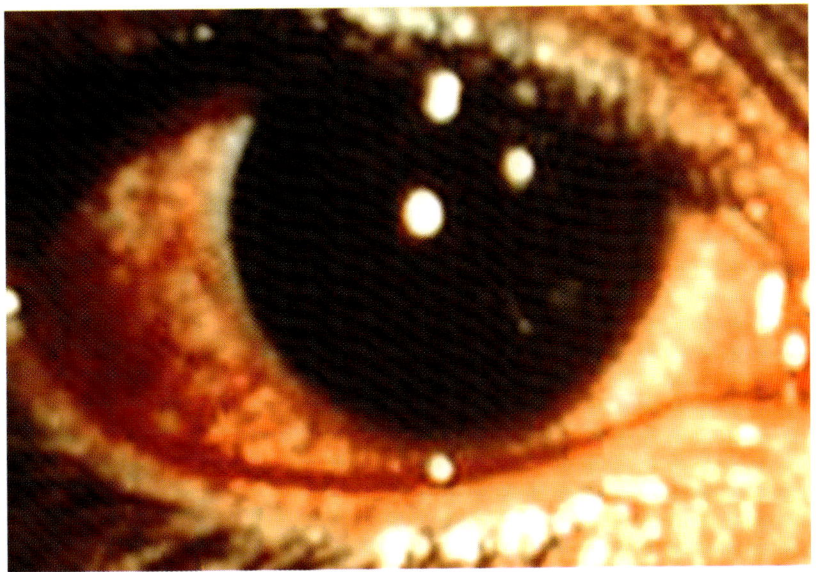

Fig. 8: Allergic conjunctivitis

Differential Diagnosis

Bacterial conjunctivitis, giant papillary conjunctivitis, viral conjunctivitis, atopic keratoconjunctivitis, superior limbic keratoconjunctivitis and keratoconus.

Treatment

Pharmacologic intervention may help alleviate the symptoms of acute allergic conjunctivitis. Various classes of medication may be effective against the symptoms of acute allergic conjunctivitis. Artificial tears provide a mechanical barrier and help to improve the first-line defense at the level of conjunctival mucosa. These agents help to dilute various allergens and inflammatory mediators that may be present on the ocular surface, and they help flush the ocular surface of these agents. Systemic and/or topical antihistamines may be given to relieve acute symptoms due to interaction of histamine at ocular H1 and H2 receptors. If well systemic antihistamines often relieve ocular allergic symptoms, patients may experience some secondary effects, such as drowsiness and dry mouth; they should be adverted about it. Topical antihistamines competitively and reversibly block histamine receptors and relieve itching and redness but only for a short time. Corticosteroids remain one of the most potent pharmacologic agents used in the treatment of ocular allergy. They act at the first step of the arachidonic acid pathway by inhibiting phospholipase, which is responsible for converting membrane phospholipid into arachidonic acid. Corticosteroids do have limitations, including ocular adverse effects, such as delayed wound healing, secondary infection, elevated intraocular pressure, and formation of cataract with a long-term use, so caution must be take in long-term use of them.

Prognosis

Generally good, but recurrences tend to occur. Chronic use of artificial tears and decrease exposure to allergens may be useful in decrease the rate of recurrences.

Giant Papillary Conjunctivitis

Introduction

Giant papillary conjunctivitis is a common complication of contact lens wearing patients. It was first described in association with contact lens use in 1974. Papillary changes occur in the ocular tarsal conjunctivae as part of an immunoglobulin E-mediated hypersensitivity reaction. Prior to the popularization of hydrogel (soft contact lenses), this reaction primarily was seen as allergic conjunctivitis or vernal keratoconjunctivitis.

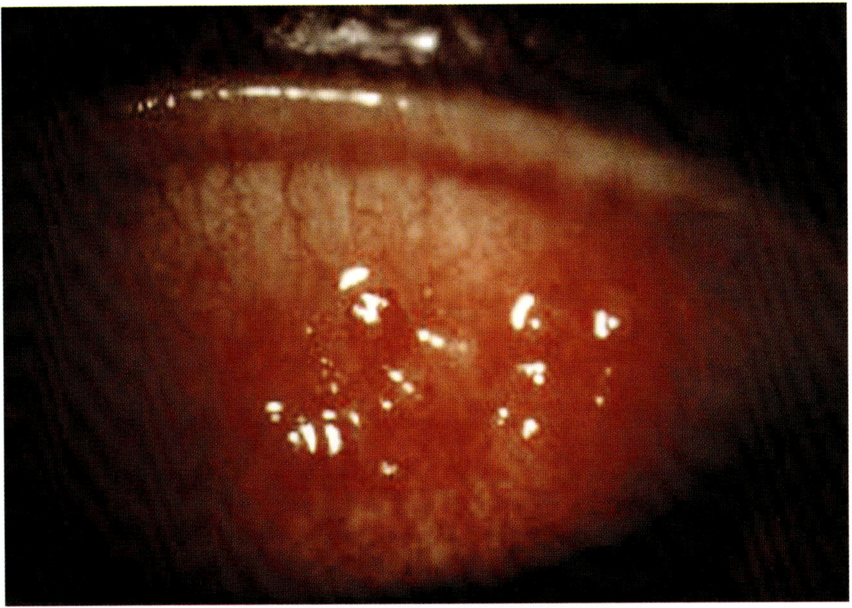

Fig. 9: Allergic conjunctivitis

Clinical Signs and Symptoms

Today, the clinical sign is generally accepted as follows: the papillae are at least 0.3 mm diameter on the tarsal conjunctiva in association with the classic allergic symptoms. Patients often report decreasing contact lens tolerance and mechanical stability, ocular itching, and mucous discharge in the tears, as well as blurred vision and conjunctival injection. Physician commonly note protein deposits at contact lenses; also they appear to ride more under the upper lids than expected. During physical examination, eversion of the lids, inflammation of the vasculature, hyperemia and papillary hypertrophy are noted.

Investigations

The antigens responsible for GPC have not been identified. From circumstantial evidence, the initiating event is believed to be mechanical irritation of the tarsal conjunctiva of the upper lids, followed by histological changes in the tissue that correspond to mast cell degranulation and typical secondary inflammatory cascade. Common tear abnormalities include elevated levels of IgG, IgE, and IgM, as well as complement factors, such as C3, factor B, and C3 anaphylatoxin. Specific antigens are thought to cause local production of these mediators. Another feature includes reduced lactoferrin levels in tears.

Differential Diagnosis

The clinician must distinguish from other diseases that cause conjunctivitis and the combination of ocular itching and mucus, that typically ocular in allergies, but also in viral and bacterial conjunctivitis and blepharitis. Other diseases must be excluded, in particular those that can cause papillary changes in the tarsal conjunctiva of the lids, like vernal and atopic conjunctivitis. Differential diagnosis must be made with other diseases that cause follicular changes, which can easily be confused with papillary changes, in the palpebral conjunctivae of the lids, like viral conjunctivitis (adenovirus and herpes), chlamydial infections, Gel-Coombs type IV hypersensitivity and toxic reactions, particularly to CL solutions. Finally from other causes of contact lens intolerance, should be excluded, such as poor fit, dry eyes, and blepharitis.

Treatment

For severe cases, patients should discontinue contact lenses for 2-4 weeks; this is a good interval of time for symptoms begin to reverse and health improves. Steroids can be used for selected cases. Combination mast cell stabilizers and antihistamine ophthalmic medications can sometimes be enough. Most patients do not require more aggressive treatment, so the physician must individualize the case. For mild-to-moderate cases the clinician must refit patients into new contact lenses; patients that use hydrogel lenses should use peroxide

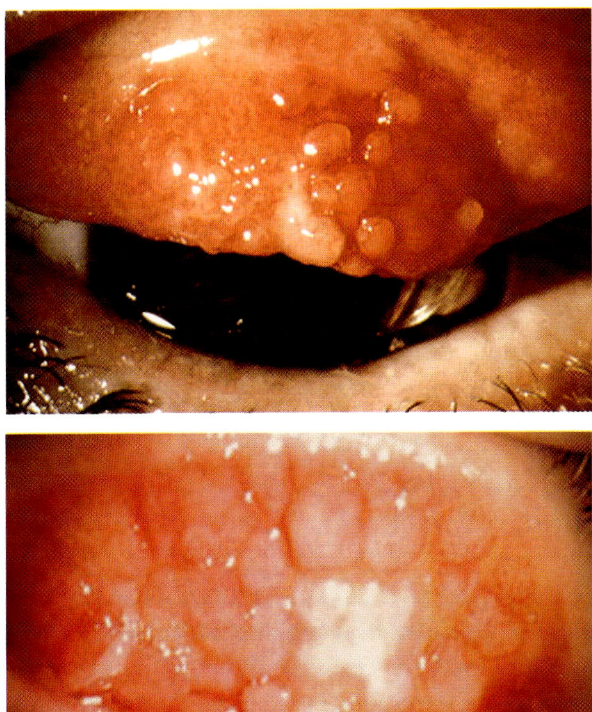

Figs 10 and 11: Giant papillary conjunctivitis

disinfecting solutions with their frequently disposable kits. Reemphasize contact lens cleaning techniques, especially rubbing with "no-rub" labeled solutions; also educate patients about the nature of this allergic disease. Topical mast cell stabilizers and antihistamine combination solutions may offer a pharmacological alternative for these patients, although contact lens cessation is the most effective treatment. Cool compresses can be added to improve symptoms.

Prognosis

The prognosis is good. Approximately 80% of patients can return to comfortable contact lenses wear with appropriate treatment. Use of long-term artificial tears can be needed.

Vernal Conjunctivitis

Introduction

Allergic conjunctivitis may be divided into 5 major subcategories. Seasonal allergic conjunctivitis (SAC) and perennial allergic conjunctivitis (PAC) are commonly grouped together. Vernal keratoconjunctivitis (VKC), atopic keratoconjunctivitis (AKC), and giant papillary conjunctivitis (GPC) constitute the remaining subtypes of allergic conjunctivitis. VKC is a chronic bilateral inflammation of the conjunctiva commonly associated with a personal and/or family history of atopic disease. Almost all patients have one or more atopic conditions, such as asthma, eczema, or allergic rhinitis.

Clinical Signs and Symptoms

As with other allergic or type I hypersensitivity disorders, itching is the most important, characteristic and most common symptom. Other commonly reported symptoms are photophobia, foreign body sensation, tearing, and blepharospasm. Ocular signs of VKC commonly are seen in the cornea and conjunctiva. The palpebral form has the presence of giant papillae in the superior tarsus; commonly the inferior tarsal conjunctiva is unaffected. Giant papillae assume a flattop appearance, which often is described as "cobblestone papillae". In severe cases, large papillae may cause mechanical ptosis. As the name implies, papillae tend to occur at the limbus and have a thick gelatinous appearance. They commonly are associated with multiple white spots (Horner-Trantas dots), which are collections of degenerated epithelial cells and eosinophils. Horner-Trantas dots are transient, with each appearance rarely lasting more than 1 week. In laboratory studies conjunctival scrapings of the superior tarsal conjunctiva and of Horner-Trantas dots show an abundance of eosinophils.

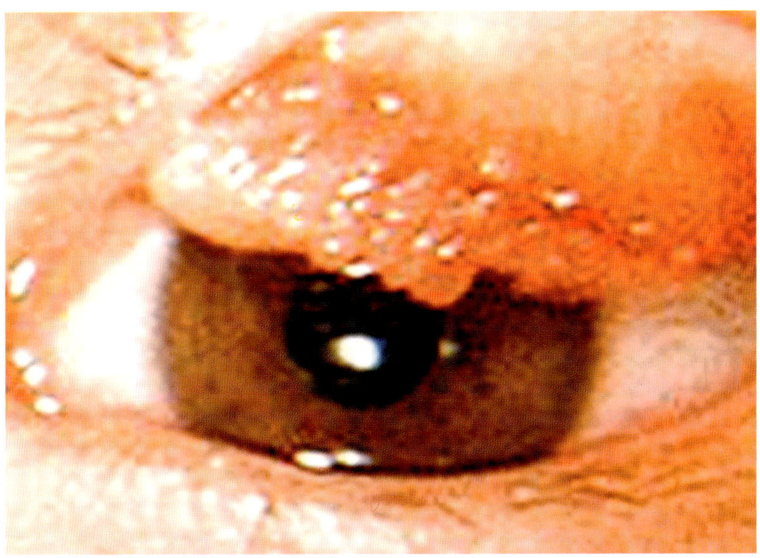

Fig. 12: Vernal conjunctivitis

Investigations

More than 90% of patients exhibit one or more atopic conditions, such as asthma, eczema, or seasonal allergic rhinitis. Another type of corneal involvement is vernal pseudogerontoxon, which is a degenerative lesion in the peripheral cornea resembling corneal arcus. Keratoconus may be seen in chronic cases, which may be associated with chronic eye rubbing.

Differential Diagnosis

Bacterial conjunctivitis, giant papillary conjunctivitis, viral conjunctivitis, atopic keratoconjunctivitis, superior limbic keratoconjunctivitis, keratoconus.

Treatment

Mast cell stabilizers are perhaps the mainstay of treatment and are safe for long-term use. However, topical corticosteroids generally become necessary for most patients with significant symptoms. Because of their potential adverse effects, topical steroids should be prescribed at the lowest effective concentration and for the shortest duration possible. Several reports have shown that topical cyclosporine may be effective in reducing some of the signs and symptoms without adverse effects. Oral aspirin has been shown to be effective.

Prognosis

Prognosis is favorable. This condition generally clears up readily but may reoccur.

Atopic Conjunctivitis

Introduction

Allergic conjunctivitis may be divided into 5 major subcategories. Seasonal allergic conjunctivitis (SAC) and perennial allergic conjunctivitis (PAC) are commonly grouped together. Vernal keratoconjunctivitis (VKC), atopic keratoconjunctivitis (AKC), and giant papillary conjunctivitis (GPC) constitute the remaining subtypes of allergic conjunctivitis. Atopic conjunctivitis is a bilateral inflammation of conjunctiva and eyelids, which has a strong association with atopic dermatitis. It is also a type I hypersensitivity disorder.

Clinical Signs and Symptoms

They may have seasonal variation with worsening symptoms during winter months. The single most common symptom is bilateral itching of the eyelids,

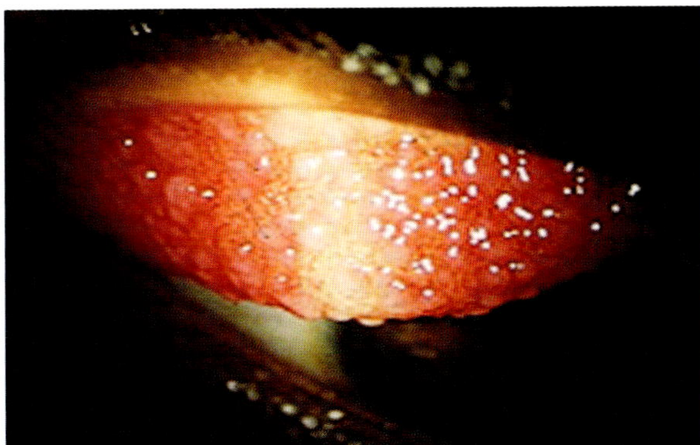

Fig. 13: Vernal conjunctivitis

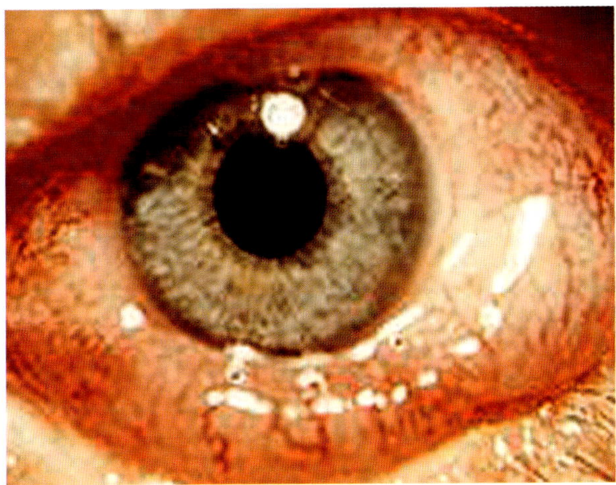

Fig. 14: Atopic conjunctivitis

but watery discharge, redness, photophobia, and pain may be associated features. The disease can affect eyelid skin and lid margin, conjunctiva, cornea, and lens. Skin of the eyelids may exhibit eczematous dermatitis with dry, scaly, and inflamed skin. Lid margins may show meibomian gland dysfunction and keratinization. Staphylococcal colonization of eyelid margins is very common and may result in blepharitis that might need treatment. Conjunctiva may show chemosis and typically a papillary reaction, which is more prominent in the inferior tarsal conjunctiva, in contrast to that seen in vernal keratoconjunctivitis. Another corneal finding, which may be associated with AKC, is keratoconus, which may stem from chronic eye rubbing.

Investigations

In 1953, the first description was made regarding the association between atopic dermatitis and conjunctival inflammation. The investigators reported cases of conjunctival inflammation in male patients with atopic dermatitis. Atopic dermatitis is a common hereditary disorder that usually has its onset in childhood; symptoms may regress with advancing age. Approximately, 3%, of the population is afflicted with atopic dermatitis, and, of these, approximately, 25% have ocular involvement. Conjunctival scrapings may demonstrate the presence of eosinophils, although the number is not as significant as that seen in vernal cases. Mast cells also may be found within the substantia propria of the conjunctiva in greater numbers. There is an increased amount of IgE in the tears. Although this disease is typically recognized as a type I hypersensitivity reaction, evidence has been found that supports some involvement of type IV hypersensitivity reaction, as is the case of vernal conjunctivitis.

Differential Diagnosis

Bacterial conjunctivitis, giant papillary conjunctivitis, viral conjunctivitis, superior limbic keratoconjunctivitis, keratoconus.

Treatment

Treatment of patients with atopic conjunctivitis is similar to that of vernal conjunctivitis cases, in that it includes controlling the environment and avoiding allergens and may require topical and systemic medications to provide symptomatic relief; topical vasoconstrictors and antihistamines may provide very limited, short-term relief; they are not the mainstay of treatment. Topical mast cell stabilizers and topical corticosteroids provide significant relief of symptoms. Mast cell stabilizers have to be used for several weeks prior to seeing a clinical effect, and, in the interim, topical steroids used in a pulsed fashion may help to control symptoms; so, many times the treatment is a combination of medication.

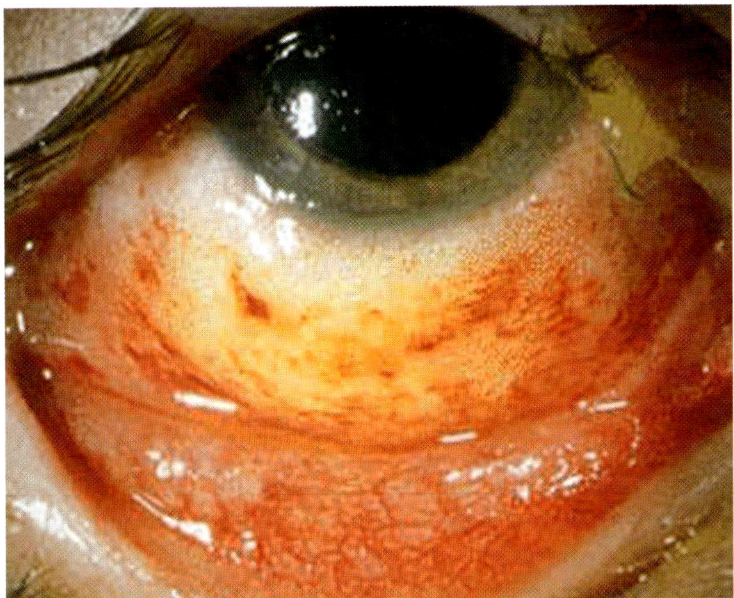

Fig. 15: Atopic conjunctivitis

Prognosis

Prognosis is favorable. This condition generally clears up readily but may reoccur; the goal should be controlling the environment and avoiding allergens.

Ocular Cicatricial Pemphigoid

Introduction

Ocular cicatricial pemphigoid (OCP) is one of the chapters of mucous membrane pemphigoid, a group of systemic autoimmune diseases characterized by T-lymphocyte deregulation, the production of circulating auto antibodies directed against a variety of adhesion molecules in the hemidesmosome-epithelial membrane complex, and the production of proinflammatory cytokines and immune system activation markers. This disease can affect the skin and other mucous membranes (oral mucosa, pharynx, larynx, trachea, esophagus, vagina, urethra, anus), in addition to its hallmark feature, chronic cicatrizing conjunctivitis.

Clinical Signs and Symptoms

Ocular symptoms include red eye, tearing, dry eye, blepharospasm, itching, grittiness, heavy eyelid, foreign body sensation, decreased vision, burn sensation, photophobia and diplopia. There are four stages of the diseases described as follows: Stage I is characterized by chronic conjunctivitis with mild conjunctival and/or corneal epitheliopathy with sub epithelial conjunctiva fibrosis, best seen at the tarsal conjunctiva as fine, white striae. Stage II is characterized by cicatrization with conjunctival shrinkage, distorted anatomy, and foreshortening of fornices. Stage III is characterized by the presence of symblepharon; subepithelial scarring alters the orientation of lashes, causing aberrant lash growth; in addition, cicatricial entropion may occur. Stage IV is the end stage, consisting of a dry eye with keratinization of the cornea and ankyloblepharon, which immobilizes the globe. Profound keratopathy can develop secondary to eyelid disorders, tear insufficiency, and corneal exposure. Corneal epitheliopathy, persistent epithelial defects, stromal ulceration, and neovascularization may be present. The cornea may become completely scarred, vascularized, and keratinized.

Investigations

A triggering agent in the genetically susceptible individual, leading to clinical manifestations of the disease, may occur in a double mechanism; human leukocyte antigen DR2 (HLA-DR2), human leukocyte antigen DR4 (HLA-DR4 [HLA-DR*0401]), and human leukocyte antigen DQw7 (HLA-DQw7

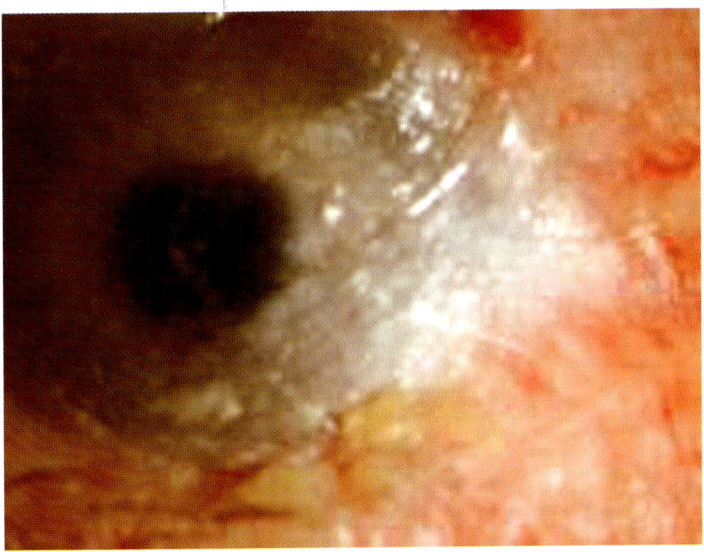

Fig. 16: Ocular cicatricial pemphigoid

[DQB1*0301]) genotypes have been identified as conferring increased susceptibility to the development of ocular cicatricial pemphigoid. Circulating autoantibodies are difficult to demonstrate by classic indirect immunofluorescence technique. Specialized radioimmunoassay and immunoblot techniques allow the circulating autoantibodies to be seen in all patients who have active conjunctivitis. The resultant inflammatory mediators that are produced induce migration of lymphocytes, eosinophils, neutrophils, and mast cells. The separation of the epithelium from the underlying tissues within the basal membrane may be the result of direct cytotoxic action or the effect of lysosomal proteolytic enzymes.

Differential Diagnosis

Definitive diagnosis of OCP is made by demonstration of linear deposition of immunoreactants (e.g., IgG, IgA, IgM, complement 3 component [C3]) at the basal membrane of biopsy specimen of inflamed conjunctiva using immunofluorescent or immunoperoxidase technique. Other histological techniques, such as hematoxylin and eosin staining, periodic-acid Schiff (PAS), and Giemsa staining, are not diagnostically specific. Only experienced laboratory technicians should process conjunctival tissue to obtain the highest possible diagnostic yield and sensitivity. A negative or inconclusive biopsy result may be secondary to poor biopsy technique or poor handling of the specimen, so be aware of a false negative result. Differential diagnosis should be made with irradiation, trauma, progressive systemic sclerosis (scleroderma), toxic epidermal necrolysis, erythroderma congenital, porphyria cutanea tarda, epidermolysis bullosa, linear IgA bullous disease, paraneoplastic pemphigus, bullous systemic lupus erythematosus, *Corynebacterium diphtheriae* conjunctivitis, sebaceous cell carcinoma, adenoviral conjunctivitis and intraepithelial epithelioma.

Treatment

No topical agent is effective in stopping OCP activity. In selected patients, subconjunctival steroid injections or subconjunctival injections of mitomycin C may be used temporarily for slowing disease progression, while systemic therapy takes effect. Use an adjuvant treatment with topical lubricants in patients with dry eye symptoms. Keratinized posterior lid margin conjunctiva also may respond to topical retinoid therapy. Systemic corticosteroids can control the activity of the disease; however, they are not as effective as other immunosuppressive drugs, and the doses required have been shown to be high and so with adverse effects. For mild-to-moderate inflammation, diaminodiphenylsulfone is the first-line agent, provided the patient is not glucose-6-phosphate dehydrogenase deficient. If therapeutic response is not satisfactory, or if the use of diaminodifenylsulfone is contraindicated, or if the

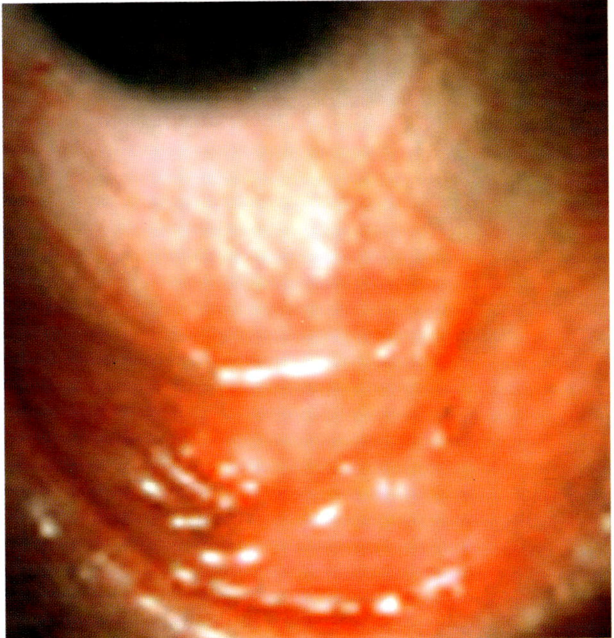

Fig. 17: Ocular cicatricial pemphigoid

patient cannot tolerate the drug, methotrexate or azathioprine can be substituted. If inflammation persists, use cyclophosphamide sequentially. For severe inflammation, initially use cyclophosphamide, and add systemic prednisone with rapid taper for a limited period of time. Patients with active conjunctival inflammation refractory to chemotherapy or patients who do not tolerate the spectrum of immunosuppressive drugs can be treated with intravenous immunoglobulin. Treatment is difficult and must be individualized.

Surgical approaches include depilation, punctual occlusion, lid surgery, entropion surgery, fornix reconstruction, corneal surgery and cataract surgery with variable results according the case.

Prognosis

Patients may be limited by visual acuity. Based on the results of one study, slightly more than one-third of patients receiving immunosuppressive therapy, according to the guidelines for use of immunosuppressive agents, respond to the therapy and remain free of inflammation following the cessation of therapy. Another one-third of patients were free of disease activity, but they continued to receive chemotherapy because their disease had been controlled for only a short time or because they had a history of relapse while on therapy. Nearly one-third of patients only responded partially to treatment. Inability to control inflammation and to stop progression of cicatrizing conjunctivitis was seen only in a few individuals; for them the prognosis is poor.

Stevens-Johnson Syndrome

Introduction

In 1922, Stevens and Johnson first described 2 patients with "an extraordinary, generalized eruption with continued fever, inflamed oral mucosa, and severe purulent conjunctivitis." In the 1990s, Bastuji and Roujeau proposed that the denomination of SJS should be used for a syndrome characterized by mucous membrane erosions and widespread small blisters that arise on erythematous or purpuric maculae that are different from classic targets.

Clinical Signs and Symptoms

Ocular symptoms include red eye, tearing, dry eye, pain, blepharospasm, itching, grittiness, heavy eyelid, foreign body sensation, decreased vision, burn sensation, photophobia and diplopia. Other affected sites include skin lesions, oral lesions, esophageal lesions, pharyngeal lesions, laryngeal lesions, anal lesions, tracheal lesions, vaginal lesions and urethral lesions. An external examination may reveal conjunctival hyperemia, entropion, skin lesions, nasal lesions, mouth lesions and discharge (i.e., catarrhal, mucous, membranous). The slitlamp examination can reveal abnormalities in different structures: in

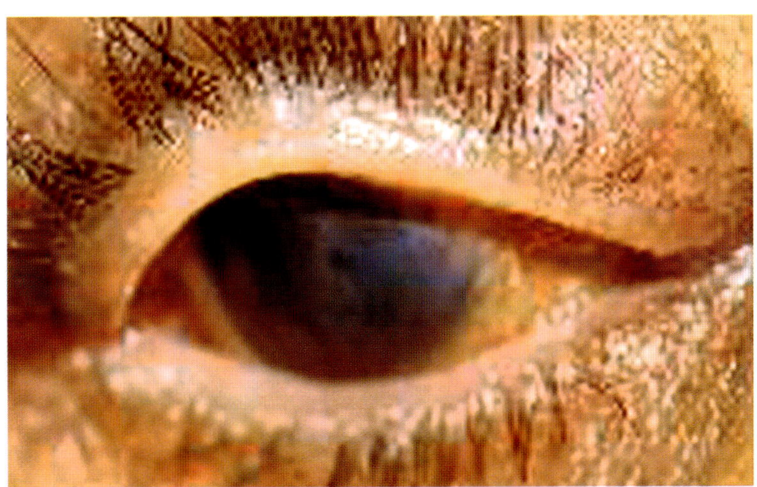

Fig. 18: Stevens-Johnson syndrome

eyelids trichiasis, distichiasis, meibomian gland dysfunction and blepharitis; in conjunctiva papillae, follicles, keratinization, subepithelial fibrosis, symblepharon and even ankyloblepharon; in cornea superficial punctate keratitis, epithelial defect, stromal ulcer, neovascularization, keratinization, limbitis, stromal opacity and even perforation. Skin biopsy is the only diagnostically helpful laboratory study.

Investigations

An idiosyncratic, delayed hypersensitivity reaction has been implicated in the pathophysiology of SJS. Certain groups of patients appear more susceptible to develop SJS than the general population. The slow acetylators, patients who are immunocompromised, and patients with brain tumors undergoing radiotherapy with concomitant antiepileptic are among those at most risk. Various etiologic factors (e.g., infection, vaccination, drugs, systemic diseases, physical agents, food) have been implicated as causes of SJS. Drugs most commonly are blamed. Reports have linked SJS to the use of drugs, rather than to other etiologic factors. Antibiotics are the most common cause of SJS, followed by analgesics, cough and cold medication, no steroidal anti-inflammatory drugs (NSAIDs), psychoepileptics, and antigout drugs. Other drugs also can be involved in the pathogenesis of SJS. Caucasians with HLA-Bw44 appear to be more susceptible to develop SJS. Antigen presentation and production of tumor necrosis factor alpha by the local tissue dendrocytes results in the recruitment and augmentation of T-lymphocytes; proliferation enhances the cytotoxicity of the other immune effector cells. The activated CD8+ lymphocytes, in turn, can induce epidermal cell apoptosis via several mechanisms, which include the release of granzyme B and perforin. Apoptosis of the keratinocytes can also take place as a result of ligation of their surface death receptors with the appropriate molecules. Those can trigger the activation of the cascade system leading to DNA disorganization and finally cell death.

Differential Diagnosis

Chemical burns, allergic conjunctivitis, bacterial conjunctivitis, viral conjunctivitis, atopic dermatitis, districhiasis, entropion, sarcoidosis, scleritis, Sjogren syndrome, trachoma and trichiasis between others.

Treatment

Supportive systemic therapy: Management of patients with SJS is usually provided in intensive care units or burn centers. No specific treatment of SJS exists; therefore, most patients are treated symptomatically. As a medical precept, the symptomatic treatment of patients with SJS does not differ from the treatment of patients with extensive burns.

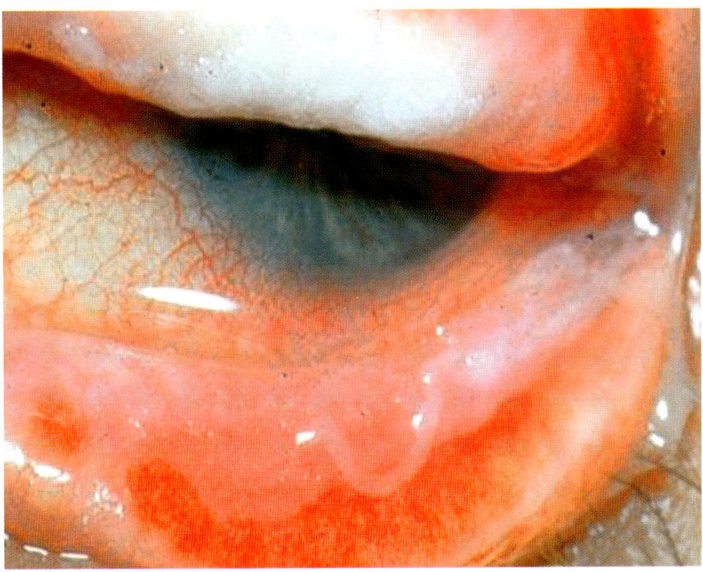

Fig. 19: Stevens-Johnson syndrome

Treatment of acute ocular manifestations usually begins with aggressive lubrication of the ocular surface. As inflammation and cicatricial changes arise, most ophthalmologists use topical steroids, antibiotics, and symblepharon lysis. In case of exposure keratopathy, tarsorrhaphy may be required. Maintenance of ocular integrity can be achieved through the use of amniotic membrane grafting, adhesive glues, lamellar grafts, and penetrating keratoplasty, either in the acute phase or in subsequent, follow-up care. Visual rehabilitation in patients with visual impairment can be considered once the eye has been quiet for at least 3 months.

Treatments of chronic ocular manifestations include, in the case of mild chronic superficial keratopathy, long-term lubrication. In addition, some patients may require a cosmetically acceptable long-term lateral tarsorrhaphy. The visual rehabilitation in patients with severe ocular involvement, resulting in profound dry eye syndrome with posterior lid margin keratinization, limbal stem cell deficiency, persistent epithelial defects with subsequent corneal neovascularization, and complete corneal opacity with surface conjunctivalization and keratinization, is difficult and often frustrating for both the patient and the physician. Limbal stem cell transplantation and amniotic membrane grafting with superficial keratectomy removing conjunctivalized or keratinized ocular surface can be performed. Patients with persistent corneal opacity require lamellar or penetrating keratoplasty. To preserve corneal clarity after the visual reconstruction, the long-term use of gas permeable contact lenses may be necessary to protect the ocular surface.

Prognosis

Of the patients with this disease, 27-50% progress to severe ocular disease.

Superior Limbic Keratoconjunctivitis

Introduction

This disorder is characterized as an inflammation of the superior bulbar conjunctiva with predominant involvement of the superior limbus and an adjacent epithelial keratitis with papillary hypertrophy of the upper tarsal conjunctiva. Factors predisposing to conjunctiva laxity include thyroid eye disease, tight upper eyelids, and prominent globes. Prolonged eyelid closure with associated hypoxia and/or reduced tear volume may be also a predisposing factor.

Clinical Signs and Symptoms

Patients present with complaints of burning and irritation of the affected eye. Some patients may present with redness. Up gaze may evidence the reason of these symptoms. Symptoms remit and exacerbate and are variable in degree,

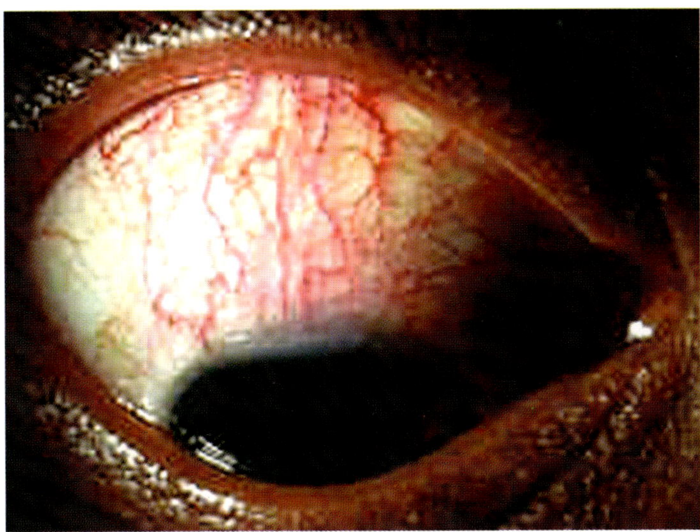

Fig. 20: Superior limbic keratoconjunctivitis

but no diurnal pattern to the worsening of symptoms exists. In most cases, the condition is present bilaterally, although one eye may be more symptomatic. Patients with filaments are usually extremely symptomatic. Commonly, a history of thyroid dysfunction can be adverted. Marked inflammation of the upper lid tarsal conjunctiva, adjacent inflammation of the upper bulbar conjunctiva, and punctate rose bengal staining of the cornea at the upper limbus, are common findings. The conjunctiva extending from the upper limbus to the insertion of the superior rectus muscle also demonstrates thickening, hyperemia, and typical rose bengal staining. Approximately, one-third of patients present with filaments on the upper cornea or along the superior limbus.

Investigations

It is believed that superior limbal keratitis is present secondary to superior bulbar conjunctiva laxity, which induces inflammatory changes from mechanical soft tissue micro trauma. In settings where the physiological tolerance of mechanical forces on the delicate ocular surface is exceeded, chronic inflammation results in thickening of the conjunctiva and keratinization; this is the cycle that perpetuates the inflammation. Eventually, a filamentary response may be induced on the affected cornea. Factors inducing conjunctiva laxity include thyroid eye disease, tight upper eyelids, and prominent globes.

Differential Diagnosis

Allergic conjunctivitis, bacterial conjunctivitis, giant papillary conjunctivitis, viral conjunctivitis, dry eye syndrome, epiescleritis, floppy eyelid syndrome, epidemic keratoconjunctivitis, thyroid ophthalmopathy and trachoma, between others.

Treatment

Several approaches have been used to speed the recovery of patients toward the resolution of symptoms. Pressure patching, placement of a bandage contact lens, silver nitrate solution application, mast cell stabilizers, and vitamin A preparations have been used with moderate success. As these approaches usually offer only temporary mitigation of symptoms, more definitive treatments often are required.

Surgical resection of the involved conjunctiva as delineated intraoperatively by the use of rose bengal staining removes the affected tissue. Folds of superfluous conjunctiva are eliminated, adhesions with underlying Tenon capsule and episclera develop, and keratinized epithelium is replaced by normal in growth. Also a conjunctival autograft can be performed.

Prognosis

Prognosis is excellent, although symptoms may last for years.

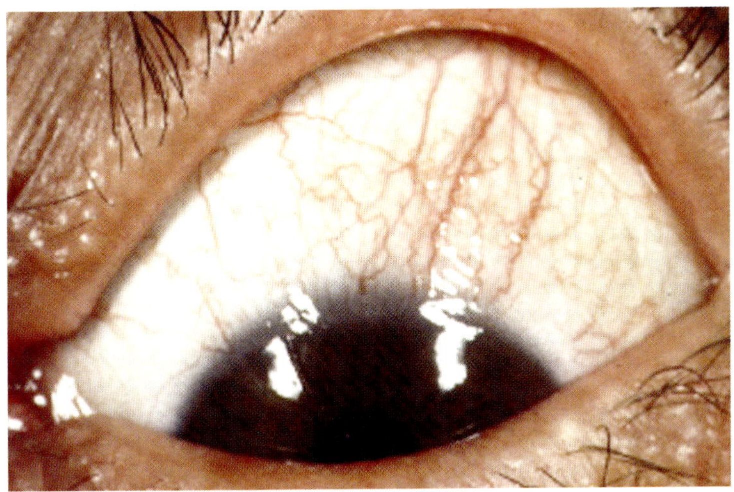

Fig. 21: Superior limbic conjunctivitis

Phlyctenular Conjunctivitis

Introduction

Phlyctenular keratoconjunctivitis is a nodular inflammation of the perilimbal tissues that occurs secondary to an allergic hypersensitivity response of the cornea and conjunctiva. The disease has a worldwide distribution and is most often seen in the first and second decades in women. The disease has been associated with systemic disorders such as Behçet's disease, tuberculosis, HIV and rosacea among others, but can be present alone.

Clinical Signs and Symptoms

Patients typically present with symptoms of tearing, ocular irritation, mild to severe photophobia and a history of similar episodes. If the underlying cause is staphylococcus, a rope-like, mucopurulent discharge may be present. The phlyctenular lesions can be present in two structures: corneal and conjunctival. slitlamp evaluation of a conjunctival phlyctenule reveals a 1 to 3 mm, hard, slightly elevated, yellowish-white nodule, surrounded by a hyperemic response, in the vicinity of the inferior limbus. The lesions tend to be bilateral because this is a hypersensitivity reaction. Corneal phlyctenules produce more severe symptoms, sometimes simulating the severity of a bullous keratopathy; they usually begin adjacent to the limbus as a white mound, with a radial pattern of vascularized conjunctival vessels on the conjunctival side; the lesion may then migrate toward the center of the cornea, producing very important pain and discomfort.

Investigations

The exact mechanism by which phlyctenules are produced is unclear. Histologically, they are composed of lymphocytes, histocytes and plasma cells. Polymorphonuclear leukocytes are found in necrotic lesions. Their formation seems to be the result of a delayed hypersensitivity reaction to tuberculin protein. Anyhow it is consider a hypersensitivity reaction.

Differential Diagnosis

Allergic conjunctivitis, bacterial conjunctivitis, giant papillary conjunctivitis, viral conjunctivitis, dry eye syndrome, epiescleritis, floppy eyelid syndrome, epidemic keratoconjunctivitis, trachoma, infiltrates secondary to chronic blepharitis, inflamed pingueculae, herpes simplex and infectious or marginal corneal ulcer.

Treatment

Ocular management of phlyctenular keratoconjunctivitis begins with patient education to improve eyelid hygiene. Lid scrubs two to three times a day, along with artificial tears and ointments may help the treatment and reverse mild and

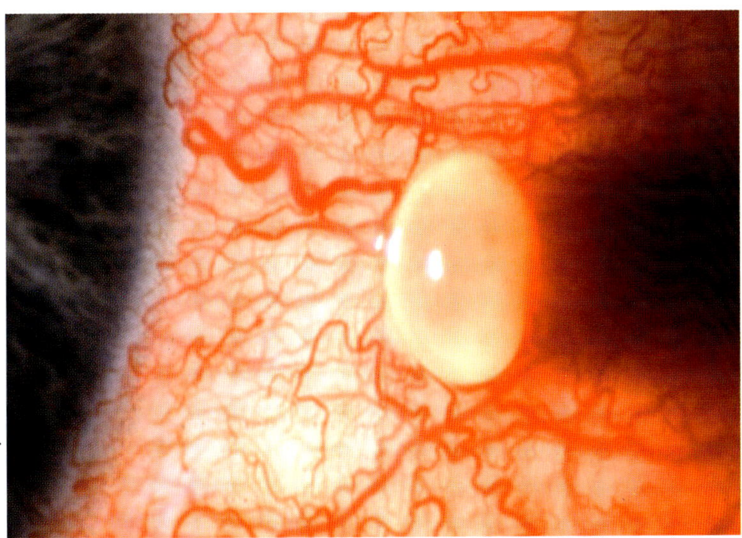

Fig. 22: Phlyctenular

some moderate cases. Moderate to severe cases require topical steroidal or steroidal/antibiotic combination medicines. If the suspected etiology is staphylococcus or rosacea, tetracycline or erythromycin, along with topical antibiotic ointments such as bacitracin or erythromycin should be added. Treatment during days of oral and topical steroids and antibiotics may continue to relieve patients' signs and symptoms. Weekly follow-up is recommended. Once significant improvement is noted, the steroid should be suspended; nevertheless the antibiotic coverage should continue. Eyelid hygiene should be maintained indefinitely.

Prognosis

Generally, good if measures are well taken; in some particular cases of poor general measures, recurrences are frequent.

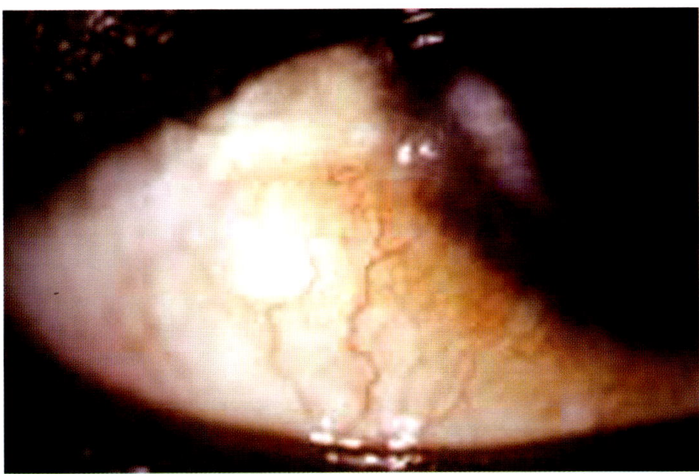

Fig. 23: Phlyctenular conjunctivitis

Neoplastic Disorders

Lymphoma

Introduction

Lymphoma is best described as malignant growth of lymphoid tissue, or cancer of elements of the lymphatic system; in this particular case the diagnosis is made when these cells are found in the conjunctival tissue. Any patient with conjunctival lymphoma deserves a complete medical evaluation to determine if systemic lymphoma is present.

Clinical Signs and Symptoms

Conjunctival lymphomas represent a mass lesion of the superficial ocular surface. The lesions have been classically described as "salmon-colored patches," and may present bilaterally in as many as 20% of patients, because systemic involvement. The lesions are fleshy and may grow rapidly. Sometimes they appear to arise from within the fornix and extend toward the cornea. Conjunctival lymphomas resemble several other benign tumors of the ocular surface, including squamous papilloma, pyogenic granuloma and lymphangiectasis. Patients with conjunctival lymphoma tend to be young to middle-aged adults. They may complain of chronic redness but rarely report ocular discomfort; because of this there can be a delay in the diagnosis.

Investigations

Lymphoma is best described as malignant growth of lymphoid tissue, or cancer of elements of the lymphatic system. Lymphoid tissue is present in most organs throughout the body, and is connected by channels and conduits to lymph nodes, located primarily in the neck, axillae, groin and abdomen. In the eye, lymphoma can manifests as a conjunctival or orbital mass, a choroidal infiltration with secondary uveitis, or an infiltrative optic neuropathy. Systemic involvement is common.

Differential Diagnosis

Biopsy is crucial in any case of suspicious conjunctival lesions. The most critical element, after establishing the presence of a conjunctival lymphoma, is differentiating between the mucosa-associated lymphoid tissue lymphoma (MALT) and non-MALT varieties, due that MALT lymphomas are less aggressive, while non-MALT lesions are considered highly malignant and invasive. In addition, any patient with biopsy-proven of lymphoma deserves a complete medical evaluation to determine if systemic lymphoma is present. This includes basic hematology, as well as examination by a hematologist and/

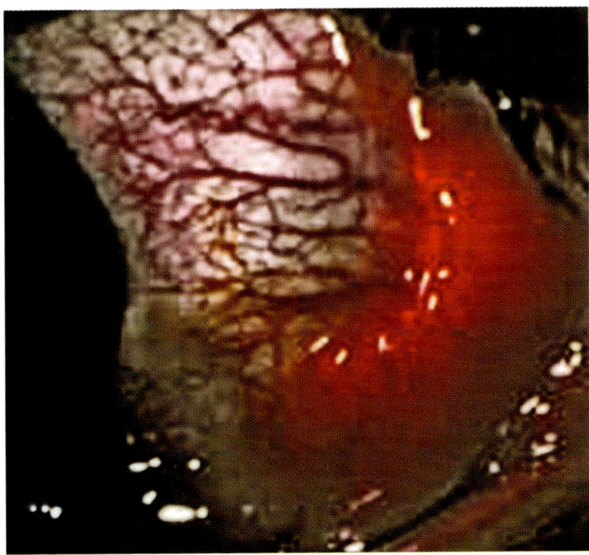

Fig. 24: Lymphoma

or oncologist. Radiographic imaging of the head, chest and abdomen are usually also obtained if systemic involvement is suspected. Differential diagnosis includes lymphoid neoplasia, benign reactive lymphoid hyperplasia, and leukemic infiltrates, benign hereditary intraepithelial dyskeratosis, angioma, lymphangioma, Kaposi sarcoma and pyogenic granuloma.

Treatment

Therapy for conjunctival lymphoma depends on the disposition of the tumor and whether there is disseminated lymphoma elsewhere in the body. Isolated conjunctival lymphoma (i.e., involving the conjunctiva but no other ocular or systemic structures) is most often treated with external beam irradiation. Despite lymphoid tumors of the conjunctiva traditionally are treated with radiation therapy, new modalities include the use of liquid nitrogen spray. Preliminary results are comparable to those with radiation therapy, indicating that cryotherapy for certain conjunctival lymphomatous tumors may be a viable option, because of fewer ocular and systemic complications and lower cost.

Prognosis

Lymphoid tumors of the conjunctiva are associated with systemic lymphoma in 31% of patients. Systemic lymphoma is found more often in those patients with forniceal or midbulbar conjunctival involvement and in those with multiple conjunctival tumors. Long-term systemic follow-up is advised, because related systemic lymphoma can manifest many years later.

Conjunctival Nevus

Introduction

The conjunctival nevus is one of the most common benign tumors of the ocular surface. The appearance of the nevus may vary with different degrees of size and pigmentation. If well most of them has not other clinical significance but the appearance, long-term follow-up is mandatory because of a possible malignant transformation.

Clinical Signs and Symptoms

The clinical features of pigmented lesions involving the conjunctiva can occasionally overlap. The nevus is brown in almost 65% of the cases and completely non-pigmented in 16%; these lesions are most difficult to diagnose. The most common locations of the nevus is at the bulbar conjunctiva, then at caruncle and in third place the plica semilunaris. Nevi are most commonly seen at the nasal and temporal portions of the bulbar conjunctiva. Intralesional

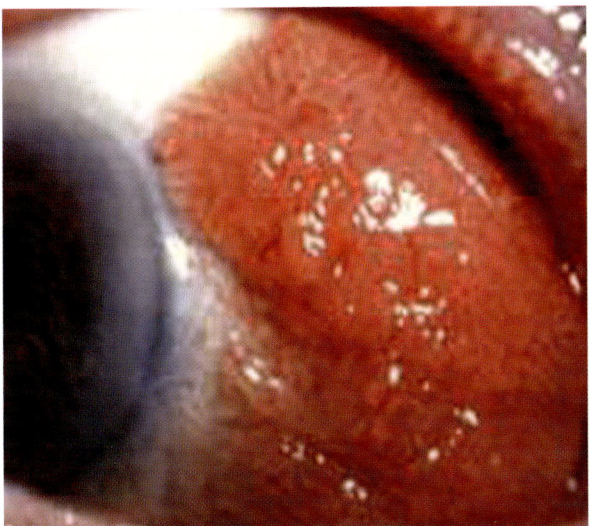

Fig. 25: Lymphoma

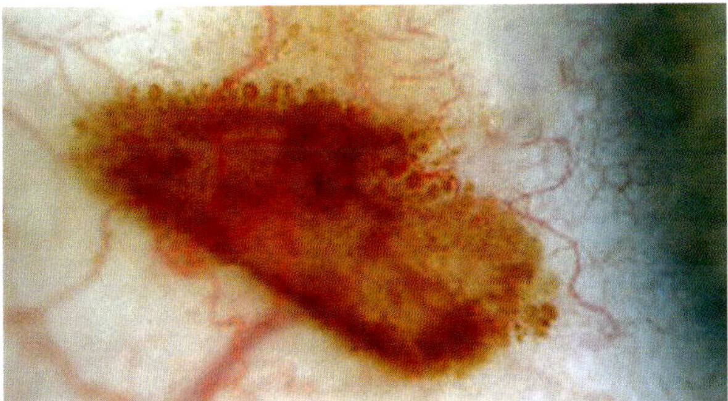

Fig. 26: Conjunctival nevus

cysts are present in a little more than half of the lesions. Conjunctival nevi can vary in appearance from darkly to lightly pigmented. The majority remain unchanged in size and pigmentation. Minor changes in color and size may occur with these benign lesions.

Investigations

The clinical features of pigmented lesions involving the conjunctiva can occasionally overlap. Many reports have provided data on the histopathologic features of conjunctival nevi; they provide clinically useful information in a large group of patients with conjunctival nevi. The infrequency of nevi involving the tarsal or forniceal conjunctiva may support the notion that pigmented lesions in these areas may not be nevi and that other conditions, such as conjunctival melanoma; it should be considered.

Differential Diagnosis

All melanic lesions of conjunctiva help to differentiate that the nevic lesions typically are present at birth, benign, situated near the limbus, cystic, brown in color (very rare, red) and move with conjunctival manipulation. It is also helpful to know that nevi may become enlarged and can be affected by hormonal changes such as in puberty, pregnancy, and with oral contraceptives. Nevi may occasionally be difficult to differentiate from melanoma and an excisional biopsy should be performed for suspicious appearing lesions.

Treatment

The mainstream of treatment is observation but in suspicious cases an excisional biopsy should be performed. If the patient wants a surgical resection for esthetic reasons, a complete pathologic study is mandatory; even so, long-term follow-up must be achieved.

Prognosis

The rate of patients that developed melanoma from a pre-existing nevus lesion is less that 1%, in large series studied over a mean of 7 years as minimum; if there is not malignant progression, the prognosis is very good.

Conjunctival Intraepithelial Neoplasia

Introduction

Conjunctival Intraepithelial Neoplasia (CIN) is the most common ocular surface neoplasm. It is a slowly progressive lesion that may evolve to squamous cell carcinoma (SCC). Males and patients older tan 70 years are more affected.

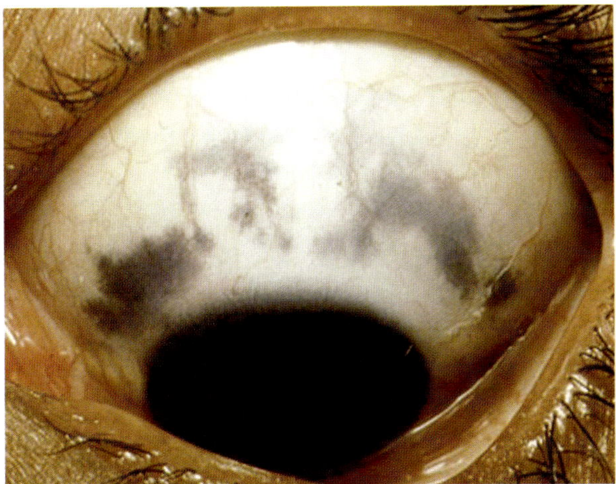

Fig. 27: Conjunctival nevus (Ota's)

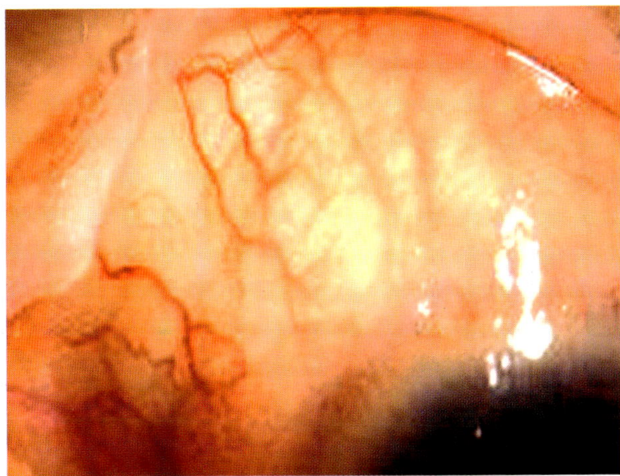

Fig. 28: Conjunctival intraepithelial neoplasia

Clinical Signs and Symptoms

Typically, CIN appears as an elevated lesion with limbal involvement. Appearance may be either leukoplakic, papilliform or gelatinous, with a characteristic tufts of blood vessels.

Investigations

Some authors have suggested that the slow cycling limbal stem cells may become hyperproliferative by stimulations, such as alterations in this anatomical site influenced by other factors (like ultraviolet radiation), which can cause abnormal maturation of the conjunctival and corneal epithelium and lead to the formation of corneal intraepithelial neoplasia. Nevertheless, the etiology and pathogenesis of corneal intraepithelial neoplasia and ocular surface carcinoma remain elusive, because there is no appropriate animal model available to study the molecular and cellular mechanisms of this disease.

Differential Diagnosis

Differential diagnosis of CIN includes a wide spectrum of ocular surface lesions, such as nevi, actinic disease, pingueculae, pterygium, pannus, conjunctival papilloma, benign intraepithelial dyskeratosis, keratinization of the corneal epithelium, and pseudoepitheliomatous hyperplasia.

Treatment

The traditional treatment of CIN is wide excisional biopsy of the tumor. Additionally, application of cryotherapy to the surgical margins in a double freeze technique, as well as external beam radiation has been advocated to reduce recurrences. More recently, coadjuvant therapy with immune modulators such as 5-fluouracil, Mitomycin C, topical vitamin A, and topical Interferon Alfa-2b have also demonstrated to be effective in treating these lesions. Recurrences rate varies from 7 to 69% in different series, and particularly occur if lesions were incompletely excised. Thus, pathologic examination of margins is very important.

Prognosis

If complete resection is done without lesion of margins and concomitant therapy is given, there is a complete cure. Recurrence can occur when incomplete treatment is applied.

Squamous Cell Carcinoma

Introduction

Conjunctival squamous cell neoplasia (CSCN) is the most common malignant tumor of the ocular surface. It represents a serious problem with a high impact

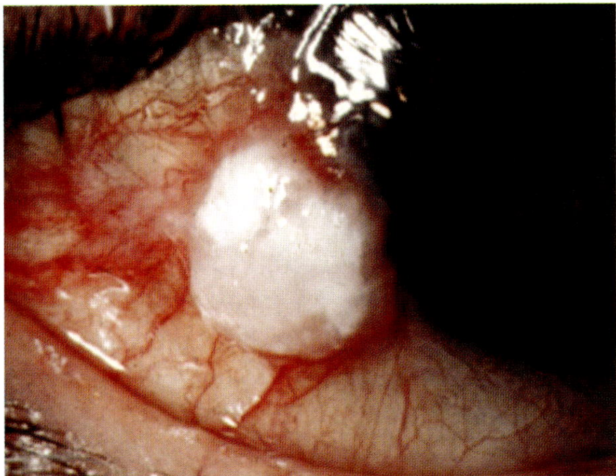

Fig. 29: Conjunctival intraepithelial neoplasia

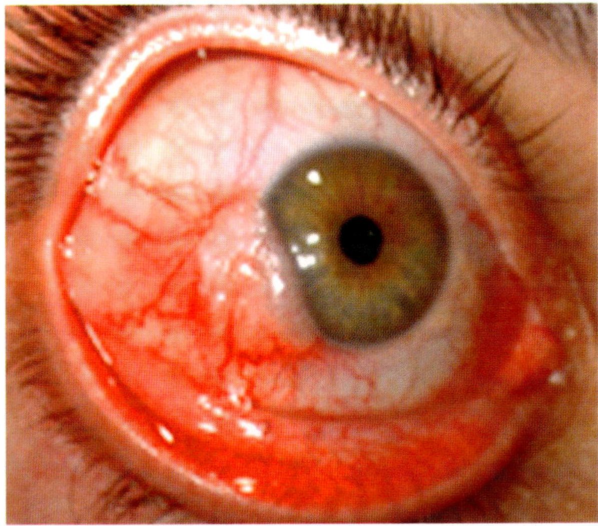

Fig. 30: Squamous cell conjunctival carcinoma

on public health owing to its relatively high prevalence and the potential to cause severe disability. The disease is prevalent in tropical areas because of the incidence of more ultraviolet radiation.

Clinical Signs and Symptoms

Clinically, the malignancy may appear as leukoplakic lesions which are white, shiny appearance caused by keratinization of the normally no keratinized conjunctival epithelium. Early manifestations are small masses at or around the limbus resembling pterygium, occurring in middle aged patients. The tumor then grows slowly, invading the nearby tissues including the ocular globe, eyelids, and orbital tissues leading to severe visual loss, loss of the eye, and severe facial deformities. Red eye (68%) and ocular irritation (57%) are the most common presenting symptoms, and 44% of the patients usually have other eye findings consistent with extensive solar exposure. The stagings of conjunctival squamous cell carcinoma are classified by the thickness of epithelial dysplastic changes and the tumor invasion into the substantia propria of the conjunctiva.

Investigations

The disease severity varies from conjunctival intraepithelial neoplasia (CIN), carcinoma in situ (CIS), to invasive squamous cell carcinoma (grade 1 dysplasia through grade 3 carcinoma in situ). When a clonal population of neoplastic cells has infiltrated through the basement membrane and invaded into the substantia propria of the conjunctiva, this becomes a squamous cell carcinoma. Multiple factors may contribute to the development of the disease; risk factors are believed to include fair skin pigmentation, atopic eczema, tobacco smoke, and mainly ultraviolet radiation due to sun exposure or other sources. A role for some infectious agents in the pathogenesis of SCC has been suggested, in particular with HPV (human papillomavirus types 16 and 18). However, the role of HPV in SCC remains unclear. Another association of SCC is with the human immunodeficiency virus (HIV). Conjunctival squamous cell carcinoma in HIV/AIDS patients presents on average at a younger age (35-40 years old) than in HIV-negative patients. Additionally, malignancy seems to be more aggressive in HIV/AIDS patients. Since HIV infection is a possible confounding factor, the investigation on HPV and HIV infections together with special characteristics on pathological figures will predict the diseases more definitely.

Differential Diagnosis

Chemical burns, limbal dermoid, conjunctival melanoma, pterygium and pseudopterygium.

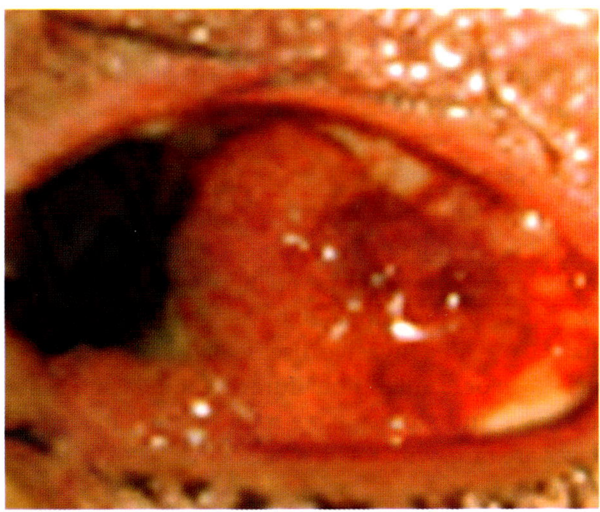

Fig. 31: Postoperative squamous cell conjunctival carcinoma

more superficial no basal portion of the epithelium in a pagetoid fashion and/or contained epithelioid cells.

Clinical Signs and Symptoms

Primary acquired melanosis appears as flat, patchy, non-cystic pigmentation in the conjunctival epithelium and can remain dormant for years or shows slow progression.

Differential Diagnosis

Differential diagnosis includes nevi, atopic melanosis, racial melanosis, and Melanoma.

Treatment

Treatment of primary acquired melanosis includes observation, excisional biopsy, alcohol epitheliectomy, cryotherapy, and topical chemotherapy. If PAM is 1 to 2 clock hours in extent, patients can be observed, although surgical excision is probably preferable. If the lesion is greater than 2 clock hours in extent, we generally recommend complete surgical excision and cryotherapy for those up to 5 clock hours and wide incisional biopsy plus cryotherapy for larger lesions. Topical mitomycin C 0.04% has also been used with a total of 6 weekly cycles of four times daily interrupted by a week's hiatus of no medication between each cycle with good results.

Prognosis

The prognosis is reasonably good for completely excised lesions.

Conjunctival Melanoma

Introduction

Conjunctival malignant melanoma is a potentially deadly tumor. Decades ago, it was believed to be one of the most malignant tumors in Ophthalmology and even small lesions with minimal growth were considered to require orbital exenteration. Today new diagnosis and treatment methods have changed this view.

Investigations

Conjunctival melanoma may arise in the context of Primary Acquired Melanosis (PAM) with atypia. In these cases, the first clinical sign of microinvasive melanoma may be a subtle thickening of PAM, but this is usually impossible to recognize clinically, thus lesions will have to be biopsied. Conjunctival melanoma may also present de novo, and vary rarely from a conjunctival nevi.

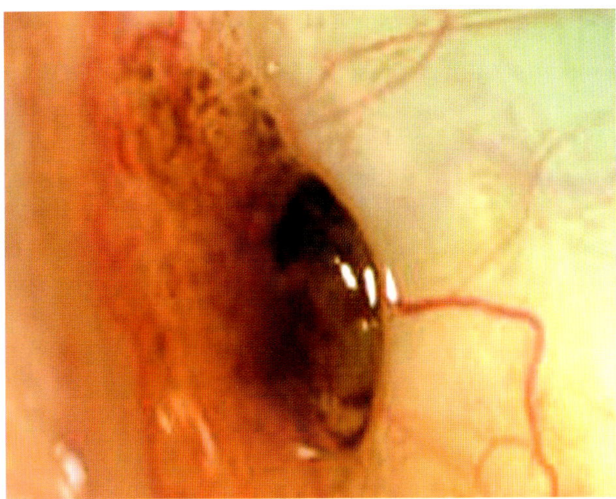

Fig. 33: Primary acquired melanosis of conjunctiva

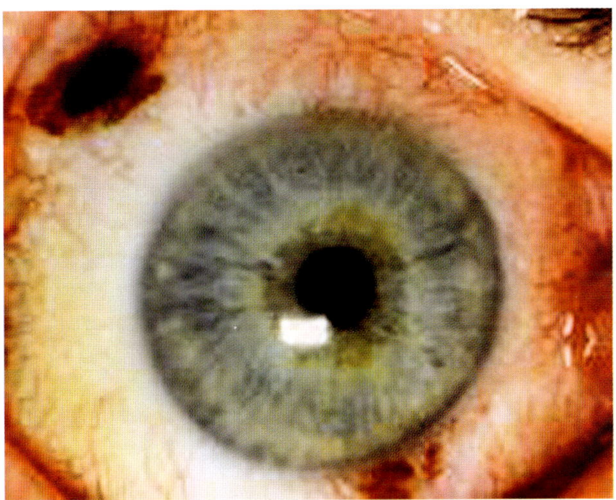

Fig. 34: Conjunctival melanoma

Clinical Signs and Symptoms

Conjunctival melanoma may present in all conjunctival areas, affecting the caruncle, plica, tarsus, fornices and lid margin. The features of a malignant melanoma are similar to those of a pigmented or nonpigmented lesion, with a smooth vascularized limbal nodule, but growth can also be elevated and pedunculated. A multifocal disease is not uncommon. Another variation of conjunctival melanoma is a lesion without pigment (sine pigmento). Corneal epithelium may also appear involved, but it is not common to have infiltration to Bowman's membrane.

Differential Diagnosis

Differential diagnosis may be difficult with numerous melanocytic lesions such as nevi, PAM, metastasis from skin melanoma. Non-melanocytic lesions like staphylomas, hematic cysts, a foreign body, and lesions from Moll's glands may be confused with melanoma.

Treatment

Treatment of conjunctival melanoma is usually surgical removing all traces of the lesion. Microsurgical excisional biopsy with the no-touch technique and supplemental alcohol corneal epitheliectomy followed by application of cryotherapy to the margins of resection is the gold standard of management. Because 26-41% of patients with conjunctival melanoma develop regional lymph node (preauricular most common) or distant metastasis, and death occurs in 13% at 10 years. Patients are recommended to have a sentinel lymph node biopsy at the time of the conjunctival tumor resection and a complete systemic work-up annually. Incisional biopsy should be avoided, because it can spread the malignant cells.

Prognosis

If a complete resection is done and there are not tumor cells at the sentinel lymph node, there is a complete cure. A good complete and systemic follow-up must be made in order to improve prognosis.

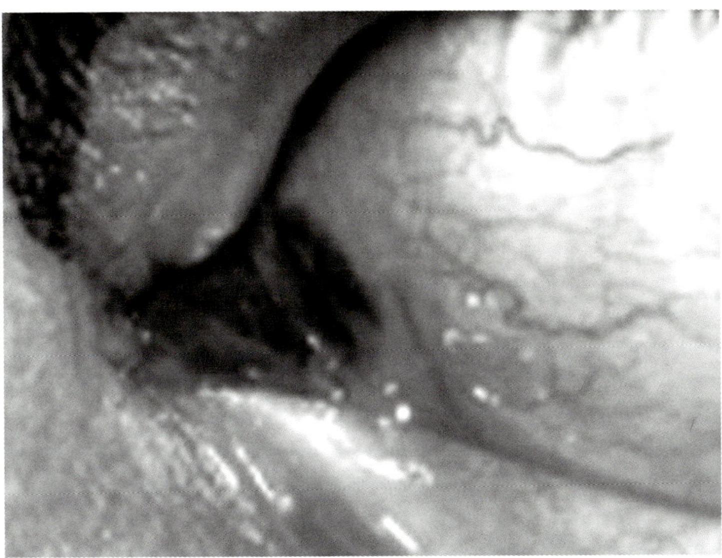

Fig. 35: Conjunctival melanoma

Limbal Dermoid

Introduction

Most of these are choristomas, which are defined as growth of normal tissue and structures in a particular site where they normally do not reside.

Clinical Signs and Symptoms

Solid dermoids that involve the cornea are yellow-white and affect the inferotemporal quadrant. Most cases are unilateral. Patients with Goldenhar's syndrome are more prone to present dermoids.

Investigations

Histologically, it reveals a thick collagenous lesion with hair, sweat glands, teeth, fat and sebaceous glands.

Differential Diagnosis

Differential diagnoses are ectopic lachrymal gland, scleral cysts, pyogenic granuloma, and more common dermolipomas. The later are more common in the temporal conjunctiva and are composed mainly by fat, and less by other structures. Management of these lesions is also surgical.

Treatment

Treatment of dermoids is difficult. It is not easy to determine either by clinical observation or by ultrasound, the depth of the lesion within the cornea. Some cases may require a lamellar or a penetrating keratoplasty at the time of excision.

Prognosis

If excision is adequate performed, either complete or incomplete, prognosis is good. Prognosis can be worst if there is some particular damage to adjacent structures.

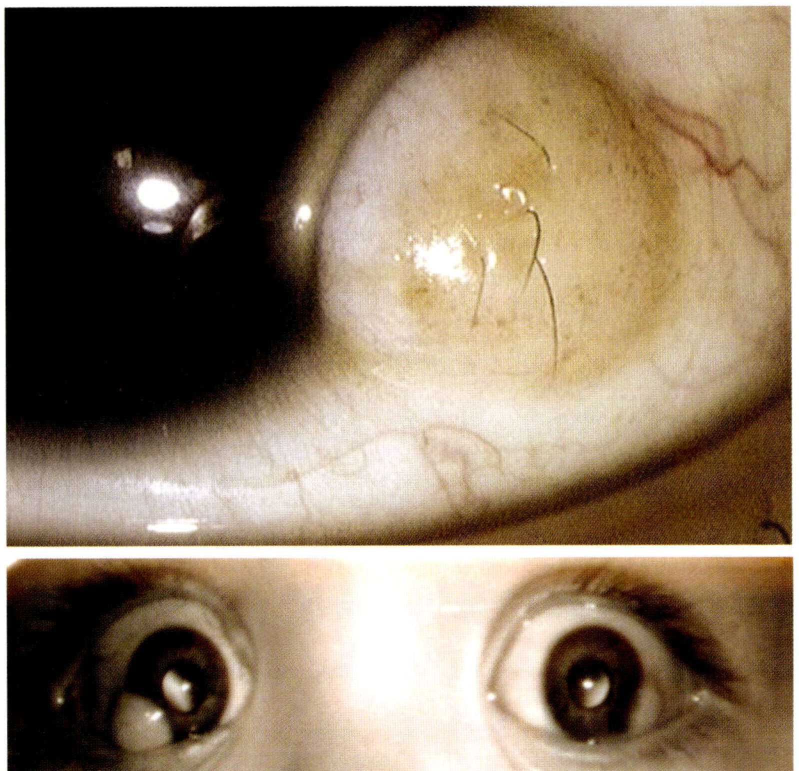

Figs 36 and 37: Limbal dermoid

Degenerations

PINGUECULAE

Introduction

- Result of bulbar conjunctival thickening because of elastoid degeneration (basophilic degeneration of collagen)
- Consequence of microtraumas and long exposure to UV light
- Prevalence increases with aging
- Not inherited
- Unilateral or bilateral.

Clinical Signs and Symptoms

- Small well defined elevated nodular lesion
- White or yellowish
- Located at limbus
- More common nasal than temporal
- Does not involve cornea
- Rarely causes symptoms. When inflammation exists it is called pingueculitis

Investigations

- Exists evidence of an association with increase age and UV light exposure
- The risk factors are outdoor work and world-equatorial residence
- The effect of UV light may be mediated by mutations in p53 gene.

Differential Diagnosis

- Conjunctival intraepithelial neoplasia. Only if it is keratinizated pinguecula
- Gaucher's diseas type I is associated with a pinguecula
- Pterygium, but it involves cornea and it is vascular.

Treatment

- Pingueculitis is treated with lubrication and if very symptomatic it responds to a short course of topical steroids or nonsesteroidal anti-inflammatory agents
- Use of hats and sunglasses are protective.

Prognosis

- Very good, but some patients must decrease sun light exposure and use eye lubricants chronically

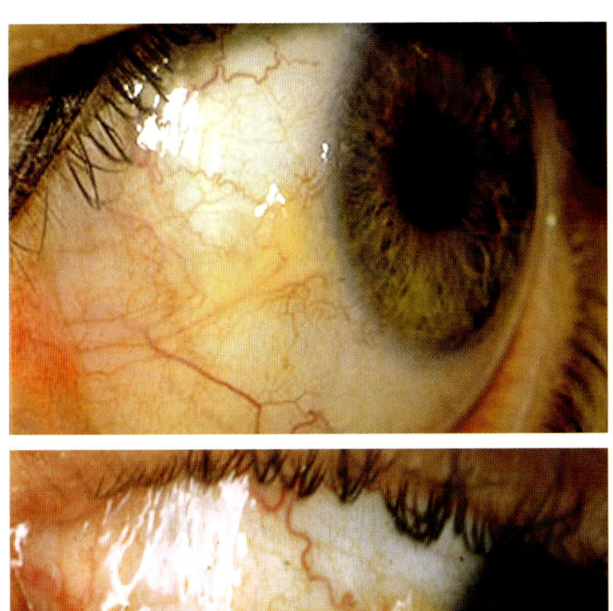

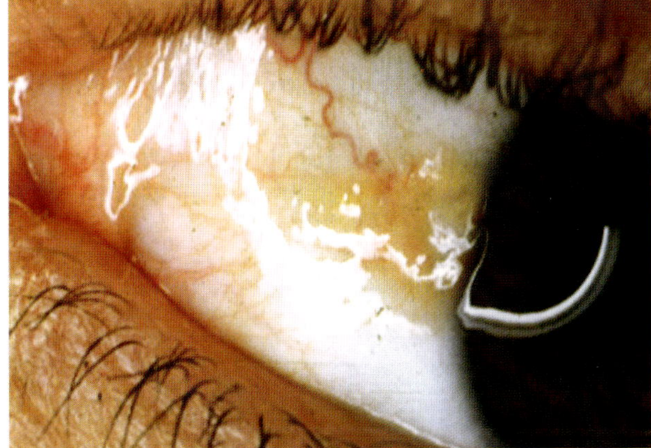

Figs 38 and 39: Pingueculae

Pterygium

Introduction

- Result of bulbar conjunctival thickening because of elastoid degeneration (basophilic degeneration of collagen). In the corneal component Bowman´s membrane is destroyed
- Consequence of microtraumas and long exposure to UV light
- Onset typically in the 20s to 40s.

Clinical Signs and Symptoms

- Fibrovascular triangular lesion extending onto the cornea in the horizontal meridian
- Thick and vascular lesion, may present an iron line central to it on cornea (Stocker´s line)
- If quiescent vessels are not dilated. If active, dilated vessels and progressive growth onto the cornea
- Unilateral or bilateral, and may be double (nasal and temporal)
- If it is too extended to the cornea may present with visual distortion or decreased acuity, or may present diplopia in lateral gaze.

Investigations

- New theories include damage to timbal stem cells by UV light and by activation of metalloproteinases
- Exists evidence of an association with increase age and UV light exposure
- The risk factors are outdoor work and world-equatorial residence.

Differential Diagnosis

- Pseudopterygium. May occur in any meridian. Usually after tauma or inflammation. Typically nonadherent to the limbus.
- Symblepharon associated with Stevens-Johnson syndrome
- Conjunctival intraepithelial neoplasia. Lack the radial orientation of pterygium
- Pinguecula. It is avascular and does not extend onto the cornea.

Treatment

- Medical therapy
  - — Ocular lubricants, vasoconstrictors intermittently for redness, short courses of topical corticosteroids if active.
  - — Use of hats and sunglasses are protective.

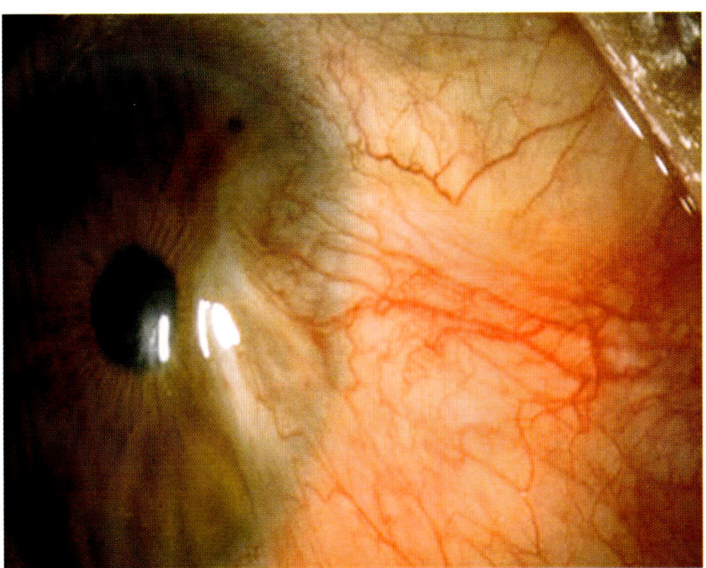

Fig. 40: Pterygium

- Surgical therapy
  - Excision indicated if decreased visual acuity because of induced astigmatism or interferes with visual axis or use of contact lens; and in case of recurrent significant inflammation.
  - It is 50% of recurrence rate but it decreases to 15% with amniotic membrane and to 5% with conjunctival autograft.

Prognosis

- As a general rule is good if recurrence does not occur; good surgical planning and good patient communication are mandatory. An aggressive recurrence may lead to symblefaron.

Conjunctivochalasis

Introduction

- Conjunctiva that is interposed between globe and eyelid becomes rounded, loose and desinserted
- More frequently lower, but may affect also upper eyelid
- It is redundant and loose
- Not edematous or inflamed
- It is probably a consequence of a mechanical factor like lid rubbing or dry conjunctiva
- Prevalence increases with age

Clinical Signs and Symptoms

- Tearing
- Irritation
- Foreign body sensation

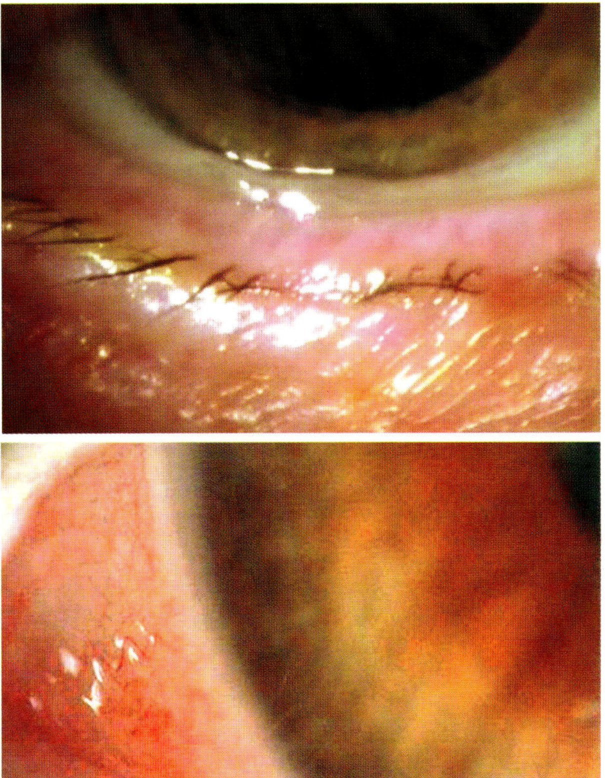

Figs 41 and 42: Conjunctivochalasias

- Obliteration of lower and upper meniscus causing instable tear film and dry eye symptoms

Investigations

- It is consequence of mechanical factors associated with aging of connective tissues.

Differential Diagnosis

- Some tumors and degenerations of conjuntiva

Treatment

- Lubrication
- If very symptomatic conjunctival resection or superficial conjunctival cauterization in cases of mild lower conjunctivochalasis.

Prognosis

- Generally good.

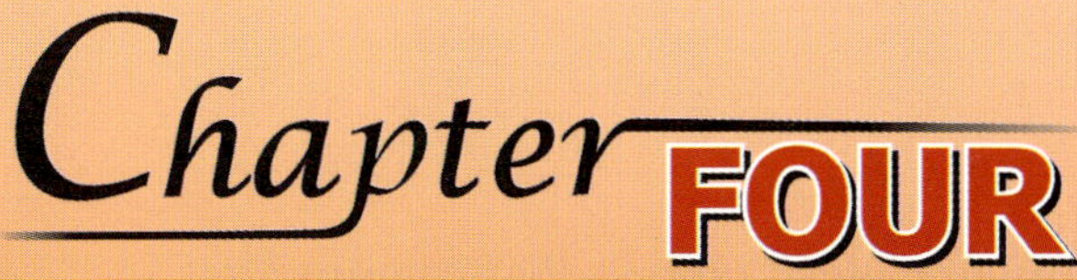

Episclera and Sclera

Arturo Perez Arteaga (Mexico)

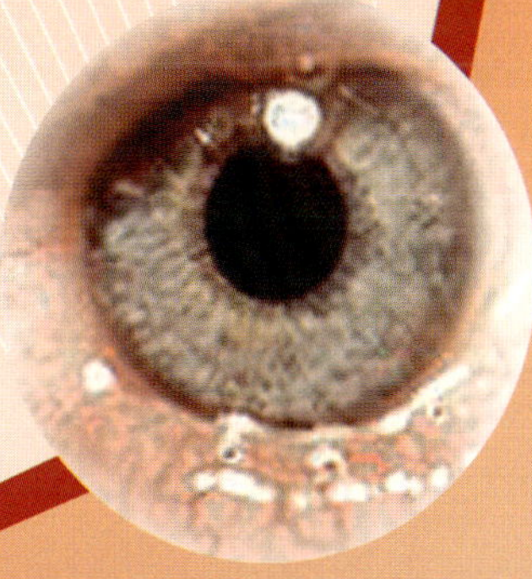

Episcleritis

Introduction

The episcleritis is an inflammatory process that compromises the laxus connective tissue between the conjunctiva and sclera.

Clinical Signs and Symptoms

The classification is between the simple (diffuse) and nodular. The simple form used to be sectorial, but sometimes can affect all the anterior segment of the eye. The inflammation is not well delimited and the affected zone is not elevated. The nodular form is characterized by an elevated inflammatory reaction localized at the interpalpebral zone; the onset is acute and the major symptoms are redness, foreign body sensation and moderate pain. Frequently the process can last 2 or 3 weeks, but sometimes it can last only days. In rare cases it can go on for months.

Investigations

Sometimes some underlying disease can be present; so if it last for more hat 2 or 3 weeks and do not respond to regular anti-inflammatory drugs, some systemic conditions should be discarded.

Differential Diagnosis

Some other inflammatory conditions of the conjunctiva and sclera like scleritis, conjunctivitis, pingueculae and pterygium.

Treatment

Local anti-inflammatory drugs; some types of cortisone type drugs are very useful; in moderate conditions nonsteroid eye drops can be very helpful, alone or in association to steroids. Remember monitoring intraocular pressure. In moderate to severe cases systemic steroids are very useful for short periods of time.

Prognosis

It is frequently good unless the inflammation is associated to systemic conditions.

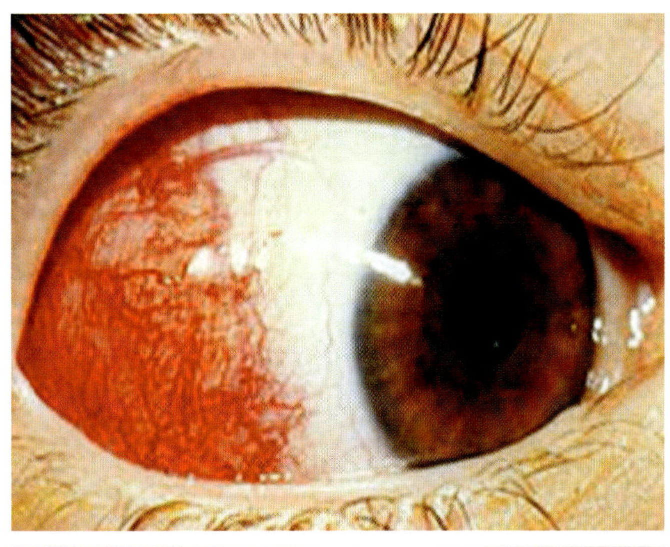

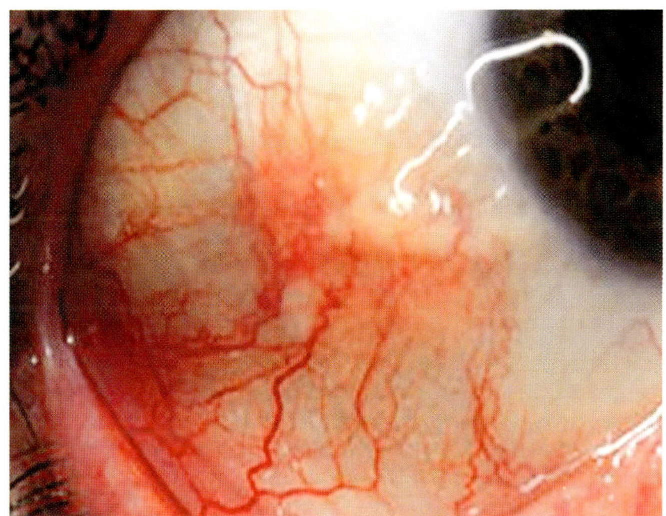

Figs 1 and 2: Epiescleritis

Scleritis

Introduction

The scleritis is the inflammation of the stroma of the sclera; this ocular structure is composed by collagen, and they are not oriented in a uniform fashion as in the cornea. It is covered by the episclera, which can also have inflammation. The scleritis can be only an isolated manifestation of some other systemic inflammatory diseases; they should be taken in count.

Clinical Signs and Symptoms

As a general rule they are unilateral and confinated to a localized area of inflammation that can be seen very congestive. Pain can be intense, accompanied by photofobia, hyperestesis and epiphora; the redness can affect a big area of the globe.

Investigations

The scleritis can be present in some autoimmune diseases like spondylitis, rheumatoid arthritis, nodous polyarteritis and lupus among others. The scleritis has terrible forms of presentation; the necrosant scleritis, the necrosant scleromalasia and the posterior scleritis; they produce a thin sclera and a translucent uveal tissue that can lead to the perforation of the globe.

Differential Diagnosis

A good method to distinguish between scleritis and epiescleritis is to produce vasoconstriction with epinephrine in drops to the episcleral vessels; when a scleritis is present there is not response of the redness, but good vasoconstriction is present in cases of episcleritis.

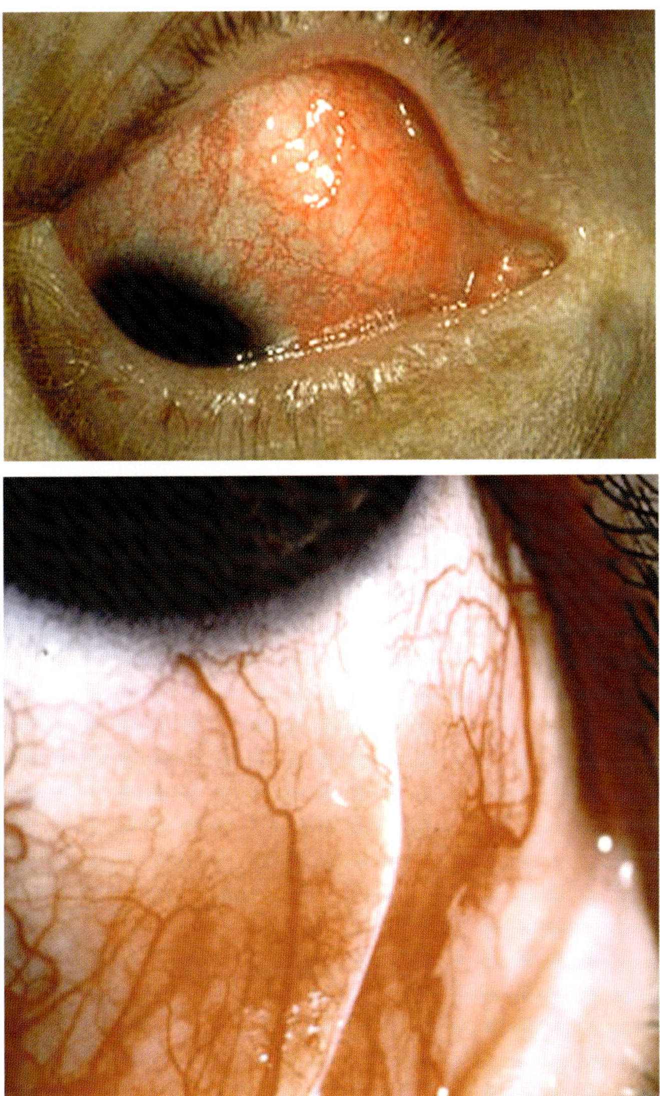

Figs 3 and 4: Scleritis

Treatment

Drops of steroids are the treatment of choice; non steroidal anti-inflammatory agents can be added either in local or systemic approach; in severe cases systemic steroids can be used. Also an intense investigation of the possible underlying disease is mandatory.

Prognosis

In the benign forms and when present isolated, frequently with no sequelae; but in the severe forms, and when accompanying systemic diseases, can be worst, and even lead to globe perforation.

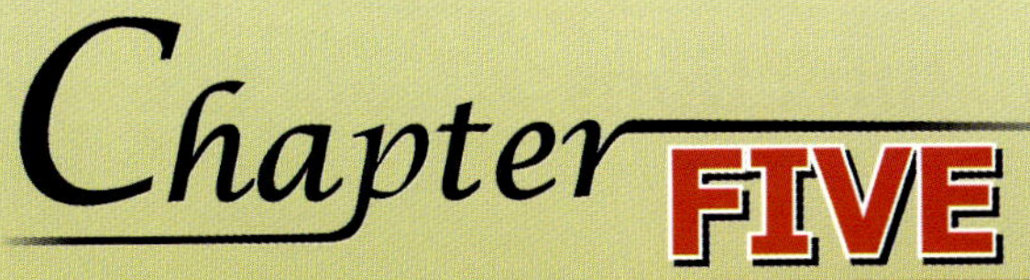

Corneal Disorders

Ashok Sharma (India)

- **Infections**
- **Inflammations**
- **Corneal Injuries**
- **Non-inflammatory Degenerations**
- **Corneal Dystrophies**

Infections

Bacterial Keratitis

Introduction

Bacterial keratitis is commonest of the corneal infections. Bacterial keratitis is potentially blinding condition. The occurrence of corneal epithelial defect is an initial event. The condition progresses fast and whole of the cornea may be involved in less than 24 hours.

Clinical Features

Patient presents with severe pain, redness, watering, photophobia and diminution of vision. Patient has marked eyelid edema, conjunctival congestion, chemosis and copious mucopurulent discharge. A classical presentation of Pseudomonas corneal ulcer is presence of infiltrate, surrounding corneal edema and hypopyon. The corneal ulcer progresses fast and progression is evident within hours. On the contrary, gram-positive infection causes localized infiltrate that progresses relatively slowly. *Staphylococcus* corneal ulcer usually occurs in the periphery of the cornea. Any surgical procedure, presence of diabetes mellitus, contact lens wear and corneal epithelial trauma may precipitate corneal infection. In the developing countries vitamin deficiency is an important risk factor.

Microbiological Diagnosis

Direct microscopic examination of the corneal smears (KOH wet mount and Gram stained) and cultures for microorganisms is the gold standard for establishing the diagnosis. In addition the newer diagnostic tests including use of fluorescent dyes, polymerase chain reaction and confocal microscopy may be helpful in selected cases. PCR has been reported to detect microbial DNA in the majority of bacterial and fungal corneal ulcers. PCR identifies potentially pathogenic organisms in a high proportion of culture-negative cases. Pseudomonas aeruginosa, *Staphylococcus aureus* and *Streptococcus pneumonae* are common bacteria causing infective keratitis. In a recent study Enterococcus faecalis keratitis has been reported in patients with abnormalities of the corneal surface and contact lens wear.

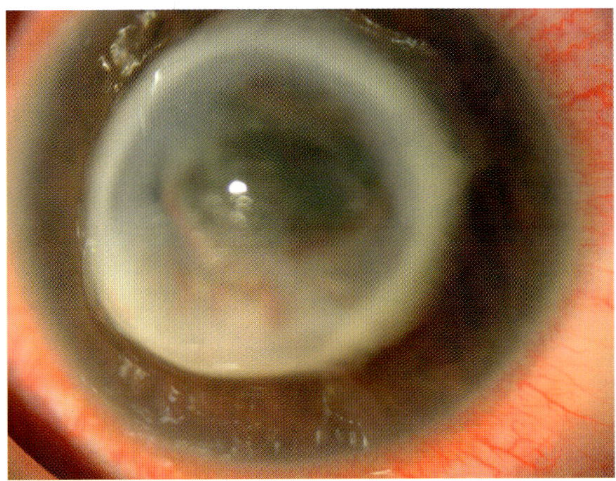

Fig. 1: *Pseudomonas* corneal ulcer

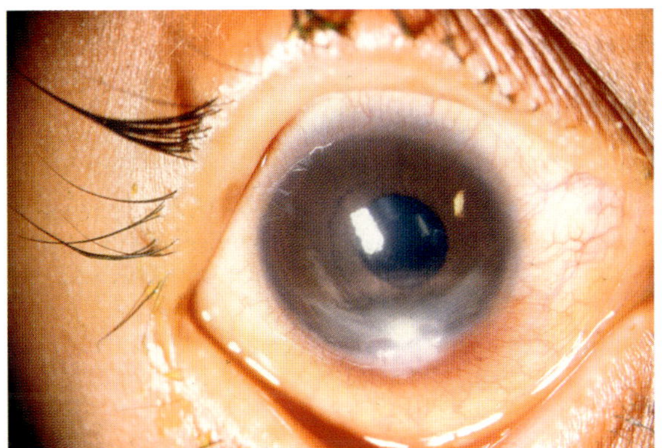

Fig. 2: Staphylococcal corneal ulcer

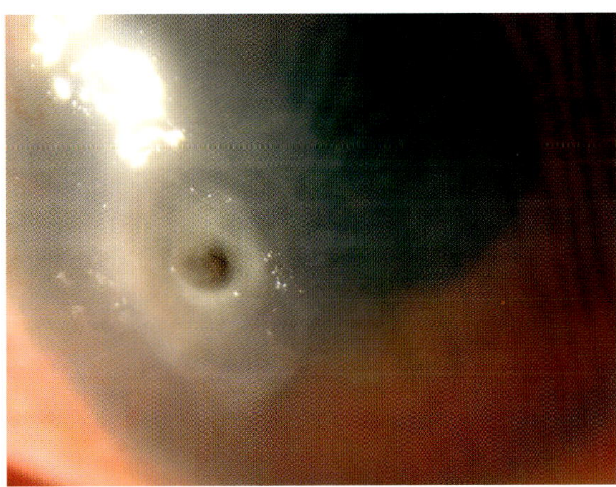

Fig. 3: Corneal perforation

Treatment

From treatment point of view corneal ulcer may be divided in nonsight threatening and sight threatening categories. Peripheral corneal ulcer and a small central or paracentral corneal infiltrate comprises the nonsight threatening group. Theses corneal ulcers may be treated with frequent instillation of fourth generation fluoroquinolone antibiotic, moxifloxacin. Large, central corneal ulcers are considered sight threatening. Combination of fortified gentamycin/ tobramycin (1.4%) and cefazolin/vancomycin (5%) is preferred in theses cases as initial treatment. Response to the initial treatment is closely monitored. In addition to the symptoms of the patient, size of the corneal infiltrate and hypopyon is considered. In case the response to the treatment is inadequate, treatment may be changed on the basis of the laboratory culture and sensitivity reports. Even if the corneal ulcer is responding to the treatment, the patients are observed for development of corneal thinning or perforation due to continued collagenolysis. Corneal perforation is confirmed by performing Siedel's test.

Corneal thinning, impending or actual corneal perforation may be treated with application of cyanoacrylate tissue adhesive. The intensive topical antibiotic treatment is continued. Patients having large corneal perforation (> 3.0 mm) or in case perforation is not responding to the cyanoacrylate tissue adhesive application, an emergency penetrating keratoplasty is considered. With the availability of the current fourth generation fluoroquinolone antibiotics and other modalities the outcome of the treatment of the bacterial keratitis has significantly improved.

Fungal Keratitis

Introduction

Fungal keratitis is a serious corneal infection occurring world wide. Recent epidemics of fungal keratitis due to contaminated contact lens solutions occurred all over the world. In the developing world it usually follows frequent corneal injuries during agriculture related activities. Indiscrinate use of topical corticosteroid drops and use of household remedies complicates the disease. In developing countries the condition is more prevalent and is a frequent cause of corneal blindness. Patients usually present late and with severe disease. Treatment of fungal keratitis is challenging as the antifungal drugs are mostly fungistatic, have narrow spectrum and limited corneal penetration.

Clinical Presentation

Fungal keratitis usually develops about a week after the initial corneal epithelial trauma. In some of the patients corneal foreign body may be present at the time of presentation. Patient are relatively asymptomatic as compared to the clinical signs. A classical presentation includes a raised, dry looking infiltrate, with

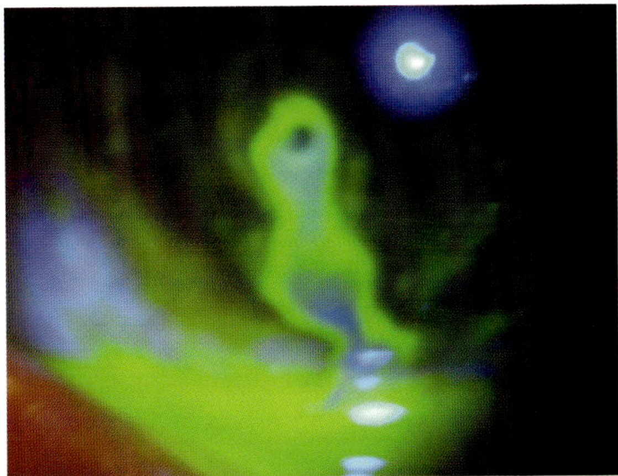

Fig. 4: Positive Siedel's test

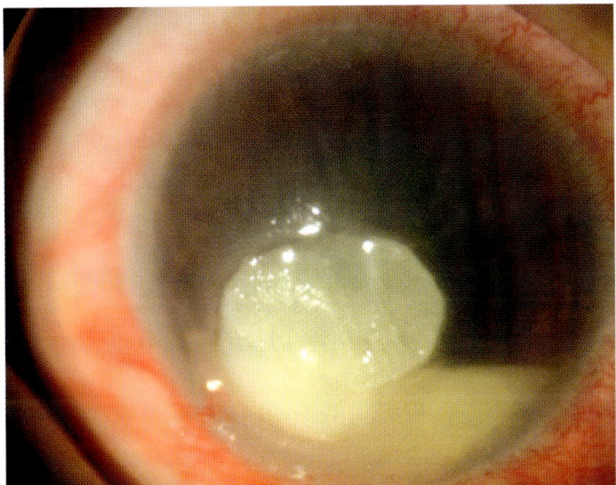

Fig. 5: Fungal corneal ulcer

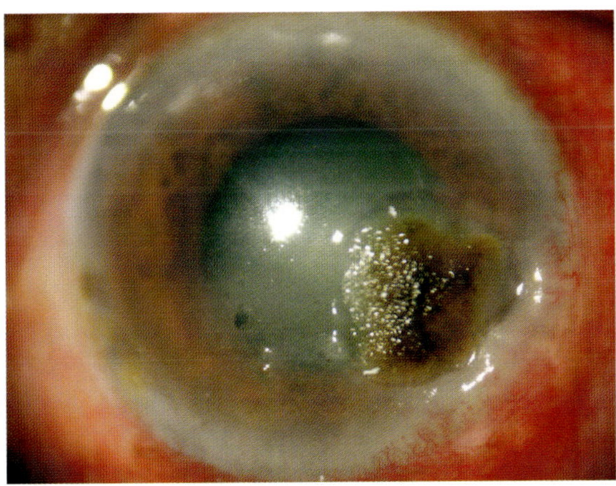

Fig. 6: Fungal corneal ulcer (Pigmentation)

hyphate margins. The presence of pigmentation in the infiltrate is considered characteristic of fungal infection. The surrounding cornea is clear. Hypopyon may be present. A detailed color coded schematic documentation of the clinical findings help in monitoring the response to the treatment. The disease usually progresses slowly as compared to bacterial keratitis. Host factors including presence of diabetes mellitus, immune compromised status and steroid exposure have an adverse effect on the outcome of the disease.

Microbiological Diagnosis

The standard protocol of management of fungal keratitis include obtaining of corneal scraping under topical anesthesia. The material obtained on corneal scrapings is subjected to the direct microscopy (KOH wet mount smear and gram stain) and cultures (bacteria and fungus). Use of fluorescent dye, Calcofluor enhances the sensitivity of the direct microscopy. Demonstration of fungal hyphae on direct microscopy or fungus growth in culture media establishes the diagnosis of fungal keratitis. Recent introduction of polymerase chain reaction and confocal microscopy has given new option to corneal specialists in selected cases. PCR has been found more sensitive than KOH wet mount and Gram's smear. *Aspergillus*, *Fusarium*, *Alternaria* and *Candida* are common fungi implicated in fungal keratitis.

Treatment

Superficial keratomycosis usually responds to the topical antifungal treatment. Topical antifungal drugs commonly used include natamycin (5%) suspension, econazole (1%), itraconazole (1%) and amphotericin (0.25%) solution. As the penetration of the antifungal drugs is limited these are not as effective in deep keratmycosis. In these cases systemic antifungal drugs including fluconazole and itraconazole 100 mg twice daily may be added to the topical treatment. It is essential to monitor liver function tests while the patient is on systemic antifungal treatment. In resistant cases intracameral and intracorneal injections of amphotercin B have been used successfully. New-generation triazoles, including voriconazole, posaconazole and ravuconazole, have been shown effective in laboratory and clinical studies. Voriconazole has been reported safe and effective against a variety of fungal pathogens.

Patients should be closely monitored and the response should be recorded. Corneal thinning, impending or actual corneal perforation may be treated with application of cyanoacrylate tissue adhesive. The intensive topical and systemic antifungal treatment is continued. Patients having a large corneal perforation (> 3.0 mm) or in case perforation is not responding to the cyanoacrylate tissue adhesive application, an emergency penetrating keratoplasty is considered. With the availability of the newer antifungal drugs including voricozole and other surgical options the outcome of the treatment of the keratomycosis has significantly improved.

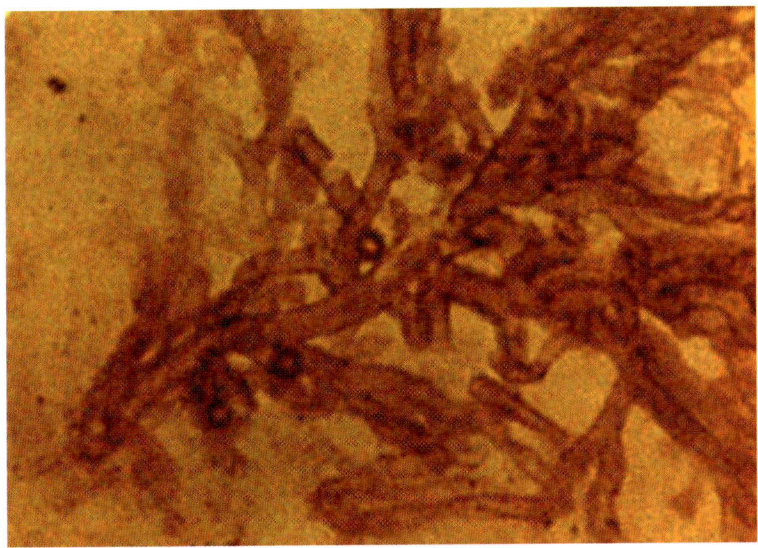

Fig. 7: Fungal hyphae in KOH wet mount smear

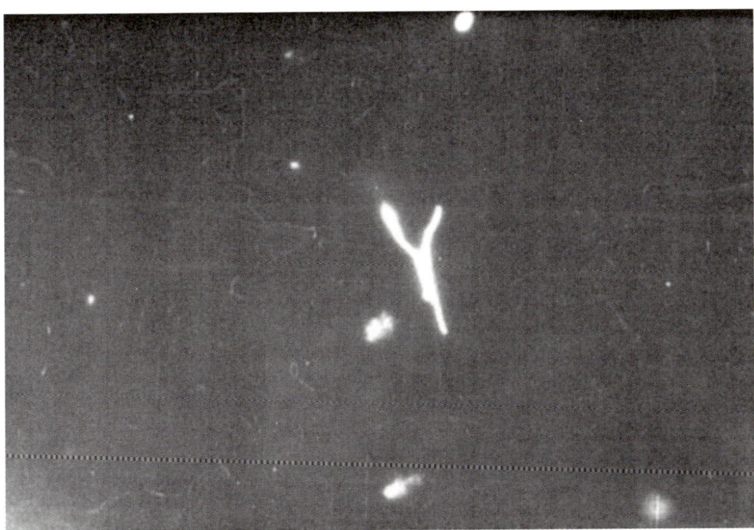

Fig. 8: Fungal hyphae in calcofluor stain

Herpes Simplex Keratitis

Introduction

Herpes simplex keratitis is common corneal infection occurring all over the world. In most of the cases infection occurs due to herpes simplex virus type 1. Ocular infection due to herpes simplex virus type 2 is rare. In more than 90% of the general population herpes simplex virus gains entry in to the body and establishes the latency by 16 years of age. The corneal involvement occurs due to reactivation of the virus in the trigeminal ganglion. In recent studies the herpes simplex virus has been reported to establish latency in the cornea after attacks of keratitis. The occurrence of fever, upper respiratory tract infection and immune suppression are some of the predisposing factors for developing recurrence of herpes simplex keratitis.

Clinical Presentation

The characteristic presentation of herpes simplex keratitis is dendritic corneal ulcer. Dendritic corneal ulcer may progress to dendrogeographical and finally to geographical corneal ulcer. The dendrites need to be differentiated from pseudodendrite of herpes zoster keratitis. The dendritic corneal ulcer due to herpes simplex infection is brilliantly stained with fluoroscein stain. In case of herpes zoster dendrite is poorly stained. Stromal keratitis, disciform keratitis, endothelitis and limbitis are other clinical presentations of herpes simplex keratitis. Corneal endothelitis is a relatively newer clinical entity characterized by corneal edema, keratic precipitates, and mild anterior chamber reaction. Corneal endothelitis has been recently classified clinically into four forms including linear, sectorial, disciform, and diffuse.

Recurrences are the hallmark of herpes simplex keratitis. In recurrent herpes simplex keratitis the corneal sensation is grossly diminished on the affected side. Metaherpetic keratitis is another presentation of herpes simplex keratitis. The condition is noninfective and does not require anti viral treatment. It is characterized by a nonhealing epithelial defect, round or oval in shape with heaped up margins of the ulcer.

Microbiological Tests

In the infective forms of the disease detection of viral antigen is possible. Histopathological examination of the corneas with recurrent herpes simplex keratitis show granulomatous reaction. On histopathology of the corneal buttons obtained during penetrating keratoplasty virus particles may be demonstrated on electron microscopic examination. Herpes simplex virus infection can also be demonstrated with polymerase chain reaction.

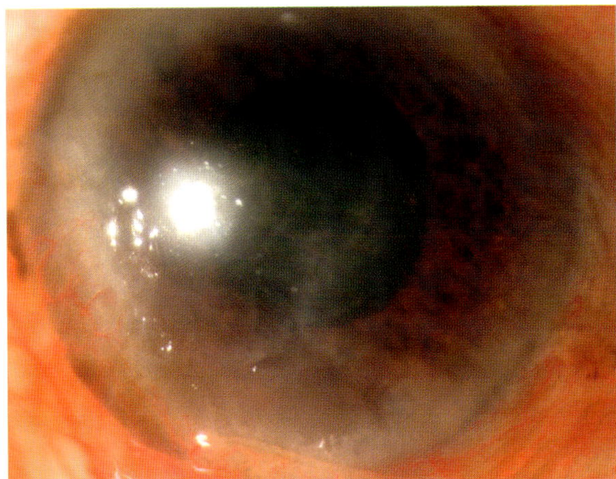

Fig. 9: Dendrogeographical ulcer

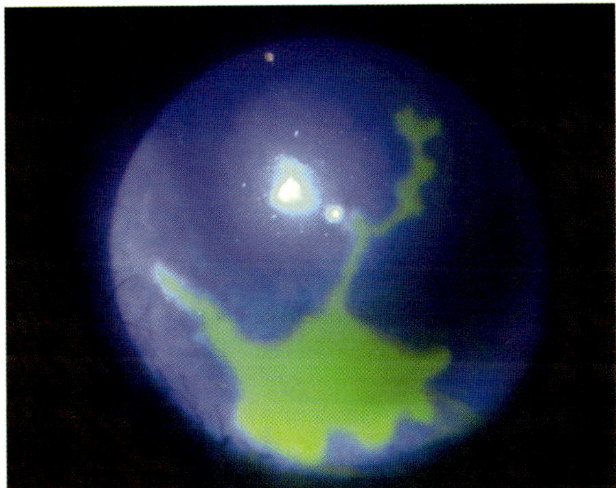

Fig. 10: Fluoroscein stained corneal ulcer

Treatment

Dendritic, dendrogeographical and geographical corneal ulcers are infective forms of the disease and are treated with topical antiviral drugs. Topical application of vidarabine, trifluridine, acyclovir or ganciclovir have resulted healing within one week of treatment in most patients. Of these antiviral agents, no treatment emerged as significantly better than the other for the therapy of dendritic epithelial keratitis. Patients who have no attendants and are unable to instill ointment themselves are given tab. Acyclovir 400 mg 5 times a day. Metaherpetic keratitis is non infective condition and does not require antiviral. Patient should be treated with prophylactic antibiotic drops, preservative free artificial eye drops, cycloplegics and bandage contact lens. Stromal keratitis, Disciform keratitis and endothelitis have both infective as well as immune component. These forms of disease are treated with combination of topical antiviral and low dose of topical corticosteroids. In case recurrence occurs within 6 months patient should be put on prophylactic dose of oral acyclovir i.e. tab acyclovir 400 mg 3 times a day.

Patients developing secondary infection should be treated with broad spectrum antibiotic drops. Patient who had multiple recurrences may develop keratolysis, corneal thinning, descemetocoele or corneal perforation. These patients should be treated with cyanoacrylate tissue adhesive application. In case the perforation is large or small perforation does not heal with cyanoacrylate tissue adhesive one may consider therapeutic penetrating keratoplasty.

Herpes Zoster Ophthalmicus

Introduction

Herpes zoster ophthalmicus is caused by Varicella zoster virus. The condition is characterized by the vesicular eruption involving frontal branch of trigeminal nerve. In case the side of the tip of the nose is involved, it indicates that the nasociliary branch is involved and Hutchinson's sign is said to positive. With Hutchinson's sign positive there are 85% chances of ocular involvement. Clinical presentation: Prodromal symptoms include headache, malaise, fever and chills followed by erythema, papules and vesicular eruptions in 2 to 3 days later. Classical presentation of herpes zoster ophthalmicus is unilateral and lesions do not cross midline. Rarely disease may occur without vesicular eruptions and may affect ophthalmic division on both sides. Corneal involvement occurs in the form of dendrites, stromal keratitis, disciform keratitis and kerato-uveitis. IOP should monitored regularly as significant number of patients may have rise in IOP.

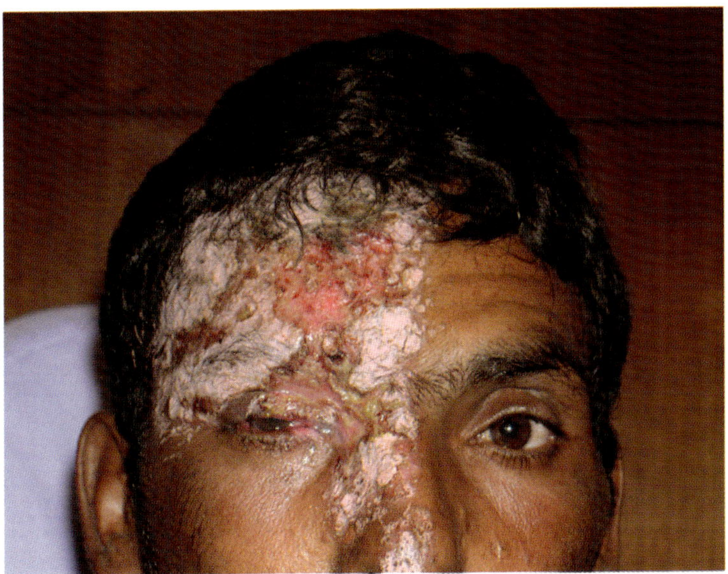

Fig. 11: Herpes zoster ophthalmicus lesions with Hutchinson's sign

Treatment

Herpes zoster should be treates with oral acyclovir 800 mg 5 times a day for 7 to 10 days. Initiation of the treatment within 72 hours of onset of symptoms is ideal. Famciclovir (500 mg/day for 7 days) and valacyclovir (1000 mg three times a day for 7 to 10 days) are the newer antiviral drug recommended in the treatment of herpes zoster. Both these drugs have more bioavailability and have been found superior to acyclovir in reducing symptoms of the disease. Oral steroid may reduce the zoster associated pain but should be used cautiously in immune compromised individuals. Topical steroid may be used in controlling corneal or scleral inflammation and also in treating keratouveitis. Topical antivirals are not recommended in the treatment of zoster. Neurotropic keratitis should be treated with, preservative free artificial drops, bandage contact lens, amniotic membrane graft and conjunctival flaps. Tarsorrhaphy is ideal in patient with severe corneal hypesthesia and decreased Schirmer values.

ACANTHAMOEBA KERATITIS

Introduction

Acanthamoeba keratitis is a rare cause of infective keratitis. Cases of infective keratitis have been reported from all over the world. *Acanthamoeba* keratitis accounts for approximately 1% of total infective keratitis patients in the tertiary eye care centers. The condition has been reported more prevalent in the contact lens wearers. From developing countries cases in non-contact lens wearing patients have been reported. Contamination of the contact lenses with tap water and access of soil contaminated water into the conjunctival sac are important predisposing factors. The condition assumes clinical importance as it poses difficulties in clinical diagnosis, isolation of the microorganism and availability of effective drugs.

Clinical Features

High index of suspicion is required to make clinical diagnosis and confirm it on the laboratory diagnostic tests. Unusual pain in a patient suffering from infective keratitis should alarm the clinician to suspect *Acanthamoeba* keratitis. Earlier ring infiltrate and radial perineuritis were considered characteristic signs of *Acanthamoeba* keratitis. In recent studies a change in the clinical features has been reported. Acanthamoeba keratitis has been reported to closely mimic epithelial keratopathy. Epithelial lesions including epithelial edema, lose epithelium and anterior stromal haze have been considered diagnostic of *Acanthamoeba* keratitis. In advanced cases corneal stromal infiltrate involves the deeper stroma. There is considerable delay of few weeks in establishing and confirming the clinical diagnosis of *Acanthamoeba* keratitis. We routinely screened patients suffering from infective keratis with unusual pain and atypical

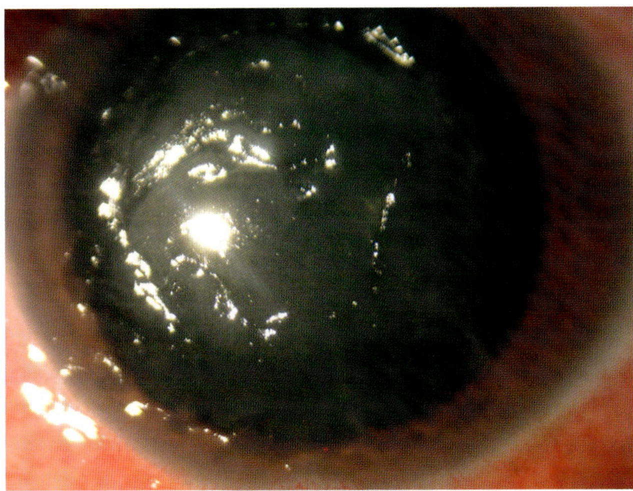

Fig. 12: *Acanthamoeba* corneal ulcer with radial perineuritis

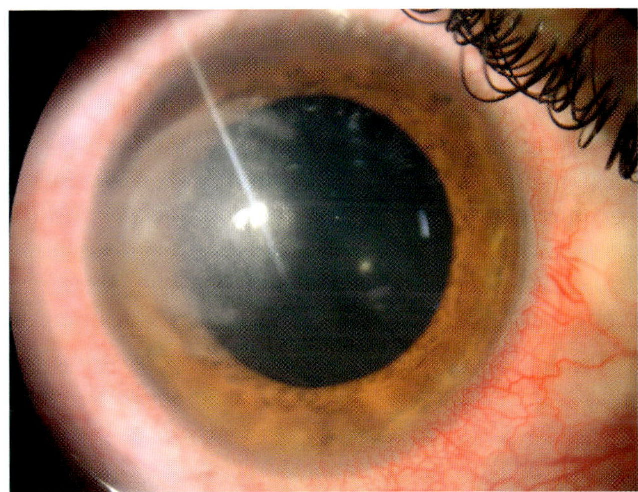

Fig. 13: Ring infiltrate in *Acanthamoeba* keratitis

presentation of herpes simplex keratitis for *Acanthamoeba* keratitis. In our experience we picked up more number of cases after screening patients with atypical presentation and resistant to conventional antiviral treatment of herpes simplex keratitis.

Microbiological Tests

Acanthamoeba keratitis may be diagnosed on direct microscopy of the corneal smears. *Acanthamoeba* cultures are considered more specific. In recent studies confocal microscopy has been used to confirm diagnosis. Confocal microscopy performed and evaluated by an experienced person, sensitive and specific in the diagnosis of *Acanthamoeba* keratitis. Real-time polymerase chain reaction has been standardized to confirm the diagnosis of *Acanthamoeba* keratitis. Polyhexamethylene biguanide has been reported to inhibit PCR and specimen collection occur prior to the use topical treatment has been advocated to avoid possible false negative results.

Treatment

Treatment of *Acanthamoeba* keratitis is initiated once the diagnosis is confirmed. Chlorhexidine (0.02%) and polyhexamethylene biguainde (0.02%) are the most effective drugs against trophozoites and cysts. Both these drugs are recommended as the first line of treatment. Propamidine isethionate 0.1%, dibromopropamidine, pentamidine and hexamidine are other drugs used in the treatment of Acanthamoeba keratitis. Neomycin, ketaconazole, clotrimazole, miconazole and itraconazole may be used in addition to primary treatment.

Reducing the incidence of *Acanthamoeba* keratitis requires multifaceted efforts. These include education of contact lens wearers, on the safe and hygienic contact lens wear, proper care of their lenses, execution of standardized and rigorous SCL solution disinfection regimens. Response to the treatment is slow as the drugs are less effective against the cysts. Treatment has to be continued for longer period after resolution of the infiltrate.

Atypical Mycobacterium Keratitis

Atypical *mycobacterium* keratitis is a rare infection. The cases have been reported in patients presenting with postcataract surgery infections and infective keratitis following LASIK. Cases of atypical *mycobacterium* keratitis without any risk factors have also been reported. A case of Mycobacterium chelonae keratitis in a patient without any previously described risk factors has been reported. The only risk factor in this patient was a rheumatoid arthritis related Sjogren's syndrome. Atypical *mycobacterium* infection may be considered in case the corneal infection show no response to regular antibacterial treatment. The clinical presentation includes diffuse corneal edema, several infiltrates with fluffy edges, surrounded by several smaller satellite infiltrates.

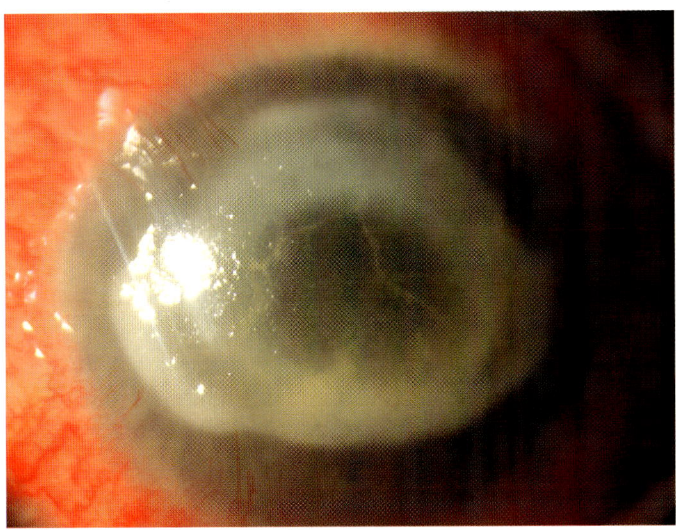

Fig. 14: Dense corneal infiltrate in *Acanthamoeba* keratitis

Microbiological Tests

Patients are subjected to corneal scrapings direct microscopy and cultures are performed. In most of the patients routine microscopic examination and culture results are negative. The corneal scrapings are repeated and cultured specifically for atypical mycobacterium. The ophthalmologist and the microbiologist should have good rapport and communication to obtain rapid diagnosis. In case the microorganism grows sensitivity test to various drugs should be performed.

Treatment

Most of the atypical mycobacteria are sensitive to fourth generation fluoroquinolone antibiotic moxifloxacin. Although rare, Atypical mycobacterial keratitis resistant to fourth-generation fluoroquinolones after laser *in situ* keratomileusis (LASIK) has been reported. Aminogycoside antibiotic, Amikacin has been used to treat atypical mycobacterium keratitis in the past. However the response to treatment has been less favorable (60%). The micro-organisms have also been found to be sensitive to ciprofloxacin, clofazimine, and clarithromycin. Systemic antibiotics, ciprofloxacin 750 mg and clarithromycin 500 mg twice daily have been used. Treatment period may be longer and some of the patients may require treatment for few months.

Post LASIK atypical mycobacterium keratitis may not respond to intensive topical antibiotic treatment. These patients may require therapeutic penetrating keratoplasty for controlling the infection or optical penetrating keratoplasty for visual rehabilitation.

Nocardia Keratitis

Nocardia keratitis is a rare cause of infective keratitis. High index of suspicion is required for making clinical diagnosis and confirmation of the diagnosis on laboratory examination. Patients suffering from Nocardia infection usually belong to the rural areas and are engaged in the agriculture related activities. History of splashing soil contaminated water into the eyes predisposes the individual to Nocardial infection. In a study comprising of 11 cases six species including Nocardia arthritidis (3), Nocardia neocaledoniensis (3), Nocardia asiatica (2), Nocardia asteroids type 4 (1), Nocardia brasiliensis (1), and Nocardia pseudobrasiliensis (1) were isolated. Nocardia arthritidis was the most important etiologic species. In another study Nocardia asteroids was found to be the commonest isolate in Nocardia keratitis. *Nocardia neocaledoniens* is isolated in the conjunctiva and might cause conjunctivitis. In one of our patients *Nocardia* keratitis was diagnosed on histopathological examination of the host cornea button after therapeutic penetrating keratoplasty. The organisms have been found to be sensitive to commonly used topical ocular antibiotics. The highest percentage (100%) of isolates were susceptible to gentamicin eye drops and most (93.55%) to ciprofloxacin eye drops.

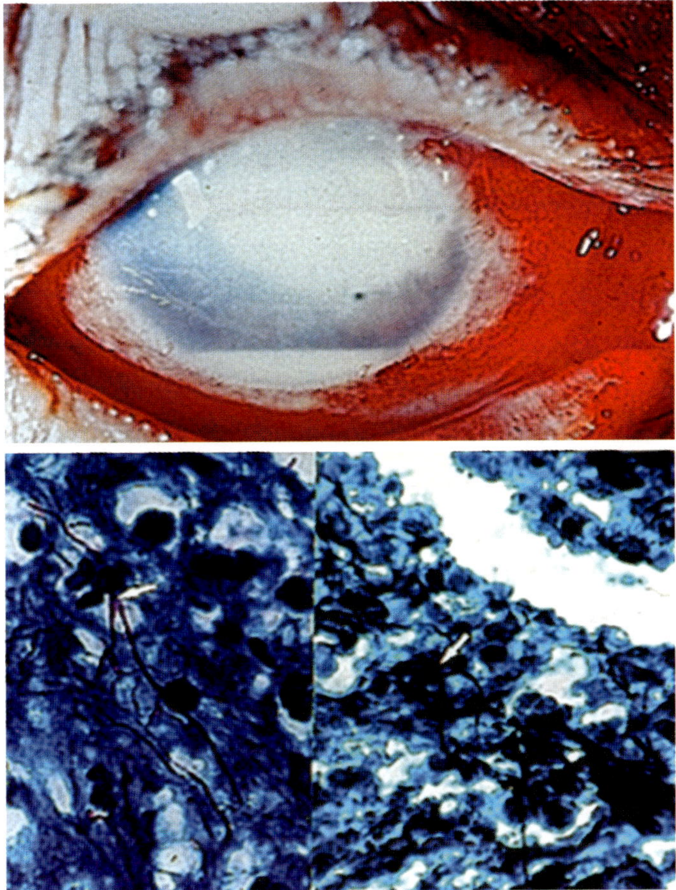

Fig. 15: *Nocardia* keratitis and *Nocardia* on histopathological examination of corneal button

Inflammations

Marginal Keratitis

Introduction

The term, marginal keratitis is used to describe the non-infectious inflammation of the peripheral cornea and the limbus. The condition occurs as a result of hypersensitivity reaction to bacterial antigen, especially *Staphylococcus aureus*.

Clinical Presentation

The condition presents as irritation, redness, photophobia and foreign body sensation. Patient usually has marked limbal and conjunctival congestion. The most diagnostic sign is peripheral corneal infiltrate. The lesion can be single or multiple. The disease may occur as unilateral or bilateral. The lesion is peripheral, parallel to the limbus and is separated by a clear zone.

These lesions invariably progress circumstantially in contrast to infective ulcers which progress towards the center of the cornea. The condition mostly occurs in middle aged adults but can occur at any age including children. Patients suffering from meibomitis, recurrent chalazia, styes and rosacea are more prone to development of marginal keratitis

In a recent report, marginal keratitis has been described as a hypersensitivity reaction to topical dorzolamide. The use of topical pilocarpine has been reported to cause marginal corneal infiltration and limbal ulceration typical of allergic marginal keratitis. Discontinuation of the offending topical medication results in complete resolution of the hypersensitivity reaction.

Marginal keratitis has also been described in association with dissecting folliculitis of the scalp. Marginal keratitis is postulated to be caused by an enhanced immune response to *Staphylococcus aureus* antigens. It is possible that a similar abnormal response to infection may play role in the pathogenesis of these two conditions.

Differential Diagnosis

The condition must be distinguished from the infective peripheral infiltrate due to *Staphylococcus* or any other bacteria. The infective infiltrate is painful, round in shape and has an overlying epithelial defect. It is invariably associated with anterior chamber reaction. The infiltrate is usually single and non-recurrent. The material obtained on corneal scraping should be subjected to Gram's stain and bacterial culture and sensitivity tests. Patient should be treated with intensive topical broad spectrum antibiotics. Peripheral dendritic ulcer and conjunctival ulcer characteristic of Herpes Simplex keratitis should be excluded.

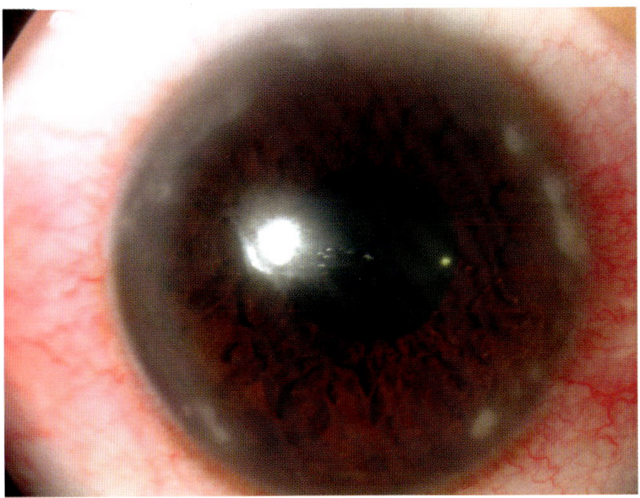

Fig. 16: Early marginal keratitis (multiple infiltrate)

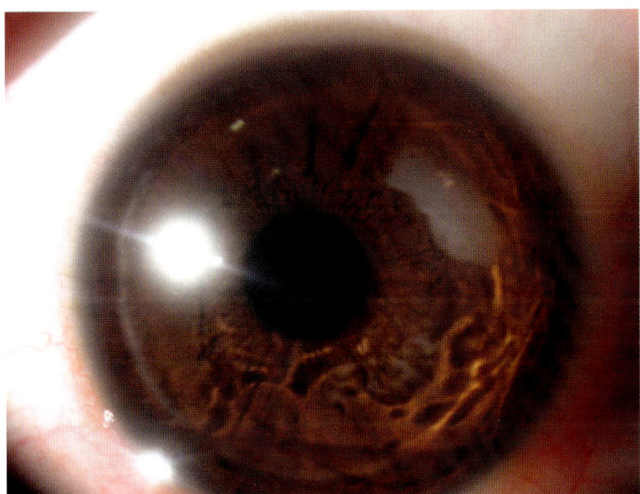

Fig. 17: Advanced marginal keratitis

Marginal keratitis should also be distinguished from keratitis associated with connective tissue disorders, dry eye, Mooren ulcer, Terrien marginal degeneration, Pellucid marginal degeneration, vernal keratoconjunctivitis and rosacea keratitis. Fuchs marginal keratitis is another condition that can result peripheral infiltrate, stromal thinning and pseudopterygium formation. Fuchs' superficial marginal keratitis may result in bilateral nasal pseudopterygia encroaching on the visual axis, reducing visual acuity in both eyes.

Treatment

In mild cases warm compresses, eyelid hygiene, broad spectrum antibiotic fluoroquinolone 4 times a day and preservative free artificial tear drops should improve the condition. In moderate and severe cases mild topical steroid should be added in addition to the above treatment. Lotepredinol 0.2% or Prednisolone 0.25%, 4 times a day may be prescribed. A broad spectrum antibiotic should be used 4 times a day. Topical steroid should not be prescribed alone. Once the condition improves topical steroid should be tapered. During the period the patient is on topical steroids IOP should be constantly monitored. Topical cyclosporine ophthalmic emulsion 0.05% (Restasis) twice daily may be added to control the limbal and eyelid inflammation. In case of recurrence oral Doxycycline 100 mg twice daily should be prescribed.

Vernal Conjunctivitis

Introduction

Vernal conjunctivitis is characterized by bilateral, recurrent inflammation of conjunctiva, occurring in children. The disease predominantly occurs in children and young adults. The onset is usually between 3-10 years. The disease is usually self limiting and severity decreases as the child grows. Vernal conjunctivitis is more often seen in hot climates in northern hemisphere. The peak incidence of the disease is between April to August, i.e. in summer months. Most of the cases shows characteristic seasonal variation, i.e. the symptoms exacerbating in the summer months and subsiding in the winder months. Inverse seasonal variation of the disease, i.e. symptoms becoming worse in the winter months has been observed in 1-2% of the patients. Patients having chronic disease may also have symptoms through out the year.

Clinical Presentation

Itching, redness, blepharospasm and photophobia are the main symptoms of the disease. Children have mucoid, ropy discharge and difficulty in opening eyes in the morning. The disease has been described to occur in three forms:

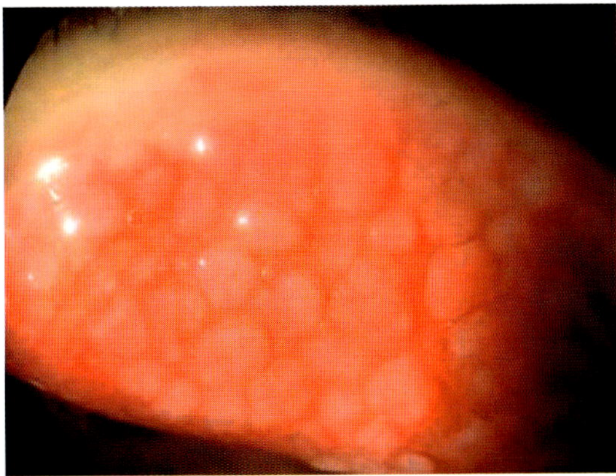

Fig. 18: Severe palpebral form of vernal conjunctivitis

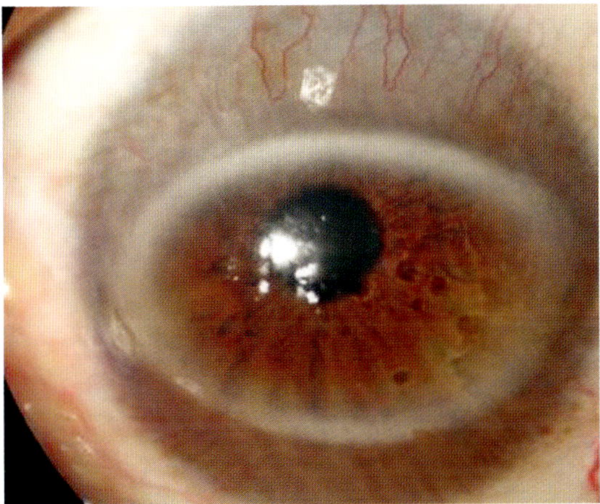

Fig. 19: Severe limbal form of vernal conjunctivitis

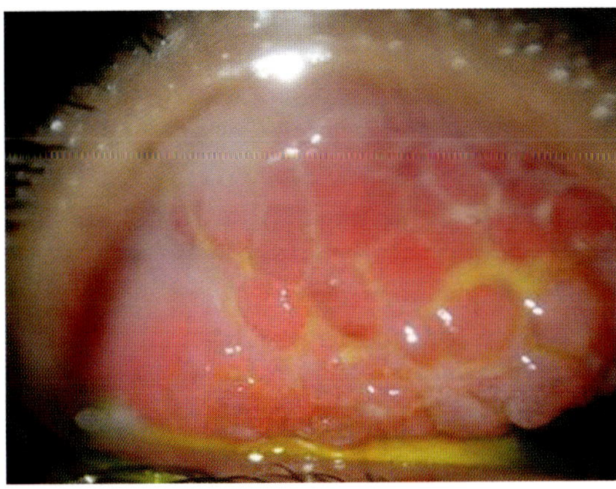

Fig. 20: Recalcitrant vernal conjunctivitis before supra tarsal injection of triamcinolone acetonide

palpebral, limbal and mixed. Palpebral form of disease is characterized by diffuse papillary hypertrophy, covered by milky layer. Papillae are localized lymphocytic proliferations with vascular tuft in the centre of the cornea. Clinically presence of central vessel which branches at the surface distinguishes it from follicle, in which vessels are absent. In severe cases papillae becomes enlarged and more confluent. Once these papillae are tight packed they assume polygonal shape and due to the pressure from the corneal surface, their top becomes flat. In severe and chronic form of disease, papillae may become extremely enlarged, teamed as "cobblestones" or "giant papillae". White dots, termed as Horner's or Trantas spots may occur on the papillae. Diffuse milky appearance of papillae may be due to fibrin deposit. It is described as sign. In case fluorescein stain is positive in the center of the papilla, it indicates that mast cells are degranulating and the disease is active.

Limbal form of the disease occurs more often in blacks. It is characterized by limbal hypertrophy diffuse of localized. It may be localized and limbal papilla formation may occur. Areas of chalky white pinpoint lesions Horner's or Tranta's dots may occur. These lesions should be distinguished from Herbert pits, which are flat, transparent and permanent. These occur in trachoma, caused by Chlamydia trachomatis. In severe limbal form of the disease micro pannus may develop and encroach peripheral cornea. Superficial punctuate erosions also described as microerosions may occur, these may continue to progress to vernal or shield ulcer.

Chronic cases develop muddy discoloration of conjunctiva. Initial stages, these children develop myopic astigmatism. Some of these may progress and develop keratoconus. Later in life. Patients with chronic vernal conjunctivitis may develop fungal keratitis even if they are not exposed to topical steroids or have no vernal ulcer.

Treatment

The best method of treatment is avoidance of allergen, which is extremely difficult. Avoidance of contact with pets, exposure to dust and heat may be avoided. Cold compresses may not only provide relief from symptoms may even cut down the necessity of medicine. Mild cases may respond to cold compresses, vasoconstrictors and nonspecific antihistaminics. Moderate cases may be treated with histamine, H_2 receptor specific against (levocabastine and emedestine), most cell stabilizers (cromolyn sodium, iodoxamide and nedocromil sodium) and drugs having both antihistaminic and most cell stabilizers usually take 2 weeks to provide symptomatic relief and drugs having both antihistaminic and must all stabilizer effect provide rapid relief. Topical NSAID drugs (ketoprofen, keratorolac) and successful in controlling symptoms. Topical steroids may be used in severe cases for short duration as pulse therapy. Topical cyclosporine (0.05 to 2%) and topical MMC local application have also been

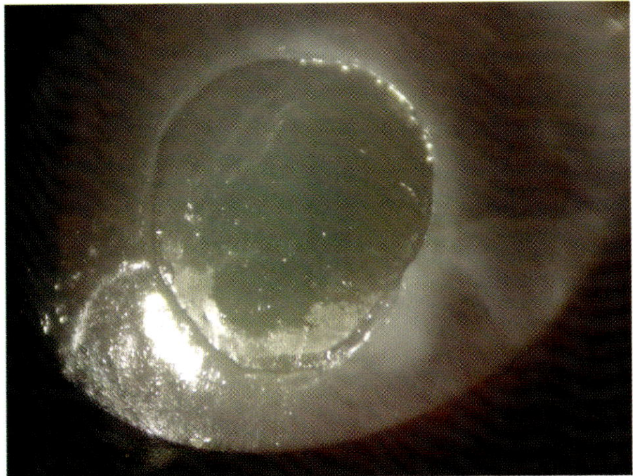

Fig. 24: Large vernal ulcer with plaque

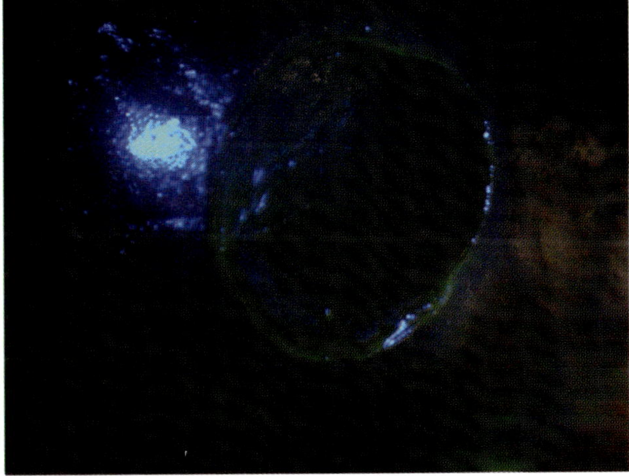

Fig. 25: Vernal plaque: staining poorly with fluorescein

to bandage contact lens, amniotic membrane has been used to promote healing. Topical cyclosporine (0.05-2%) has also been used to treat shield ulcers. Supra tarsal injection of triamcinolone acetonide (20 mg) into either side may be considered as an adjuvant in recalcitrant vernal ulcers in addition to surgical debridement and bandage contact lens application. Vernal ulcers or plaques should be treated on emergency basis as they are known to cause amblyopia in children.

Vitamin A Deficiency

Vitamin A deficiency is the leading cause of childhood blindness worldwide. Majority of those afflicted reside in the developing world. According to World Health Organization estimate 228 million children are affected by moderate to severe Vitamin A deficiency. In addition 500,000 cases of vitamin A deficiency with new active corneal lesions occur every year.

Vitamin A deficiency occurs when the body stores of Vitamin A are exhausted and daily intake does not meet the body requirement. Neonates, who get adequate breast feed usually get protection as mothers milk provide adequate vitamin A. However children born to mothers, who have poor reserve of vitamin A and insufficient intake during pregnancy, usually develop vitamin A deficiency. Biological stressors such as diarrhea or measles precipitate vitamin A deficiency in infants and neonates.

In vitamin A deficiency, the organs and tissue where there is rapid turn over including skin, mucous membranes, conjunctiva and cornea are affected the most.

Definition of Xerophthalmia, Keratomalacia

According to WHO classification of new signs of vitamin A deficiency have been divided into various stages. World Health Organization reclassification of xerophthalic signs.

Classification	Ocular Sign
XI A	Conjunctival xerosis
XI B	Conjunctival xerosis with Bitot's spots
X 2	Corneal xerosis
X 3A	Corneal ulceration + keratomalacia (1/3rd cornea)
X 3B	Coreal ilceration + keratomalacia (≥ ½ cornea)
X S	Cornea scar
X N	Night blindness
X F	Xerophthalmic fundus

It is not must that the vitamin A deficiency progresses stage wise. Patient may develop keratomalacia without developing corneal or conjunctival xerosis.

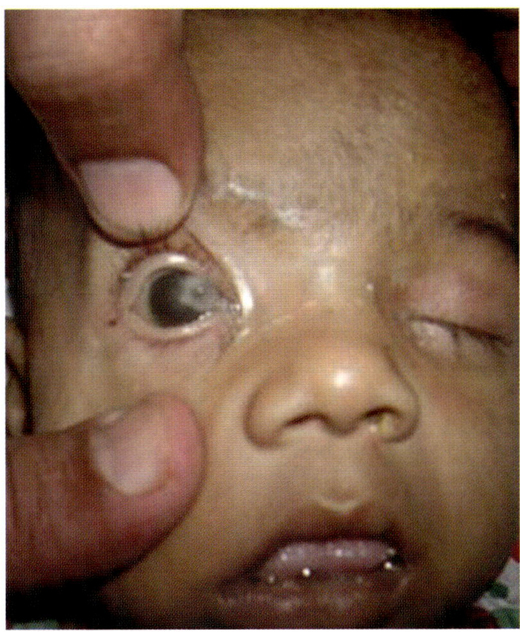

Fig. 26: Neonates (20 days old) with bilateral superadded bacterial infection following vitamin A deficiency. Active *staphylococcal* keratitis (RE)

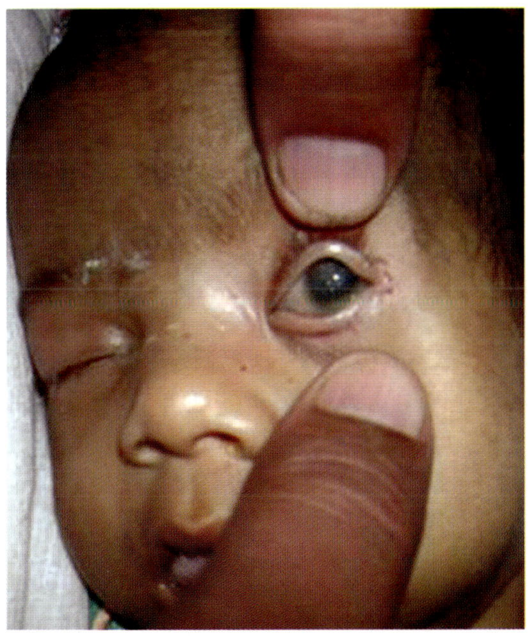

Fig. 27: Active *staphylococcal* keratitis (LE)

Secondary bacterial infections due to *Staphylococcus* and *Pseudomonas aeruginosa* are common. Experimental studies have shown that vitamin A deficiency increases adherence of *Pseudomonas aeruginosa* on ocular surface including cornea. Thus even subclinical vitamin A deficiency may predispose children to the development of bacterial keratitis.

Pathophysiology

Vitamin A is a fat-soluble vitamin ingested in the diet in two forms: retinal itself from animal sources such as milk, fish, meat, liver and eggs or as the provitamin, carotene from plant sources such as green leaf vegetables fruits, yellow fruits and red palm oil.

Vitamin A serves two important functions in the human body. As a precursor to photosensitive visual pigments it participate to initiate or neural impulses from photoreceptors. The second it is required for conjunctival epithelial cell RNA and glycoprotein synthesis which helps to maintain conjunctival mucosa and corneal stroma.

Xerophthalmia is a problem when the combined deficiency of vitamin A and protein occurs. Xerophthalmia is common in Asia and in some parts of Africa. Xerophthalmia can affect any age group, most common affected children aged between one to six years.

Ocular Manifestation

The clinical signs of xerophthalmia were reclassified by WHO in 1982. These signs and symptoms include the following.

Night Blindness

Night blindness is the earliest end the most common symptoms of vitamin A deficiency. Electroretinography and dark adaptation studies can detect the impaired retinal function even at the stage of subclinical vitamin A deficiency. Night blindness is the earliest sign to recover (24-48 hours) to systemic administration of vitamin A.

Conjunctival Manifestations

Xerosis (XIA) is the term used to describe dryness. Xerosis clinically represents as dry granular patch that exhibit thickening wrinkling, loss of pigmentation and transparency. It stains brilliantly with rose bengal.

Bitot's Spots: (X1B)

Bitot's spots are triangular, grey patches of keratinized conjunctival debris overlying an area of conjunctival xerosis, in the interpalpebral conjucntiva. Some times these patches appear in malnourished individuals in whom

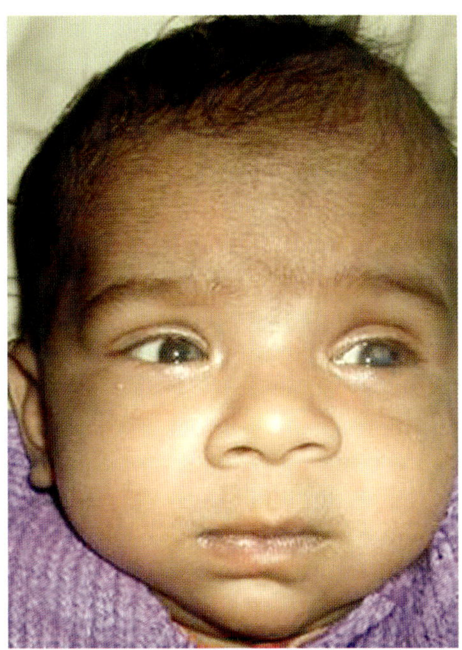

Fig. 28: Bilateral corneal opacity following healing of corneal ulcer and vitamin A deficiency

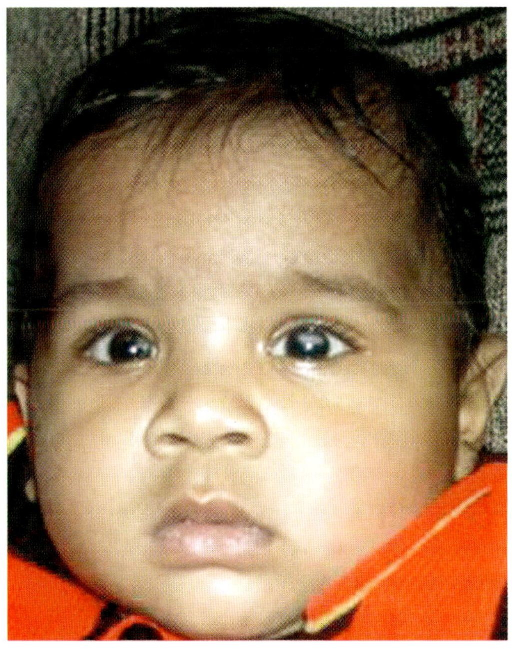

Fig. 29: Child after 2 years of follow-up

vitamin A levels are normal. In individuals with vitamin A deficiency these spots will disappear immediately after intiation of therapy.

Corneal Manifestations

Keratomalacia is defined as full thickness liquefícative necrosis of cornea clinically it appears as well defined, opaque, grayish yellow appearance. Stroma can slough leaving bare descemet's membrane or in severe cases corneal perforation. Keratomalacia is often associated in the systemic stressors such as measles, diarrhea or respiratory infection or comitant severe protein energy malformation.

Xerophthalmic Fundus

Xerophthalmic fundus represents of yellow and while dots in retinal periphery. Fluoroscein angiographs reveal these dots to be focal retinal pigment epithelial defects.

Diagnosis

Clinical diagnosis can be confirmed on conjunctival impression cytology. It is a non invasive method of obtaining superficial conjunctival cells. Microscopic examination of the stained slides reveal squamous metaplasia, enlarged irregular cells, keratinized epithelial cell, and loss of goblet cells.

Treatment

Vitamin A

The oral dose 200,000 IU of vitamin A in oil followed by 200, 000 IV of additional dose next day is given. Children with severe protein deficiency should receive an additional oral dose every 2 weeks till their protein deficiency improves. In case the child is suffering from malabsorption or severe corneal involvement 100, 000 IU water miscible vitamin A intramuscularly is preferred.

Prevention

Vitamin A prophylactic dose for newborn is 50000 IU, children younger than 1 year 100,000 IU every 4-6 months and children more than 2 years 200,000 IU every 4-6 weeks.

The most important step in the prevention of nutritional blindness due to vitamin A deficiency is to ensure that children take adequate amounts of carotene containing foods including cereals, vegetables and fruits.

Corneal Edema

Normal cornea is transparent with corneal thickness 520 to 560 μm in the center. Corneal endothelial cells keep a cornea in a state of relative dehydration because of endothelial pump functions. In case endothelial cell count decreases

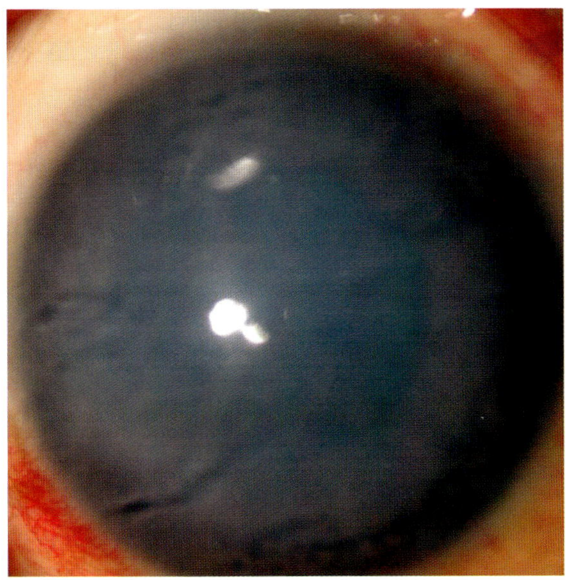

Fig. 30: Patient with corneal edema due to silicone keratopathy

below a critical value of 500 cells / mm^2 endothelial cell function is inadequate to maintain normal transparency of cornea and corneal edema occurs. Clinically corneal edema can be diagnosed on slit-lamp biomicroscopy which reveals increased corneal thickness. It is useful to compare corneal thickness with that in the normal eye. In case of localized corneal edema, one should compare it with corneal thickness in the area above or below the edema. Ultrasonic pachymetery is a convenient rapid and provides accurate quantitative estimation of corneal thickness. Specular microscopy is useful in providing details of endothelial cell density, polymorphism and pleomorphism. In cases with severe corneal edema and scarring confocal microscopy may delineate details of corneal endothelial cells count, shape, size and variation.

In children corneal edema may be due to congenital hereditary endothelial dystrophy, infantile glaucoma with corneal endothelial cell decompensation, following penetrating eye injuries, complicated cataract surgery and rarely toxic endothelitis due to bee sting injury. Patient suffering from congenital hereditary endothelial dystrophy may have associated raised intraocular pressure. Patients have buphthalmos with secondary corneal endothelial cell decompensation have increased corneal diameter in addition to raised intraocular pressure. Patients suffering penetrating eye injury, under go multiple surgeries including primary repair, cataract surgery, vitreoretinal surgery for retinal detachment and secondary scleral fixated PCIOL. Patients may develop corneal endothelial cell decompensation in case he develops severe uveitis. In adults complicated cataract surgeries with severe intraocular inflammation, mechanical touch of the instruments and surgeries without viscoelasitc substance may cause corneal endothelial all decompensation and may lead to corneal edema. Children having undergone pars plana vitrectomy and lensectomy for retinal detachment may develop corneal decompensation and corneal edema due to silicone oil keratopathy. Rarely complication like descemet's membrane detachment may be responsible for persistent corneal edema. Fuchs dystrophy is another important cause of corneal edema. Patient are usually diagnosed of Fuchs dystrophy at the time of evaluation for cataract surgery. In case patient is not diagnosed as Fuchs dystrophy before cataract surgery, he may develop corneal decompensation after cataract surgery.

Treatment

Corneal edema of inflammatory origin, i.e. toxic endotheliatis or herpetic origin is treated with topical and systemic steroids. Patients having corneal edema due to herpes simplex virus infection need topical or oral acyclovir. Patients with non-inflammatory corneal edema are evaluated thoroughly. Retina evaluation and ultrasonography is performed to rule out retinal detachment. Patients are put on topical or systemic steroids to cut down inflammation and anti glaucoma medication to reduce IOP. Topical hyperosmotic agents, use of hair drier may provide symptomatic relief for a brief period. In case patient

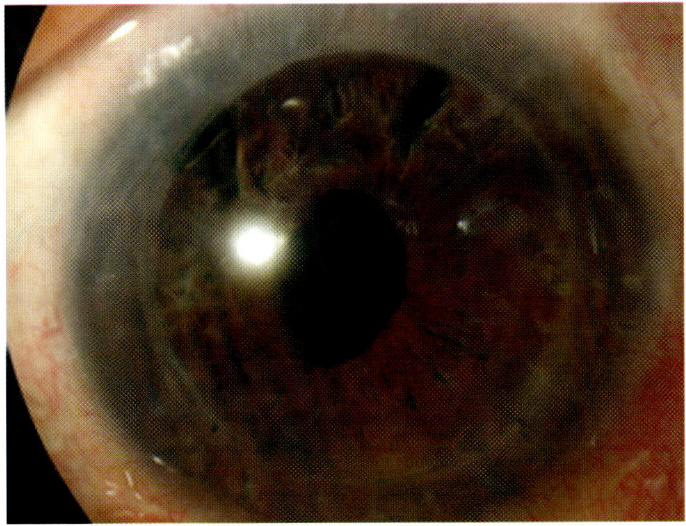

Fig. 31: Patient following penetrating keratoplasty and IOL exchange

suffering from postsurgery corneal edema is improving, one should wait for 3 months before considering surgical management. Penetrating keratoplasty with IOL exchange or secondary PCIOL is the definite treatment for corneal edema. Patients suffering from Fuch's dystrophy or pseudophakic corneal edema are currently considered for Descemet's Stripping Automated Endothelial Keratoplasty (DSAEK) or Descemet's Stripping Endothelial Keratoplasty (DSEK). The DSAEK surgery provides rapid visual rehabilitation, higher UCVA/ BSCVA and lower astigmatism. Both DSAEK and DSEK are preferred surgical options endothelium decompensation. The dislocation of the donor disc has been reported significantly higher in the DSAEK group.

Numular Corneal Opacities

Numular sub epithelial corneal opacities are frequent in chronic stage of adenoviral keratoconjunctivitis. The pathogenesis of numular keratitis includes postimmune reaction to the persistent virus particles in the subepithelial keratocytes. There is no consensus in the literature on the treatment of numular keratitis. Asymptomatic patients should be prescribed preservative free artificial eye drops and kept under observation. Of symptomatic group, in most of the patients spontaneous resolution of the opacities and symptoms occur over a period of time. Patient who develop decrease in vision due to corneal inflammation treatment become necessary. Topical steroids suppress host immune reaction and resolution of the numular corneal opacities occur rapidly. However these opacities invariably re-appear once topical steroids are discontinued. Long-term topical steroids are hazardous. The use of topical steroids over prolonged periods may cause cataract, glaucoma and dry eye. In our experience even careful and prolonged tapering of corticosteroids failed to prevent recurrences of corneal opacities. Even without treatment in most of these cases spontaneous disappearance of opacities has been observed within a year. Topical cyclosporine is a potent immune suppressant is commonly used in prevention of transplant rejection. Cyclosporine has been found in to cure numular corneal opacities in nearly 66% of the patients. Response to the topical cyclosporine is slow. The drug is well tolerated. Patients may have mild stinging sensation following instillation of topical restasis. Topical cyclosporine (0.05%) has been found safe even on long-term use. Recurrences of nummular keratitis following stopping of topical cyclosporine (0.05%) are known. These patients usually respond to another course of topical cyclosporine application.

Dry Eyes

Dry eye is common and yet under diagnosed condition. The understanding of newer concepts in the pathogenesis of dry eye has virtually revolutionized the management of the disease. The better under standing of the role inflammation

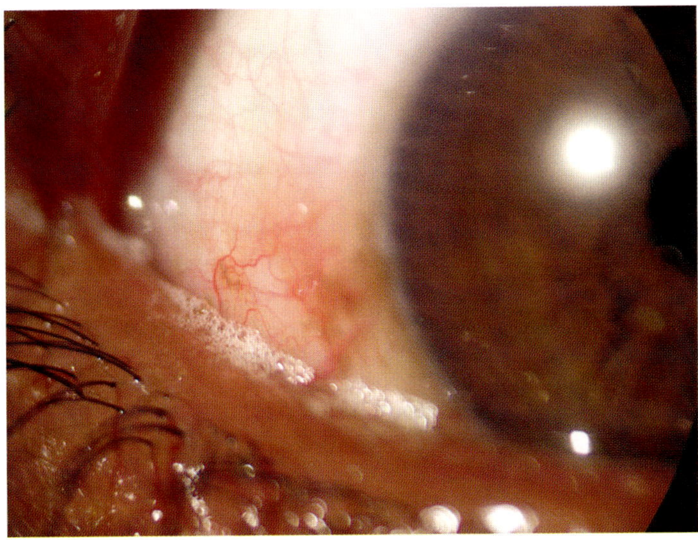

Fig. 32: Frothy discharge in dry eye

of lacrimal gland tissue and ocular surface has changed the concept of the disease. Previous definitions of the disease purely based on the decrease in the amount of tear secretion are no longer valid. Any disturbance in the anatomical and physiological well being of the normal ocular surface is considered dry eye. Various component aqueous deficiency, mucin and lipid deficiency are well described. Several condition including meibomian gland disease and blepharitis are commonly associated with dry eye syndrome. Several drugs anti-depression and anti-histaminics specifically enhances dry eyes.

Clinical Presentation

Dry eye is likely to go undetected unless specifically looked for. Patients before cataract surgery should be routinely screened for dry eye. The incidence of the dry eye increases as the age advances. Females in the post menopausal age should also be screened for dry eye. Young adults working overtime on computers may also develop relative dry eye due to infrequent blinking and continuous exposure to airconditioning specially if humidity is not controlled. Rarely patient present with complaint of infrequent tearing. Excesive watering a paradoxical complaint by many patients should also be kept in mind. Patients may also present with complication of dry eye following cataract surgery. Patient also present with infective keratitis due to secondary infection. Dry eye rarely occurs in children. Children suffering from juvenile rheumatoid arthritis are also predisposed to develop dry eyes.

Diagnosis

Diagnosis of dry eye in children requires high index of suspicion. Frothy discharge from the eye particularly from the outer angle is characteristic. Evaluation of tear meniscus height and presence of debris in tear film are helpful in establishing clinical diagnosis. In addition to Schirmers test, Tear Film Break up time and vital dye staining, a simple mucus ferning test has been found useful. Patients should be investigated for presence of associated autoimmune disorder such as rheumatoid arthritis.

Treatment

Frequent instillation of preservative free artificial tears remains the mainstay of the treatment. Use of hypotonic solution to counter the desiccation effect of hyperosmotic tears on corneal epithelium has been recommended. Recent introduction of an emulsion used as a vehicle in cyclosporine has been reported beneficial in dry eye (Refresh endura). The constituents of emulsion glycerin and polysorbate 80 act in unison to stabilize ocular surface and prevent evaporation of tear film. In addition spectacles with side shields may improve comfort and moistened sponge may increase the humidity may be helpful in some patients. Punctal occlusion is a useful option to retain tears. This can be

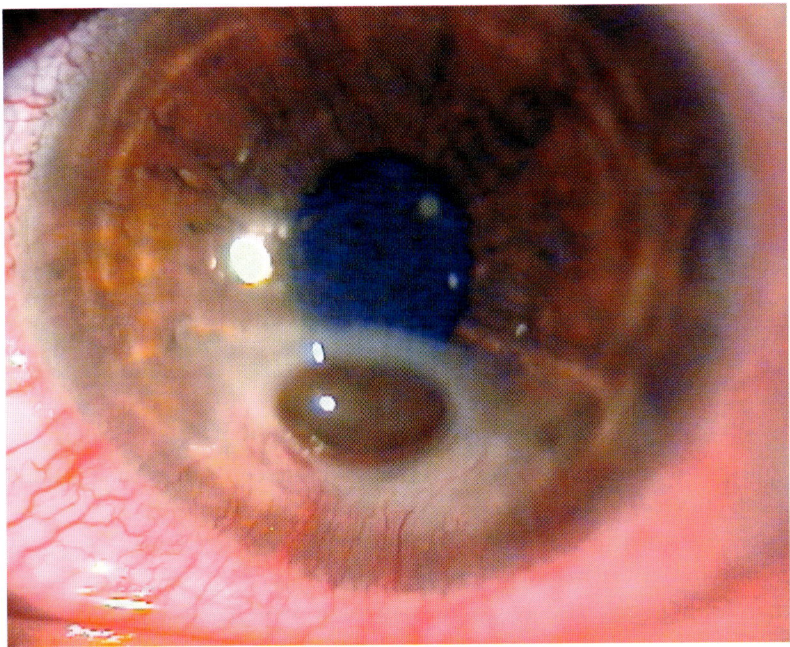

Fig. 33: Paracentral corneal perforation in a patient with dry eye and rheumatoid arthritis

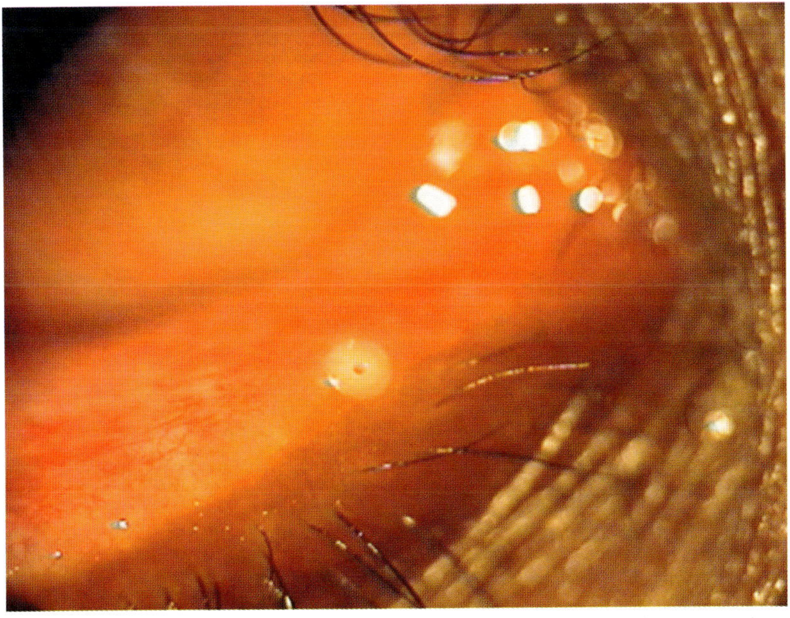

Fig. 34: Punctal occlusion with punctal plug in dry eye

achieved by punctual cautry, laser application or inserting punctual plugs. Oral pilocarpine (Salagen, MGI - Pharma) and cevimelin (Evoxac; Daiichi Pharma cortical) have been used to increase tear secretion.

One of the most exciting additions in the treatment of dry eye is use of topical cyclosporine 0.05% (Restasis Allergan). The drug is a potent immunosuppressive agent and has selective action of T cells. It avoids the side effects of long term use of steroids. There has been found safe and effective in clinical trials. We have an extensive experience of using this drug with encouraging results. The drug is most effective in moderate cases.

Hormonal replacement therapy has not found favor with clinicians, because of risk of developing malignancy. Autologus serum therapy may be beneficial in cases in whom other modalities have not been found effective. We have found this modality particularly useful in patients with SPK. Autologus serum provides protein peptides, nutrients and growth factor those help in healing and protection of ocular surface.

Currently corneal specialists are currently better equipped with various modalities to treat patients suffering from dry eye. In future more promising treatments are likely to evolve for the benefit of dry eye patients.

Meibomian Gland Disease

Meibomian gland disease is common in general population. Several studies have reported prevalence rate up to 39% in general population. Despite high prevalence of the disease, it is frequently overlooked in eye out patient departments. Condition has been described to occur in association with contact lens intolerance and meibomian gland disease. In addition treatment of meibomian gland disease has been associated with improvement of contact lens intolerance. Meibomian gland disease has high prevalence in dry eye patients. Disease has also high prevalence up to 84% in patients with blepharitis.

Clinical Presentation

Patients present with irritation, redness and watery eyes. Slit-lamp biomicroscopy reveals mild conjunctival congestion and few SPK. Some patients have mild moderate dry eye. Meibomian glands openings may be blocked and few patients may cystic appearance of the opening. Expression of meibomian glands gives turbid secretion and in some of the glands thick secretion while few of them may be blocked. Mild eyelid erythema and vascularization of eyelid margin is considered characteristic.

Pathophysiology

Meibomium gland was first described by Henrich Meibom in 1666.1 Meibomian glands normal provide lipid component to the tear film. The lipid component provides stability to the tear film and prevent evaporation. In meibomian gland

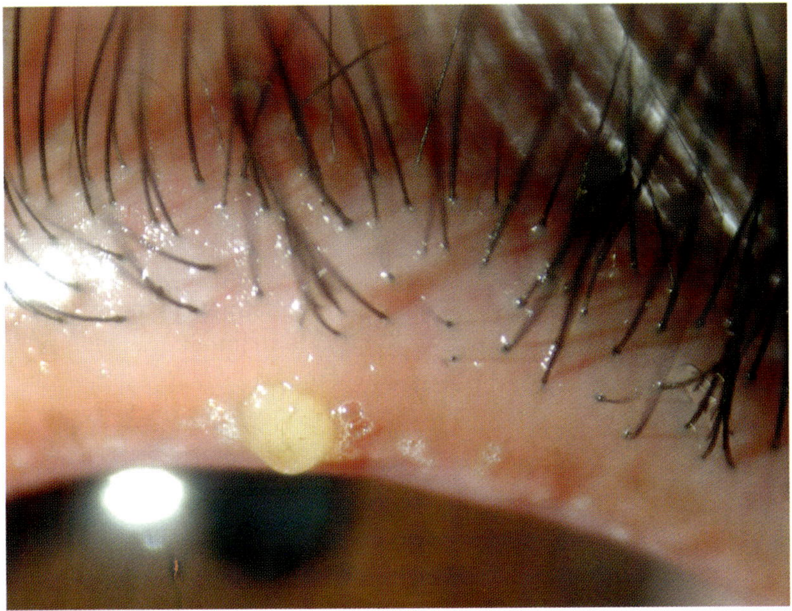

Fig. 35: Meibomian gland disease (cystic appearance)

disease the lipid secretion in altered both qualitatively and quantitatively. The deficiency leads to unstable tear film and ocular surface inflammation. Release of mediators of inflammation may initiate squmous metaplasia of the ocular surface and opening of the ducts of the meibomian glands. The progressive changes may cause stenosis and finally occlusion of the openings of meibomian glands.

Treatment

Treatment of meibomian gland disease requires treatment of the condition and associated conditions. The most important is to maintain the patency of the ducts by digital massage. Hot fomentation of the eyelid before digital massage liquefies the secretions. The glands are expressed of the thick secretion and normal secretion follow.

In addition topical antibiotic, preservative free artificial tear drops and mild topical steroids are prescribed to control ocular surface inflammation. Steroid ointment may also be used during the massage of eyelids. Azithromycin, a broad-spectrum antibiotic with potent anti-inflammatory activities, has been found effective to treat meibomian gland disease. In severer cases oral doxycycline 100 mg twice daily is given for three weeks. Doxycycline improves the quality of the lipid secretion of the meibomian glands.

In addition patient needs to take case of ocular hygiene. Cleaning of the eyelid margins with Johnson buds dipped in the Johnson baby shampoo help in cleaning of eyelid margins and removing cellular debris of the eyelid margin. Treatment is required to be continued for several months.

Neurotrophic Keratitis

Neurotrophic keratopathy is caused by the loss of corneal sensation. The condition occurs secondary to impaired trigeminal nerve function. Associated deficiency of tear film aggravates the condition and worsens the prognosis. In ophthalmic practice the condition is commonly observed after recurrent herpes simplex keratitis and herpes zoster ophthalmicus. Approximately 10 to 20% of patients with herpes zoster will develop herpes zoster ophthalmicus (HZO). In neonates the condition rarely occurs due to congenital anesthesia. Neurotrophic keratitis is also seen after surgery for neurosurgical operation for tumors.

Clinical Presentation

Punctate keratitis, epithelial haze and pin point epithelial defect are early signs of neurotrophic keratitis. Classical neurotrophic corneal epithelial defects are round or oval with heaped up margins of the ulcer. The condition frequently progresses to corneal ulceration, perforation, and loss of vision. A secondary infection may occur at any stage and progresses rapidly despite treatment.

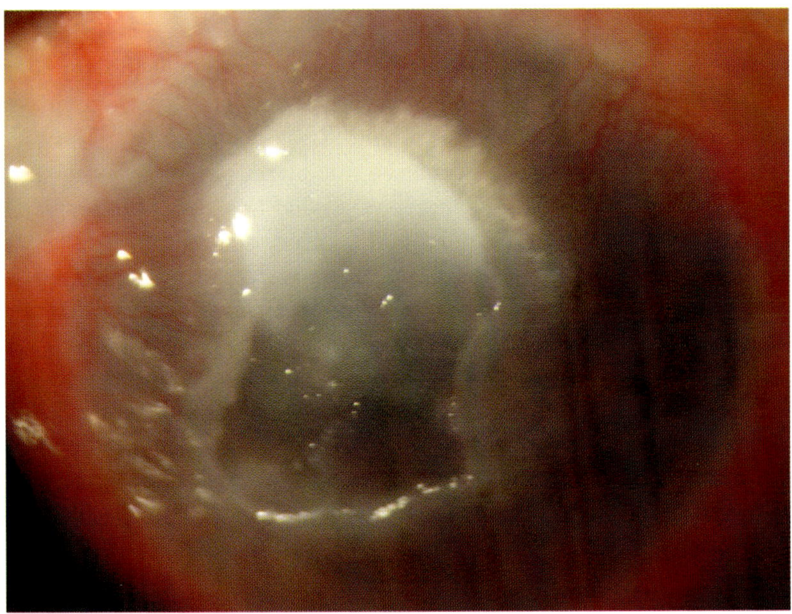

Fig. 36: Neurotrophic ulcer and ciprofloxacin deposit

Treatment

Early and aggressive treatment is required to prevent vision threatening complications following neurotrophic keratitis. The treatment of early neurotrophic keratopathy includes a bandage contact lens, antibiotic drops and frequent instillation of preservative free artificial tears. Restasis (0.05% cyclosporine ophthalmic emulsion; Allergan) bid has been found effective in the treatment of persistent epithelial defect. Once the epithelial defect heals patient may be kept on Restasis and preservative free artificial tear drops for few months. In a prospective noncomparative case series, topical umbilical cord serum (20%) was effective in treatment of refractory neurotrophic keratitis. Umblical cord serum has been found to contain many neurotrophic factors including substance P, insulin like growth factor 1 (IGF-1), and nerve growth factor (NGF) . Umbilical cord serum (20%) eyedrops have been recommended in the treatment of neurotrophic keratitis. In case neurotrophic keratitis does not respond to these measures tarsorrhaphy may be considered to heal the corneal ulcer and prevent complications.

Patient presenting with impending or actual corneal perforations or with extensive corneal scarring may require surgery. Success rate for tectonic or optical penetrating keratoplasty is low due to poor healing in total anesthetic cornea. Control of pre-existing ocular inflammation, increased intraocular pressure, lagophthalmos, dry eye, exposure, or neurotrophic keratitis before performing corrective surgery may improve the success rate significantly.

HZO is associated with poor healing, as evidenced by a high occurrence of ulceration, superinfection, and surgical failure. In another study a Boston keratoprosthesis was successfully used to replace the severely damaged cornea, and extracapsular cataract extraction of a mature cataract was also performed at the same sitting. The Boston keratoprosthesis procedure successfully salvaged and restored vision in this high-risk herpes zoster eye in which standard keratoplasty would almost certainly have failed.

Management of neurotrophic keratopathy requires urgent decisive action. Early treatment intervention is important to help avoid severe complications developing at later stage of the disease. The use of immunomodulating agents (topical cyclosporine) in the early stage of management should be considered to prevent and heal epithelial changes in neurotrophic keratitis following Herpes Zoster Ophthalmicus.

Ocular Surface Disease and Limbal Stem Cell Deficiency

Ocular surface disorders constitute a major cause of ocular morbidity and poses a challenge to the ophthalmologists. The options of management in the past were limited and outcome used to be less favorable. The management of ocular surface disorders has undergone a complete revolution in the recent years.

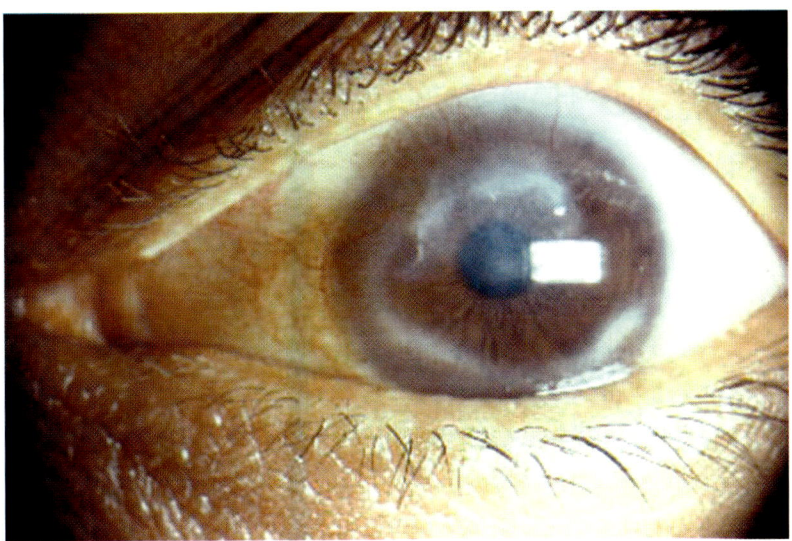

Fig. 37: Early limbal stem cell deficiency

Newer concepts on the role of limbal stem cells in the corneal epithelial cell homeostasis and ocular surface disease have been introduced. With the result newer surgical procedures including limbal stem cell transplants and amniotic membrane grafts have been added to the corneal specialist's armamentarium. The present review article aims at reviewing the basic concepts of limbal stem cells, present clinical features and classification of limbal stem cell disorders and finally describes the role of limbal stem cell transplants, amniotic membrane grafts, cultured corneal epithelial or stem cell transplants in these disorders.

Normal Ocular Surface

Corneal Epithelial Cell Homeostasis

Normal tear film, corneal and conjunctival epithelium constitute healthy ocular surface. Normal corneal epithelial mass is maintained by continuous centripetal movement of peripheral corneal epithelium towards the visual axis. In Thoft's XYZ hypotheses, X represents the proliferation of basal epithelial cells, Y is the proliferation and centripetal migration of the limbal cells and Z the epithelial cell loss from the surface. For a state of equilibrium to be maintained X+Y must equal Z. It is estimated that the corneal epithelium is constantly renewed every 7 to 10 days. The half time of corneal epithelial replacement is nine weeks, while the time required for 95-99% replacement is 9-12 months, i.e. the rate of exfoliation of epithelial cells is consistent with their production from limbal cells.

Basic Concept of Stem Cells

The existence of stem cells responsible for cellular maintenance has been identified for the number of other cells population including the limbus, epidermis and intestinal epithelium. Stem cells, by definition are present in all self-renewing tissues. These are long lived, have great potential for clonogenic cell division and are ultimately responsible for cell replacement and tissue regeneration. The stem cells are least differentiated cells in the tissue and lack markers which indicate greater differentiation. In contrast to stem cells, transient amplifying cells (TAC), that are derived from stem cell mitosis, are characterized by a high mitotic rate but a limited proliferative capacity. All post mitotic cells now theoretically are non-proliferative and are committed to cellular differentiation. The ultimate expression of the functional aspect of the tissue is achieved by the terminally differentiated cells. All cells except stem cells have limited life span and are destined to die. Location of corneal epithelial stem cells has been identified as pallisades of Vogt.s in the basal limbal epithelium.

Role of Limbal Stem Cells in Ocular Surface Healing

Following cornel epithelial injury recovery is dependent upon centripetal movement of the most proximal, viable epithelium. For small corneal epithelial

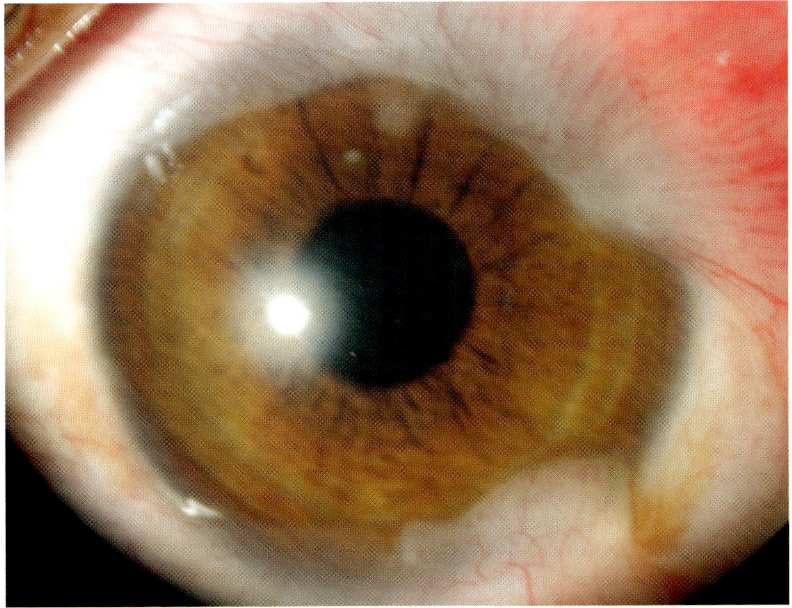

Fig. 38: Limbal stem cell deficiency

defects, adjacent corneal epithelium fills the defect. A complete corneal epithelial defect requires epithelium from the limbus, whereas in extensive corneal and limbal injury, the surrounding conjunctival epithelium provides the only source for epithelial regeneration. The rate of re-epithelialization and the ultimate functional competence of the ocular surface depends upon the source of regenerating epithelium. Following complete corneal and limbal epithelial damage, the surrounding conjunctival epithelium resurfaces the cornea.

Conjunctival Transdifferentiation, not a Reality

Conjunctivilization of corneal surface is a feature of severe limbal stem cell deficiency. Conjuctival epithelium is phenotypically different from corneal epithelium and shows neither goblet cells nor corneal epithelial based cells. Earlier theory that on long term, with the absence of vascularization and vit A deficiency, the conjunctival epithelium acquires characteristic of cornea epithelium. The process described as conjunctival transdifferentiation, is no longer believed to occur. This process of transdifferentiation, was exploited in the development of conjunctival autografts as a means of ocular surface reconstruction in the chemically injured eyes.

Limbal Stem Cell Deficiency

Limbal Stem Cell Disorders

Primary limbal stem cell deficiency occurring in aniridia is rare. Secondary limbal stem cell deficiency occurs in chemical injury, thermal injuries, radiation injury, cicatricial pemphigoid, Stevens-Johnson syndrome, pterygium. Iatrogenic limbal stem cell deficiency may occur following chronic medication, local application of mitomycin C and repeated surgical procedures at limbus.

Clinical Presentation

Conjunctivalization of the corneal surface is extreme. Conjunctival epithelium growth into the cornea vascularized pannus formation progress from the awe of limbal stem cell deficiency and finally affect the vision. Associated dry eye is due to unstable tear film. Limbal stem cell deficiency can be total or partial. In partial limbal stem cell deficiency, limbal stem cell hypo function may result in non-healing epithelial defect.

- Primary limbal stem cell deficiency
  Aniridia
- Secondary limbal stem cell deficiency
  Stevens-Johnson syndrome
  Ocular cicatricial pemphigoid
  Chemical eye injury
  Thermal eye injury

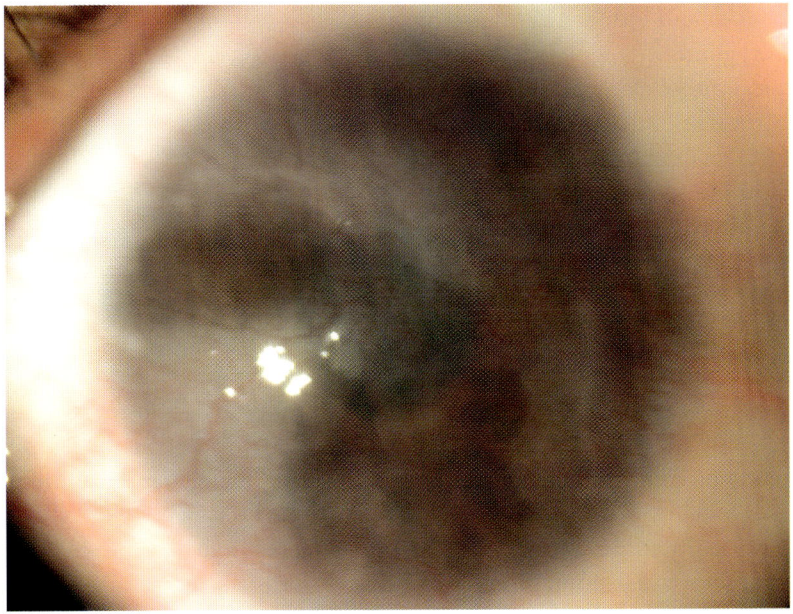

Fig. 39: Total limbal stem cell deficiency and conjunctivilization

Contact lens induced keratopathy
Pterygium
Intraepithelial neoplasms

- Iatrogenic limbal stem cell deficiency
  Antimetabolites (MMC)
  Multiple ocular surgeries
  Stem cell hypofunction in PK
  Repeated peritectomies
  Drug induced deficiency

Diagnosis

Conjunctivalization of the cornea, the hallmark of limbal stem cell deficiency, needs to be documented to make diagnosis. A severe form of conjunctivalization is usually obvious to the clinician. Whereas subtle changes in the epithelium texture, permeability, recurrent erosions may be detected on slit-lamp biomicroscopy using fluorescein dye. Impression cytology of the cornea and histopathological examination of the excised fibro-vascular tissue may show the presence of goblet cells. Impression cytology can be performed by applying nitrocellulose filter paper onto corneal surface. All cytologic specimens are processed and stained with periodic Acid-Schiff reagent and a modified Harris hematoxylin-eosin stain. Under a microscope with a 40× objective, the area with the highest cell density is counted at five different areas with each equivalent to 5625 um^2, while that of goblet cell density is measured in a similar manner but at an area equivalent to 10000 um^2. These data are then converted to number of cells per millimeter squared and are compared using the Student paired (match) t test.

The ocular adenexa should carefully examined and corrective measures for trichiasis, entropion, ectropion and other abnormality if necessary should be taken before considering ocular surface rehabilitation.

Currents in Surgical Management of Ocular Surface Disease

Treatment of Ocular Surface Disorders

In the seed, soil and rain theory ocular surface is equated to a beautiful flower. The seed represents limbal stem cells and soil is the microenvironment necessary for the survival of stem cells. Ocular surface diseases with focal or diffuse complete stem cell loss require limbal stem cell transplants. Amniotic membrane grafts improve ocular surface for better survival of limbal stem cells in partial deficiency or in limbal stem cell transplants.

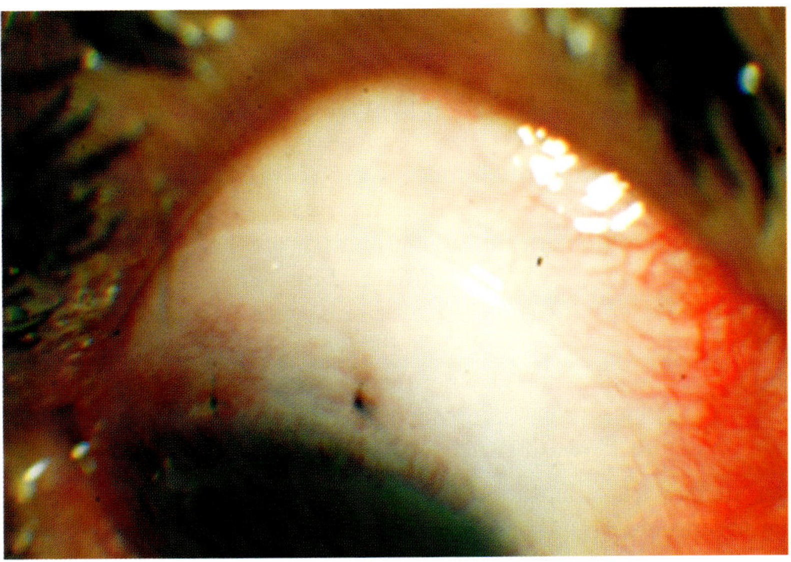

Fig. 40: Severe chemical injury before amniotic membrane transplant

Adjunct Treatment

Medical measures in promoting corneal epithelialization include preservative free artificial tears, bandage contact lenses, autologous serum eye drops and topical retinoic acid. In severe cases we can go in for punctual occlusion may it be temporary or permanent Fibronectin a glycoprotein present in the extra-cellular matrix promotes cell-cell and cell-matrix adhesion but does not influence cell mitosis or migration. Epidermal growth factor (EGF) a polypeptide that stimulates the uptake of DNA, RNA and protein processors by corneal epithelium and enhances the rate of epithelial migration by inducing hyperplasia. Both fibronectin and EGF have been shown to be beneficial in promoting epithelialization in experimental alkali injuries.

Ocular Surface Reconstruction

Ocular surface transplantation techniques described earlier conjunctival/ Tenon'advancement (Tenoplasty), glued on rigid gas permeable contact lenses, conjunctival and mucous membrane transplants. These surgical procedures have been based on the principle of conjunctival transdifferentiation. The phenomenon is no longer believed to occur and surface epithelial changes are ascribed to the functional recovery of limbal stem cells. Keratoepithelioplasty was originally introduced by Thoft as a procedure for ocular surface rehabilitation in the bilateral chemical eye injuries. The first attempt to restore ocular surface epithelial function with limbal stem cell transplantation was using allogenic corneal donor limbal epithelium. Unfortunately, this is technically difficult and has failed to produce convincing results.

Newer Surgical Procedures

Contrary to the earlier surgical procedures, newer procedures are based on the concept of limbal stem cell transplants and correcting microenvironment.

- The limbal stem cell transplants
  Autolimbal
  Live related
  Allolimbal
- Amniotic membrane transplants (AMT)
- Combined limbal stem cell and AMT
- Cultured corneal epithelial cells
- Cultured limbal stem cells.

Rationale of Newer Surgical Options

For those ocular surface and disorders characterized by the absence and aplasia of limbal stem cells, transplants of limbal stem cells are required. This is particularly feasible for those disorders, which have unilateral involvement.

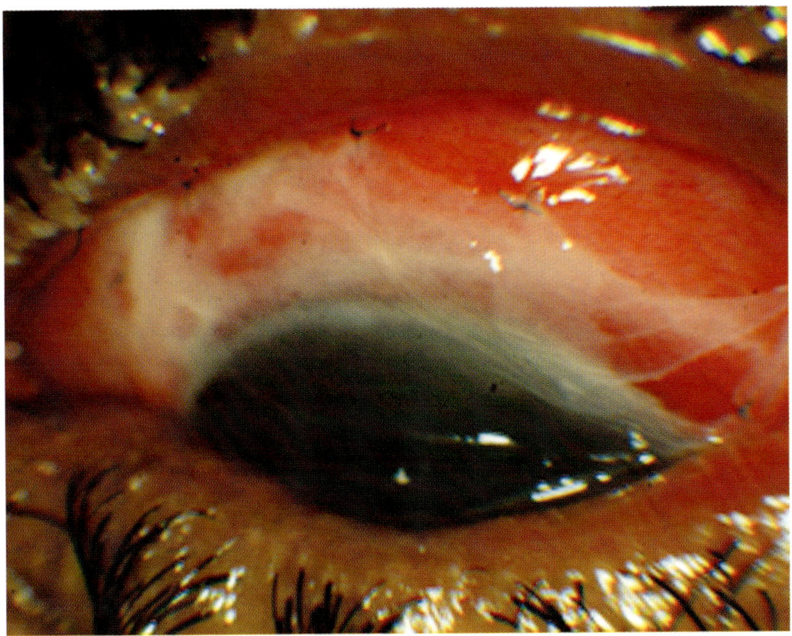

Fig. 41: Severe chemical injury after amniotic membrane transplant

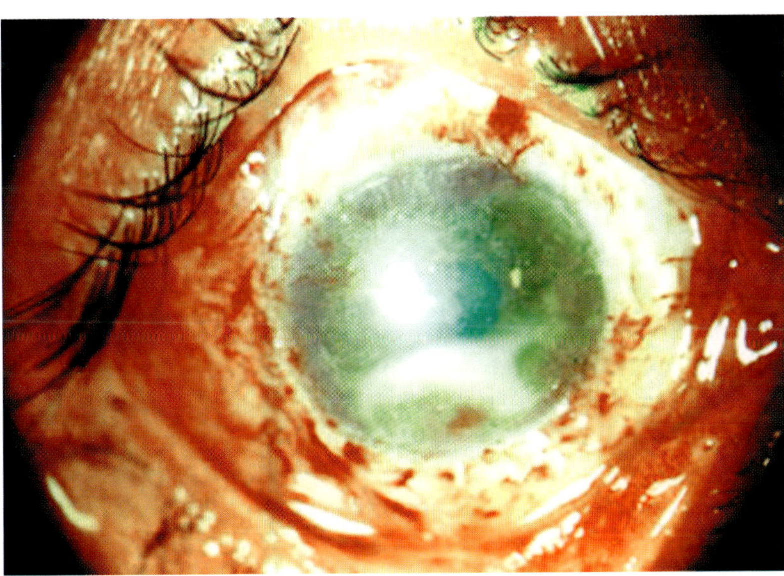

Fig. 42: Corneal epithelial cell surfacing cornea after limbal stem cell transplant

When the limbus is focally involved in one eye, an autograft can be obtained from the ipsilateral eye. In pterygium for example, excision of the lesion together with antimetabolites or beta irradiation gives recurrence rates ranging from 4.3 to 50 percent. The use of an autologus source of bulbar conjunctiva for transplantation has been reported to yield better success with a recurrence rate of 5.3 to 6 percent. The use of an autograft including limbus has been reported to decrease the recurrence rate to 3 percent.

Bilateral severe limbal stem cell deficiency due to chemical injuries, cicatricial pemphigoid and Stevens-Johnson syndrome need limbal stem cell transplants. In bilateral cases limbal stem cell transplants from either live related or donor eyes are performed. Adequate immune suppression is required in case cadaver eyes are used as source of limbal stem cell transplants. The procedure may be combined with amniotic membrane transplants. In few reports combined limbal stem cell grafts with penetrating keratoplasty have shown encouraging results. Several authors prefer single stage surgery as the stem cell population may get depleted in two-staged procedure.

Routine use of limbal stem cell transplants and AMT have improved the prognosis of penetrating grafts in patients with severe limbal stem cell deficiency. In partial limbal stem cell deficiency patients, vision may improve even without penetrating keratoplasty. With the use of cultured limbal stem cell on AMT the problem of immune suppression required for allo limbal stem cell transplants may be taken care off.

In acute chemical injuries of eye extent of limbal ischemia corresponds to stem cell loss. In persistent ephithelial defect without associated limbal stem loss usually response to measures promoting epithelial healing is seen. In persistent epithelial defects without limbal stem cell deficiency, epithelial healing has been achieved with the use of cultured corneal epithelial cells. In recent studies limbal stem cell cultures have been used to promote repopulation of limbal stem cells. Amniotic membrane grafts and cultured epithelial and limbal stem cells are newer surgical options. Amniotic membrane provides various growth factors, reduces inflammation and decreases symblepharon formation. Amiotic membrane transplants (AMT) may be used in persistent epithelial defects not responding to conventional therapy, patients with partial limbal stem cell deficiency may also improve with amniotic membrane transplants. Amniotic membrane transplants have also been recently found useful in shield ulcers, pterygium surgery and ocular surface reconstructive procedures, such as symblepharon release, excision of squamous cell carcinoma.

Unilateral limbal stem cell transplants (Auto) may be performed by taking graft from the fellow eye. A minimum of 50% of limbal stem cells need to be preserved to prevent any stem cell deficiency in the donor eye. Patients with total limbal stem cell deficiency, need limbal stem cell. Limbal stem cell transplantation is a modification of the original conjuntival transplantation

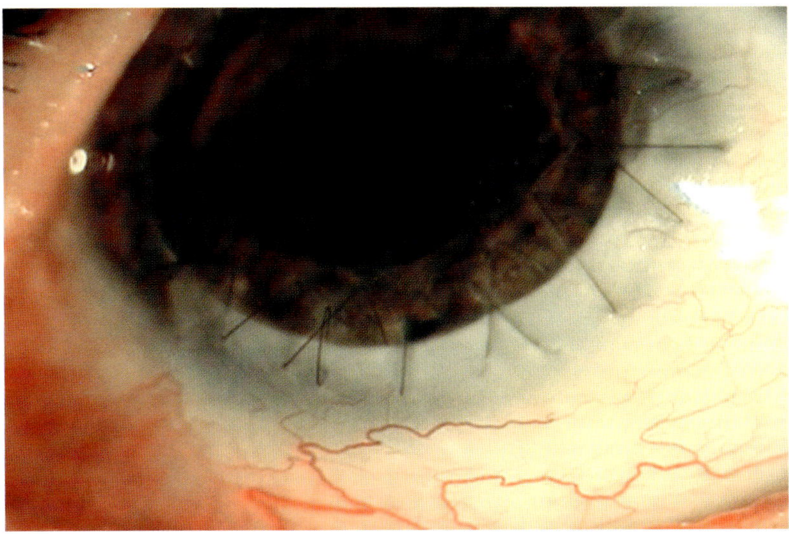

Fig. 43: Penetrating keratoplasty following limbal stem cell transplant (clear graft)

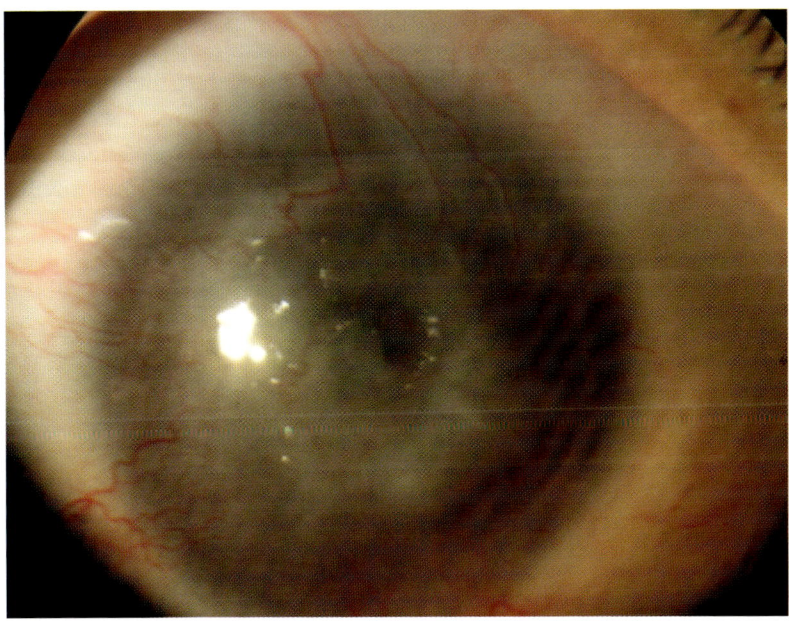

Fig. 44: Limbal stem cell deficiency before cultured limbal stem cell transplant

technique by Thoft. It restores the normal corneal epithelial phenotype after injury and is the only currently available technique to re-establish a normal corneal phenotype. The technique involves harvesting two crescents of peripheral corneal limbal epithelium with a corresponding section of conjunctiva from the limbus of the patients uninjured or less injured contralateral eye (autograft), or from a close relative (allograft). The technique has been especially of help in chemical injuries. In grade IV injuries, propr extension of an appropriate vascular supply to the limbal region by tenonplasty, either before or at the same time as limbal stem cell transplantation is mandatory to insure graft survival.

In cases of bilateral chemical injuries, limbal allograft transplantation or the use of cultured limbal stem cells may be an alternative. The survival of donor cells is presumed by the stabilization of ocular surface and regression of the features of limbal insufficiency.

Surgical Technique

Limbal Stem Cell Transplant

Surgery may be performed under local or general anesthesia. All donor surgeries in live related donors are performed under peribulbar anesthesia. Donor and recipient surgeries are scheduled simultaneously in adjacent operating theaters. Donor limbal tissue is harvested from the superior and inferior limbus of the nondominant eye of the donor or from the fellow eye in auto limbal transplants. Each graft is 2 to 3 clock hours in length and extended 2 mm on the conjunctival surface and 1 mm on the comeal epithelium. The grafts are transferred to two bowls of sterile Ringer lactate solution, taking care to identify the superior and inferior graft. The donor sites are left unsutured. After pannus excision in the recipient cornea, the grafts are anchored with one interrupted 10-0 nylon suture at each circumferential end. The conjunctival portion of the graft is anchored to the underlying episcleral tissues with a 10-0 nylon mattress suture. The corneal edge of the graft is left unsutured.

After surgery, the recipient eye is treated with betmethasone eyedrops one drop every 2 hours, methylcellulose eyedrops one drop every 3 hours and ciprofloxacin eye drops twice daily. Topical steroids are discontinued after 4 to 6 months, and tear substitutes are continued for 3 months. Oral prednisolone (1mg/kg body weight) is used in the first week after surgery and reduced gradually in the next 4 weeks.

Preparation of Preserved Human Amniotic Membrane

Human amniotic membrane is prepared and preserved using following method. The human placenta is obtained shortly after elective cesarean delivery when human immunodeficiency virus, human hepatitis type B and C, and syphilis

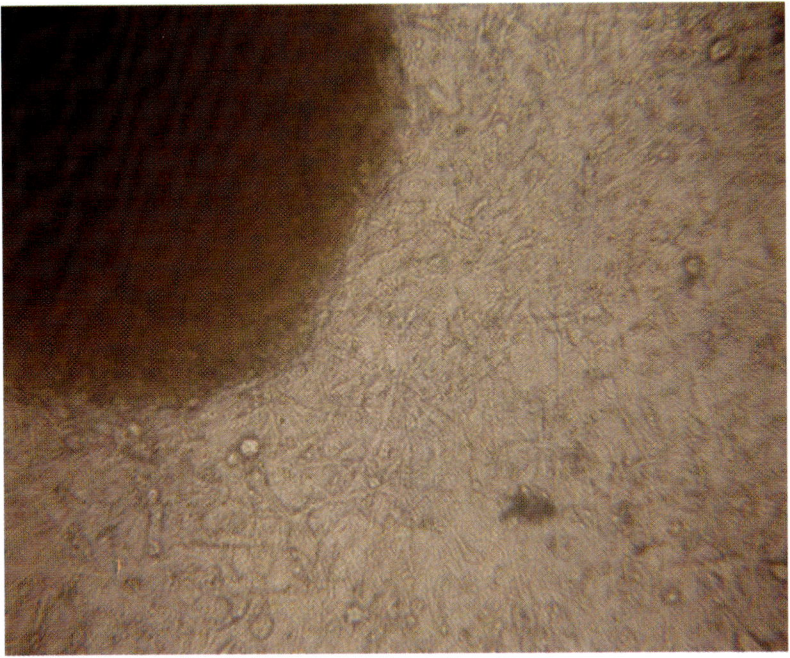

Fig. 45: Cultured limbal stem cells on amniotic membrane

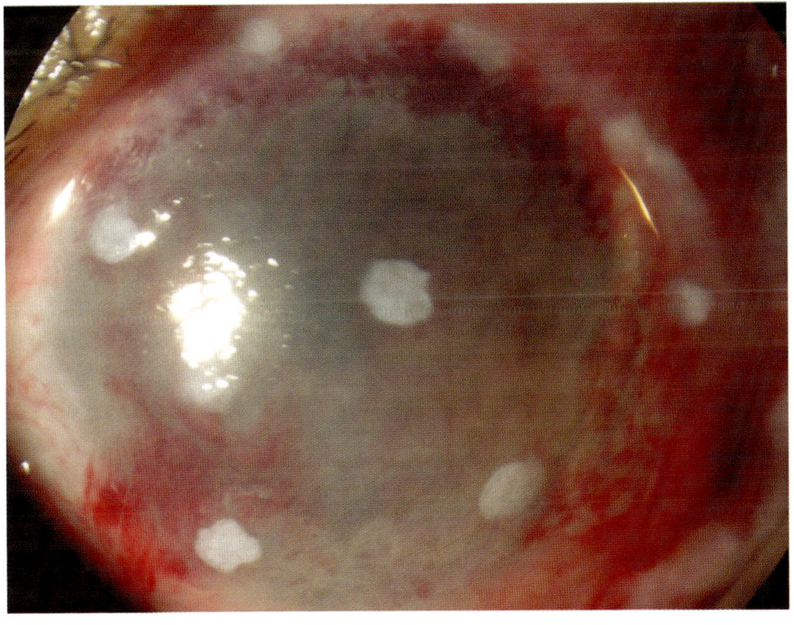

Fig. 46: Cultured limbal stem cell transplant after one week

had been excluded by serological tests. Under a lamellar—flow hood, the placenta is cleaned of blood clots with sterile Earle's Balanced Salt Solution (Life Technologies Inc, Gaithersburg, Md) containing 50 ug/mL penicillin, 50-ug/mL streptomycin, 100 ug/mL neomycin, and 2.5 ug/mL amphotericin B (Life Technologies Inc). The amnion is separated from the rest of the chorion by blunt dissection through the potential spaces situated between these 2 tissues, and flattened onto a nitrocellulose paper with a pore size of 0.45 ug (Bio-Rad, Gainesville, Fla), with the epithelium/basement membrane surface up. The paper with the adherent amniotic membrane is then cut into 3 × 4-cm disks and stored before transplantation at - 80" C in a sterile vial containing Dulbecco's Modified Eagle Medium (Life Technologies Inc) and glycerol (Baxter Healthcare Corporation, Stone Mountain, Ga) at the ratio of 1:1 (vol/vol).

Amniotic Membrane Transplantations

All surgeries in adults are performed under local anesthesia. Following the thorough removal of the conjunctival, limbal lesion and/or corneal pannus, the amniotic membrane is removed from the storage medium, peeled off the nitrocellulose filter paper, transferred to the recipient eye, and fitted to cover the defect by trimming off the excess edges. In the patients with limbal deficiency, the amniotic membrane covered the entire corneal surface and the perilimbal area extending 5 to 7 mm from the limbus. This fashioned membrane is then secured to the corneal edge of the defect by interrupted 10-0 nylon sutures if the covered limbal circumference is less than 2 clock hours, or by a purse-string running suture at the limbal area if it is more than 2 clock hours, and to the surrounding conjunctival edge with interrupted 9-0 Vicryl sutures with episcleral bites. This is followed by topical application of ciprofloxacin 0.3%, and betamethasone drops. After surgery, all patients receive prednisolone acetate eye drops every 2 hours while awake and ciprofloxacin twice daily. Sutures are removed at 3 weeks.

Combined use of limbal stem cells and amniotic membrane transplants have vastly improved the prognosis of penetrating keratoplasty in ocular surface disorders with severe limbal stem cell deficiency. We have been performing limbal stem cell transplant and some of these patients may be rehabilitated by performing penetrating corneal transplants subsequently. Recent literature describes successful management of patients suffering from end stage bilateral chemical eye burns, Stevens-Johnson syndrome and ocular cicatricial pemphigoid. One should carefully select cases for limbal stem cell and amniotic membrane transplants to get satisfactory results. However, these patients require not only multiple surgical procedures but also aggressive management for associated tear film and adenexial dysfunctions. With the introduction of cultured corneal epithelial and limbal stem cell transplantation, using amniotic membrane as carrier, there appears to be a new ray of hope at the horizon for

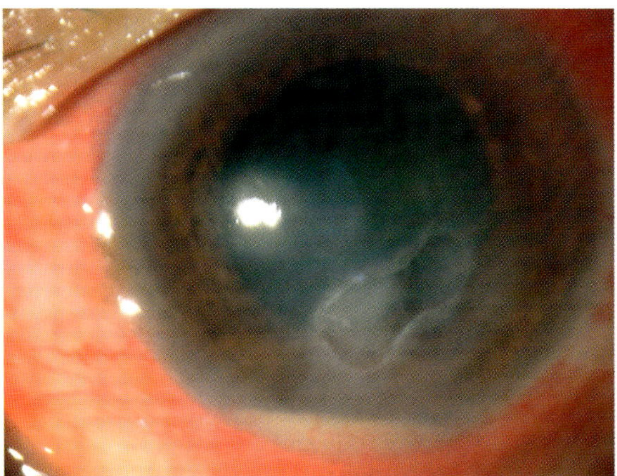

Fig. 47: Neurotrophic ulcer

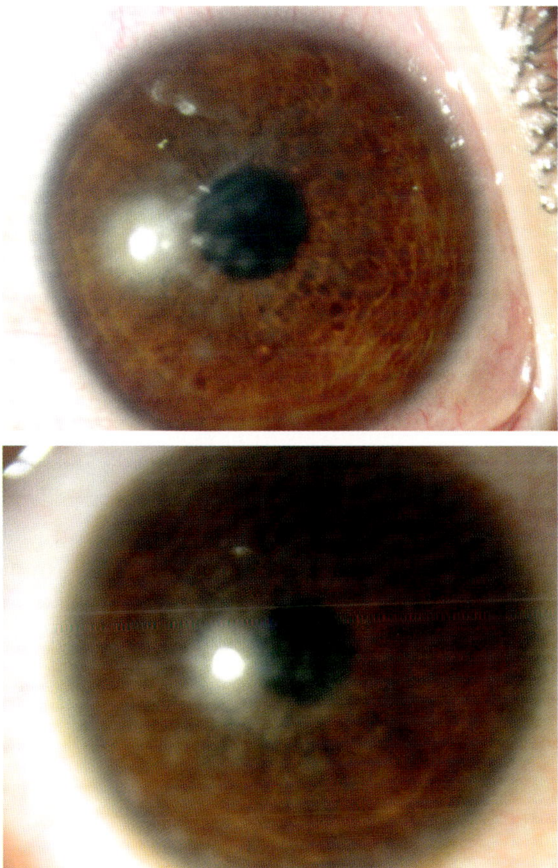

Figs 48 and 49: Adenoviral keratitis

ocular surface disease. Our early experience of performing cultured limbal stem cell transplants is encouraging. The facility for culture of limbal stem cells is provided by Reliance life sciences, India.

Mooren's Ulcer

Mooren's ulcer is a chronic, bilateral, progressive, painful, peripheral corneal ulceration. The disease progresses circumferentially initially, radially towards center and into the deeper corneal stroma at later stage of the disease. Several predisposing factors including previous trauma, history of surgical procedure and infections have been found to be associated with onset of the disease. The disease is known too occur in two forms. In younger adults it presents as a bilateral, severe and extremely painful condition. This variety of disease is known have worse prognosis. In the second variety the old individuals are affected and the condition is less severe, less painful and has better prognosis. Clinically to begin with, Mooren's ulcer presents as small epithelial defect in the peripheral cornea and marked episcleral congestion the adjoining area. As the disease progresses the peripheral corneal melt occurs and the ulcer rapidly deepens. The central edge of the ulcer is undermined. Infiltrate may be present in the advancing edge. Fluorescein stain, stains the advancing edge in the active Mooren's ulcer. The ulcer does not involve the sclera. The disease progresses both circumferential and deeper into the corneal stroma.

Differential Diagnosis

The exact etiopathogenesis is not known. Autoimmune mechanisms have been postulated to be the underlying cause the disease. The diagnosis of Mooren's ulcer is based on its classical clinical appearance and exclusion of various systemic disorders associated with development of peripheral ulcerative keratitis. Laboratory tests are performed to rule out rheumatoid arthritis, systemic lupus erythematosus, Periartritis nodosa and Wegener's granulomatosis. In a study hookworm infestation has been found a risk factor for development of Mooren's ulcer in South India. All patients suffering from Mooren's ulcer should be subjected to detailed microbiological work up. In case a microorganism is isolated broad spectrum antibiotic should be given. In contrast to Mooren's ulcer, the infective keratitis in the peripheral cornea progresses towards center.

Treatment

Patient is immediately put on topical and systemic steroids. Prophylactic broad spectrum antibiotics are given. Once the patient has been put on the treatment he needs close monitoring. Infiltrate on the advancing edge and epithelial defect should be monitored. The resolution of the corneal infiltrate and corneal epithelial defect indicate that the Mooren's ulcer is healing. Patients developing vascularization of the cornea approaching the margin of the ulcer should be

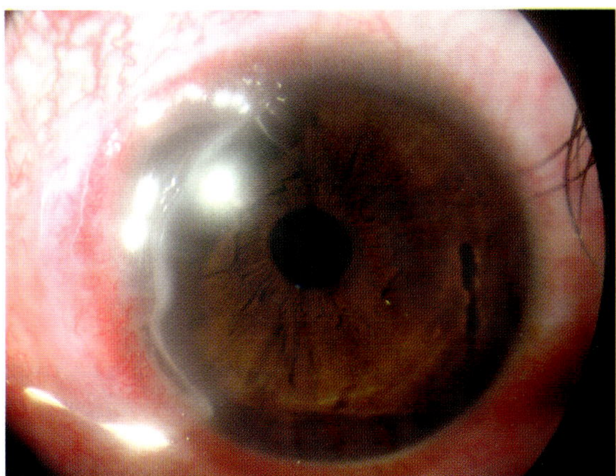

Fig. 50: Mooren's ulcer

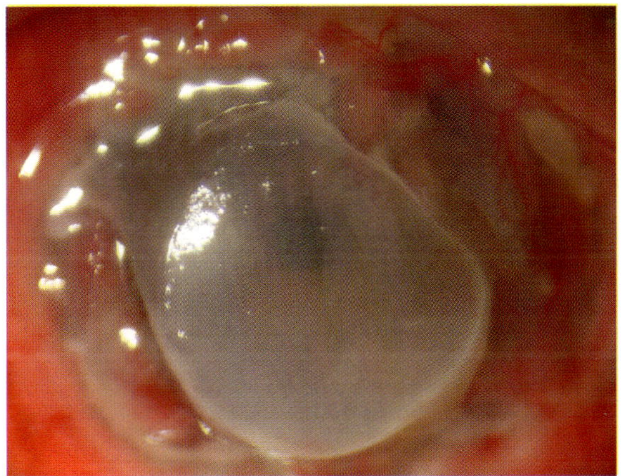

Fig. 51: Mooren's ulcer (Advanced)

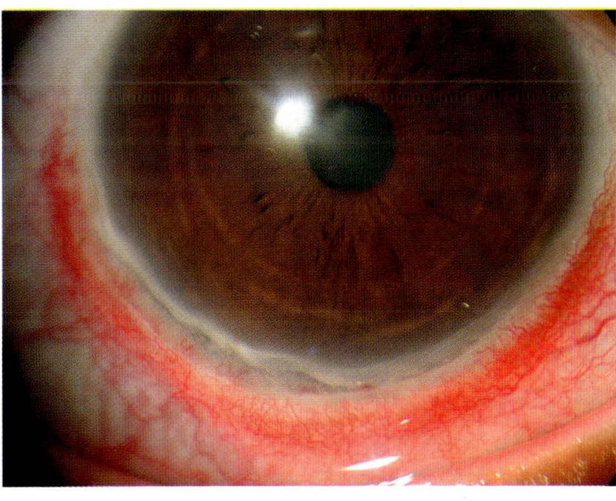

Fig. 52: Mooren's ulcer before treatment

considered for repeat peritectomy otherwise the patient will develop recurrence of the disease. Patients having significant corneal thinning need, peritectomy, cyano acrylate tissue adhesive and bandage contact application. In a recent report patients suffering from Mooren's ulcer who underwent tectonic penetrating keratoplasty have been successfully treated with topical cyclosporin 0.05% and no recurrence was observed in the follow up period. Topical 0.1% FK506 alone or in combination with keratoplasty has also been found safe and effective therapy for patients with recurrent Mooren's ulcer. In cases of advanced disease with corneal perforation actual or impending deep anterior lamellar keratoplasty, lamellar keratoplasty, penetrating keratoplasty may be performed. Patients with resistant and progressive disease require systemic immunosuppressive treatment.

Peripheral Ulcerative Keratitis

Peripheral ulcerative keratitis is common in occurrence. The disease usually starts with episcleritis and scleritis. Corneal involvement occurs once there is peripheral epithelial breakdown. Scleritis may also present in the ulcerative form. The clinical presentation finally may be as ulcerative sclerokeratitis. Scleritis and peripheral ulcerative keratitis (PUK) have been reported to present as isolated conditions. The condition clinically resembles to Mooren's ulcer. It can be differentiated due to scleral involvement, that does not occur in Mooren's ulcer. The disease relentlessly progresses despite treatment. Ulcerative scleritis is invariably considered of autoimmune origin unless proved otherwise. Author has treated a patient suffering from peripheral ulcerative keratitis presenting with scleral abscess, ulcerative scleritis and peripheral corneal ulcer. Patient had active tuberculosis and secondary bacterial infection. Rarely primary infective ulcerative sclerokeratitis may occur. *Pseudomonas aeruginosa* and *Aspergillus* have been reported to cause ulcerative sclero-keratitis. Rarely patients may get secondary infection by the microorganism.

Investigations

Any patient presenting with ulcerative sclerokeratitis should undergo complete microbiological work-up including direct microscopy of smears (KOH wet mount and Gram stained) and cultures (bacterial and fungal).

Systemic work up of these patient is necessary. Patients should undergo complete medical examination to rule out collagen vascular disorders. Rheumatoid arthritis is most common cause of peripheral ulcerative keratitis. Various other disorders known to cause peripheral ulcerative keratitis include systemic lupus erythematosus, poly arthritis nodosa, and Wegener's granulomatosis. In developing countries active or healed pulmonary tuberculosis is also an important cause of peripheral ulcerative keratitis. In a study chronic HCV virus infection has been found associated with Mooren-

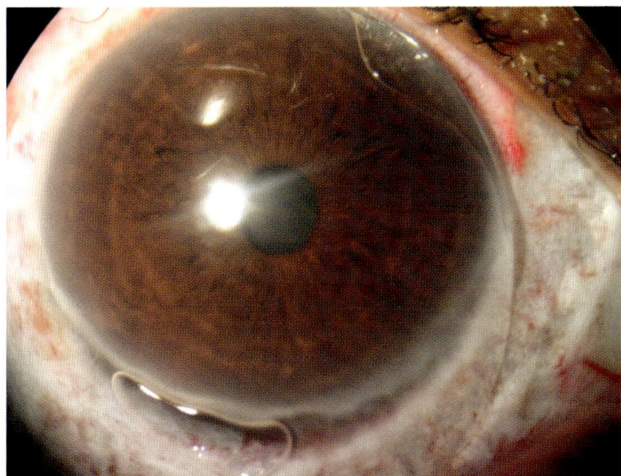

Fig. 53: Mooren's ulcer treated

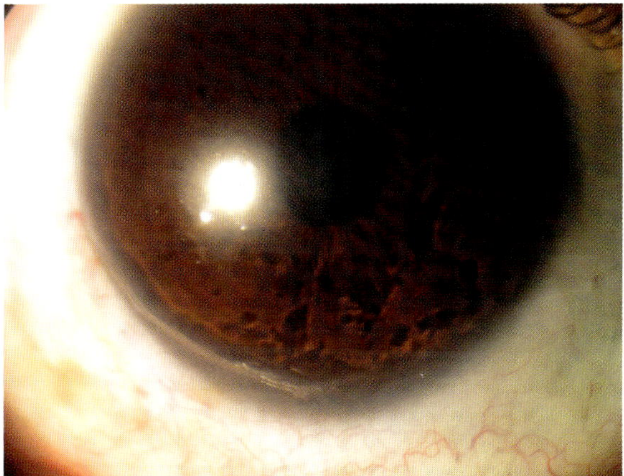

Fig. 54: Mooren's ulcer (after treatment)

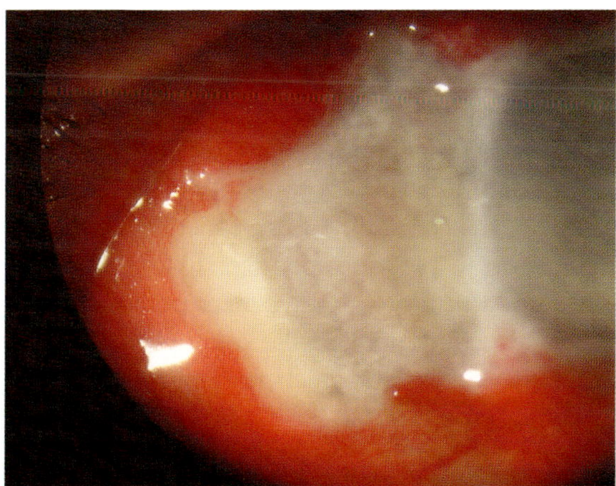

Fig. 55: Peripheral ulcerative keratitis

type ulcers. Authors suggested that all patients with Mooren-type ulcers should be tested for evidence of HCV infection in consultation with a liver specialist. However in a recent study nineteen (90%) of 21 patients with the clinical diagnosis of Mooren ulcer were found to have no evidence seropositive for hepatitis C. In a recent report HIV infection in young patients presented as PUK. The authors suggested that young patients presenting with PUK should be investigated for HIV infection. In another report hard contact lens (CL) retained in the superior fornix for over 16 years presented as PUK. Patient improved after removal of the embedded CL. A superior forniceal conjunctival pedicle graft was performed to prevent corneal perforation. The patient was managed postoperatively with a combination of topical steroids and antibiotics. The use of systemic immunosuppressive therapy was not required in this case. Micro-trauma and micro-keratitis as a result of the mechanical effect of the CL was suggested as possible etiopathogenesis.

Patients should get complete hemogram, renal and liver function tests. A montoux test and X-ray chest PA view should be ordered. X-ray chest may reveal hilar enlargement, multiple nodular or cavitary pulmonary lesions. X-ray paranasal sinuses is an important investigation in these patients. X-ray PNS may reveal mucosal thickening in maxillary sinus. In advanced cases clouding or complete opacification of ethamoidal, frontal and sphenoidal sinuses may be observed. Patients should also be subjected to Reumatoid factor, L E cell phenomenon, anti-nuclear factor and autoantibody ANCA. In a recent study patients with early RA, pANCA were found to be associated with specific serologic markers of RA and predict rapid radiographic joint destruction.

Treatment

Local treatment of the eye condition alone is not sufficient. The disease is known to progress with local treatment alone. Treatment of the underlying systemic disorder with immunosuppressive agents is the definitive treatment of the condition. Adjunct local treatment of the eye condition is necessary till the systemic immunosuppression is achieved. Depending upon the stage of the disease various measures including peritectomy, cyanoacrylate tissue adhesive application, bandage contact lens application may be necessary. Patients should also be put on topical antibiotics and anti-collagenolytic agents. In a recent study peripheral ulcerative keratitis has been successfully treated with topical application of cyclosporine 0.05%. In advanced cases presenting with extreme corneal thinning, impending or actual corneal perforation various surgical procedures including deep anterior lamellar keratoplasty, lamellar keratoplasty, penetrating keratoplasty and scleral patch graft may be required on emergency basis.

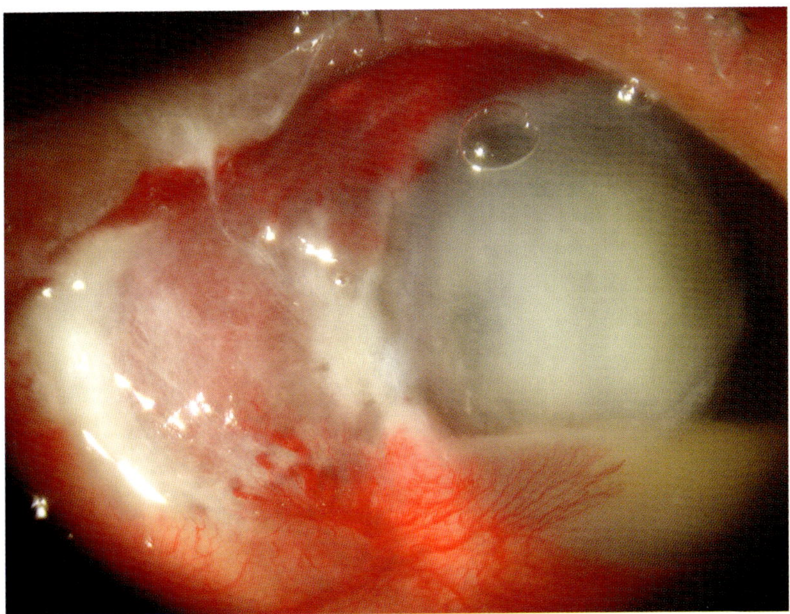

Fig. 56: Peripheral ulcerative keratitis (Response to treatment)

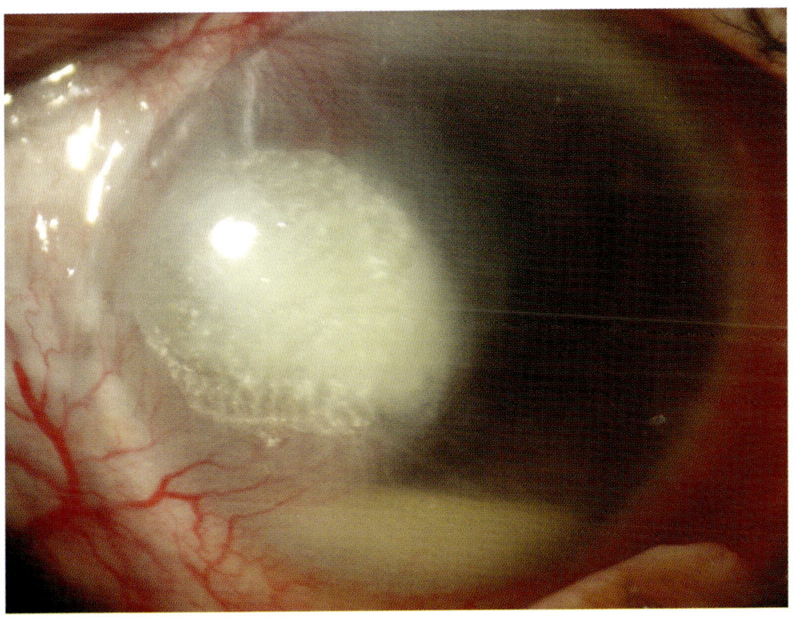

Fig. 57: Peripheral ulcerative keratitis (Glue application)

Corneal Injuries

Management of Corneal Injuries

Penetrating eye injury, perforating eye injury, globe rupture and corneal laceration are commonly used terms to describe anterior segment trauma. The ocular trauma classification group has developed a classification system for mechanical injuries of the eye. Open globe injury classification has been described as under.

Open-globe Injury Classification

Type

A. Rupture
B. Penetrating
C. Intraocular foreign body
D. Perforating
E. Mixed.

Grade

1. $\geq$ 20/40
2. 20/50 to 20/100
3. 19/100 to 5/200
4. 4/200 to light perception
5. No light perception.

Pupil

Positive: Relative afferent papillary defect present in affected eye
Negative: Relative afferent papillary defect absent in affected eye.

Zone

I. Isolated to cornea (including the corneoscleral limbus)
II. Corneoscleral limbus to a point 5 mm posterior into the sclera
III. Posterior to the anterior 5 mm of sclera.

Management of acute corneal injury: OGI needs emergency management. Brief history including mode of injury, causative agent and prior treatment should be recorded. Ophthalmic examination should aim at ascertaining whether or not the patient requires surgical intervention. In case the patient requires surgical

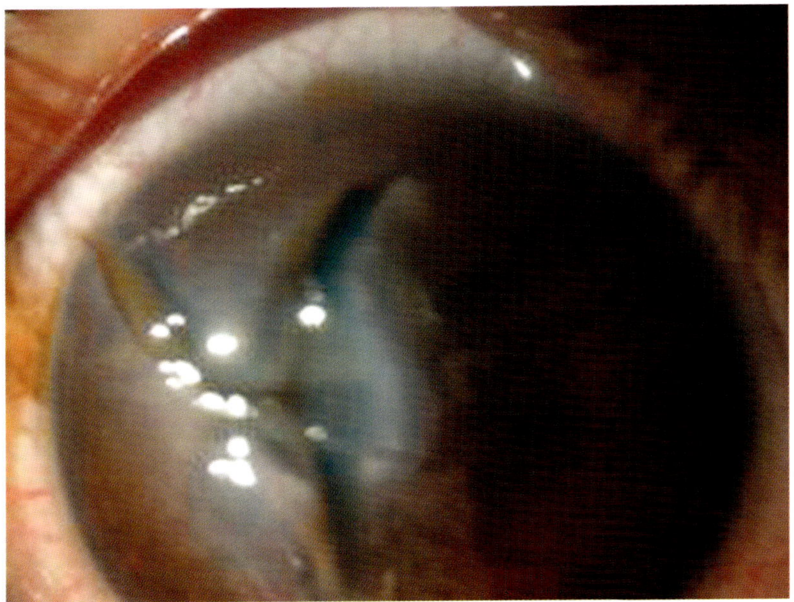

Fig. 58: Full thickness corneal laceration

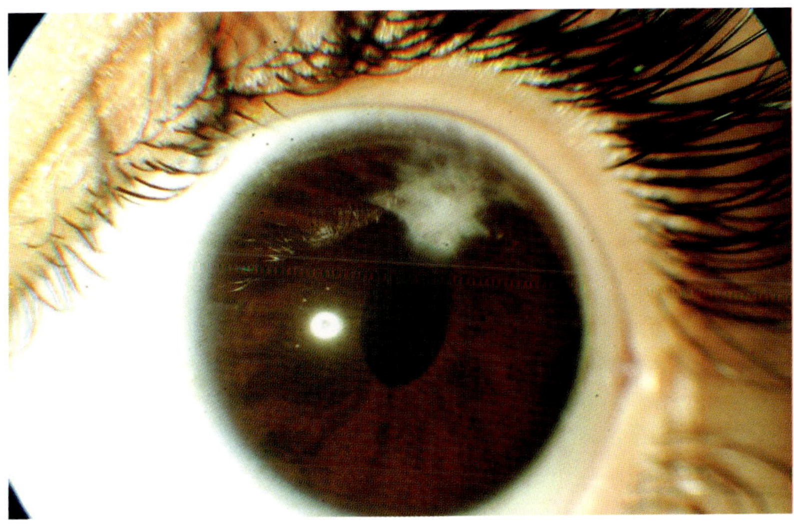

Fig. 59: Corneal laceration repair followed by cataract extraction and PC IOL implantation

intervention he should be prepared for general anesthesia. Tetanus prophylaxis should be administered. In case there is suspicion of retained intraocular foreign body, an X-ray orbit (AP) and lateral view should be done. Primary repair of the corneal injury should be performed as early as possible.

Slit lamp biomicroscopy and indirect ophthalmoscopy are preferred and ideal methods of examination and should be performed on all the co-oprerative patients. The findings of the clinical examination should be recorded in detail. Clinical signs on slit lamp biomicroscopy may be recorded by drawing schematic color coded diagrams. Photographic documentation of the clinical findings should also be done.

Anesthesia: Primary repair in cases with open globe injuries is always performed under general anesthesia. In a recent study regional anesthesia with monitored anesthesia care has been found a reasonable alternative to general anesthesia for selected patients with open globe injuries.

Principles of Repair: Principles of Surgical Repair

Extent of corneal injury should be measured and possible extension to the sclera should be ruled out. Recent iris prolapse presenting within few hours should be reposited. Old iris prolapse, torn iris and iris with possible focus of infection should be abscised. In case of ciliary body prolapse, it should not be abscised. Ciliary body can be reposited. Light cautry may be applied to small portion if required. Anterior chamber fluid should be sent for microbial cultures.

It is good practice to divide the corneal scleral laceration into corneal and scleral components. Even scleral or corneal laceration can be further subdivided by putting sutures in between at certain landmarks such as pigmentary lines on the corneal epithelium. Corneal sutures should be deep upto 80-90% of corneal thickness. Corneal sutures with shallow bites cause posterior wound gap. Corneal surgeons use adequate number of sutures in the peripheral cornea and less number of sutures near the visual axis. Corneal sutures produce compression of the corneal wound on either side of the corneal suture. The length of the wound compression is equal to half of the suture length. Corneal sutures should be placed in such a way so that the compression zone around the corneal sutures just overlap each other.

Corneal laceration with tissue loss: Approximation of corneal laceration with tissue loss is extremely difficult. Various modalities include, purse string suture, cyanoacrylate tissue adhesive application and penetrating keratoplasty.

Infective corneal laceration may also be treated with application of cyanoacrylate tissue adhesive application in addition to topical antibiotics. Lamellar corneal injuries with tissue loss may be treated with cyanoacrylate tissue adhesive application, deep lamellar keratoplasty and multi-layered amniotic membrane transplant.

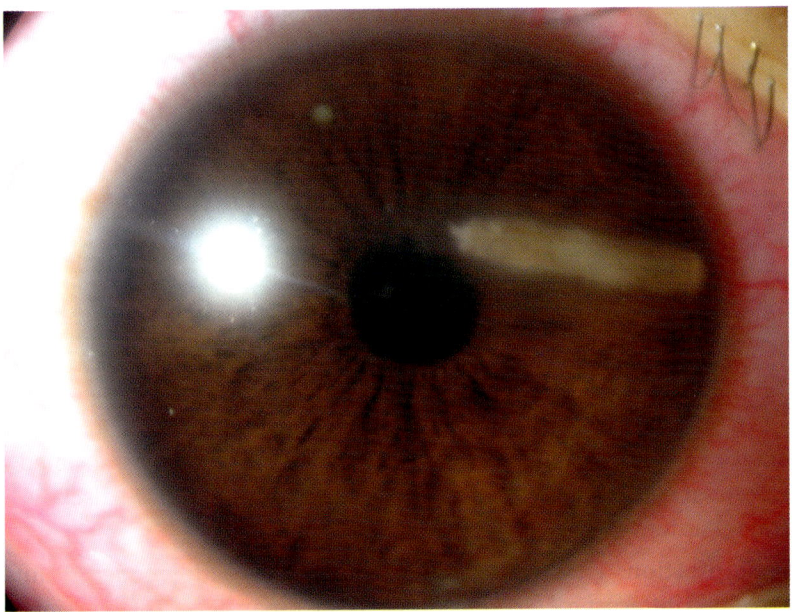

Fig. 60: Corneal injury with foreign body

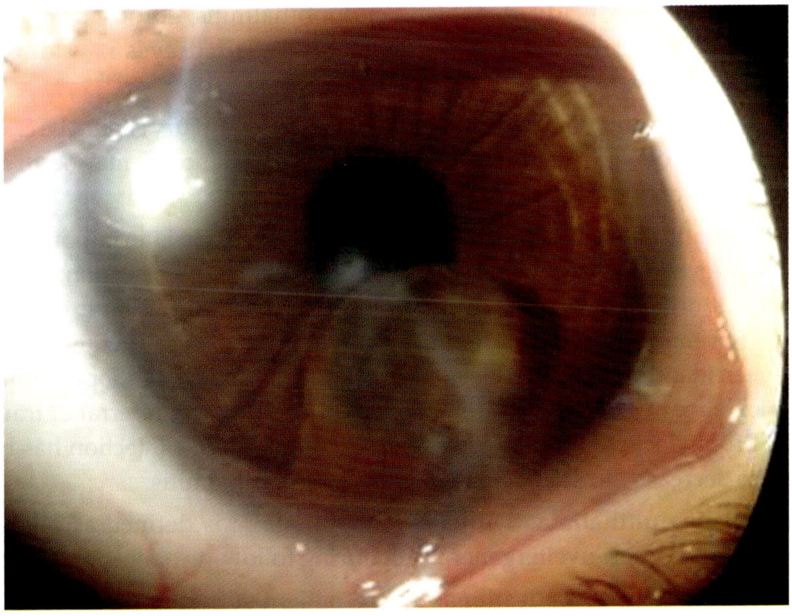

Fig. 61: Iris cyst following repair of corneal laceration

ultrasonography should be performed. Ultrasound biomicroscopy is provides accurate details of the angle structures including zonular status, angle recession, cyclodialysis, and the detection of small superficial and intraocular foreign bodies. IOP should be recorded by applanation tonometry. Avoid gonioscopy until a week or 10 days as it may be painful and the patient may not be able to co-operate.

Severity grades of hyphema: Grade 1: Hyphema less than one-third of the anterior chamber. Grade 2: Hyphema one-third to one-half of the anterior chamber. Grade 3: Hyphema one-half to less than total. Grade 4: Hyphema total clotted hyphemas. Total clotted hyphema is often referred to as black-ball or eight-ball hyphema.

The source of blood into the anterior chamber is a tear at the iris or ciliary body, usually at the angle structures. A tear at the anterior aspect of the ciliary body is the most common site of bleeding. The resolution of hyphema occurs through trabecular meshwork and Schlemm's canal or the juxtacanalicular tissue.

Raised Intraocular Pressure

Raised IOPs (above 21 mm Hg) may accompany hyphemas of any grade. Severe and persistent elevations of IOP are associated with near total or total hyphemas. The initial period of elevated IOP within 24 hours is often followed by a period of either normal or below normal pressure during the second to the sixth day. The initial raised IOP is probably the result of trabecular clogging by erythrocytes. This is followed by a period of reduced pressure due to decreased aqueous production. Subsequently with the recovery of the ciliary body function the intraocular pressure rises. Significant number of patients may present with persistent raised intraocular pressure.

Secondary Hemorrhage

Secondary bleed into the anterior chamber results in a markedly increased incidence of complications and worse prognosis. Secondary hemorrhage may occur in nearly 20% of all patients with hyphema. The incidence of secondary hemorrhage is higher in hyphemas of grades 3 and 4. Secondary bleed usually occurs on the third or fourth day, but may occur anytime from the second to the seventh day. Several studies documented that secondary hemorrhage occurs more frequently in African American patients. In a study four (40%) of the 10 patients with secondary hemorrhage had positive sickle cell trait or SA hemoglobin. Secondary bleed is attributed to lysis and retraction of the clot that has occluded the injured vessel. The secondary bleeding may result in raised IOP and corneal blood staining. Secondary bleed is associated with a poorer visual prognosis.

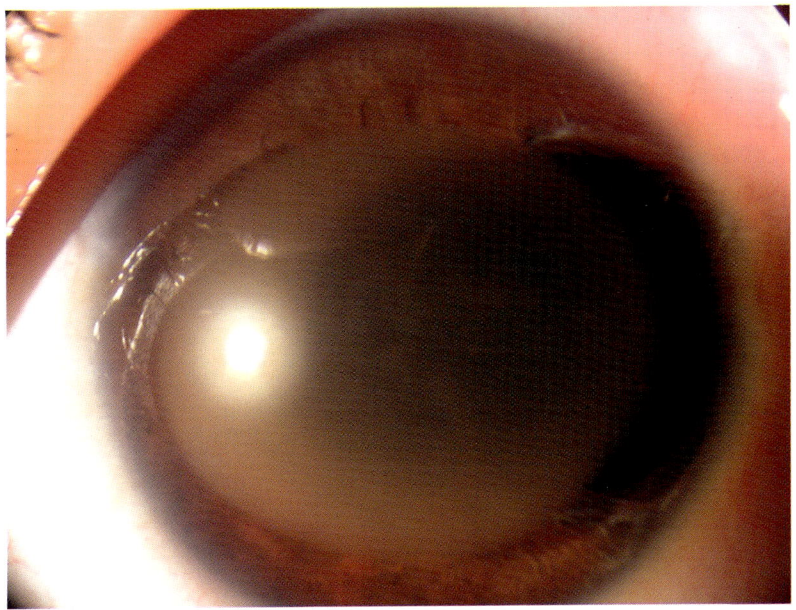

Fig. 65: Spontaneous resorption (Partial) of corneal blood staining

Complications of Hyphema: Complications from traumatic microhyphema treated with standard measures are few. Hyphema may cause posterior synechiae, peripheral anterior synechiae, corneal blood staining, and optic atrophy. Optic atrophy may result from acute rise of IOP or persistent high IOP. Posterior synechiae may secondary to iritis or iridocyclitis. Peripheral anterior synechia occur more frequently in patients who had under gone surgical intervention. Closeness of follow-up may be determined by IOP on presentation.

Medical Management

Standard protocol for traumatic microhyphema includes atropinization, bed rest, shield and restriction of antiplatelet medications. Bilateral patching, complete bed rest and sedation are not recommended. Patient remains ambulatory and mild sedation can be given to apprehensive patients. Patient should be advised to keep the head elevated at 30-45° as it allows the hyphema to settle inferiorly. Superior angle remains free for the aqueous drainage. This also allows proper monitoring of the progress and also allows early recognition of rebleed. The antiplatelet effect of aspirin tends to increase the incidence of rebleeding in traumatic hyphema and should be avoided. Non-steroidal anti-inflammatory drugs such as mefenamic acid, also share this antiplatelet effect. Systemic ACA should be used in patients with hyphemas that occupy 75% or less of the anterior chamber since the clot may persist in the anterior chamber for an increased period during administration of the drug.Topical ACA appears to be a safe, effective treatment to prevent secondary hemorrhage in traumatic hyphema. It is as effective as systemic ACA in reducing secondary hemorrhage. Some studies have investigated the application of intracameral tissue plasminogen activator (t-PA) in the management of traumatic hyphema. A potential risk with t-PA is the associated risk of developing rebleeding of the initial wound. The application has been considered in resolving hyphemas that either fail to clear spontaneously or are associated with malignant IOP.

Surgical Intervention

Immediate surgical intervention is indicated in case the IOP remains elevated at 50 mm Hg or higher for 4 days. In case the surgical intervention is delayed optic atrophy may occur.

Paracentesis causes little surgical trauma and reduces the elevated IOP. Paracentesis is especially beneficial in patients with sickle-cell trait or disease. However, the decrease in IOP may be transient, and there may be no appreciable reduction in the amount of the formed clot.

Irrigation: Using a one- or two-needle technique, the surgeon must be particularly careful to have direct visualization of the anterior chamber, but this technique has some disadvantages. Maintaining the position of the needle tip in the anterior chamber may be difficult during the procedure. A hazardous situation

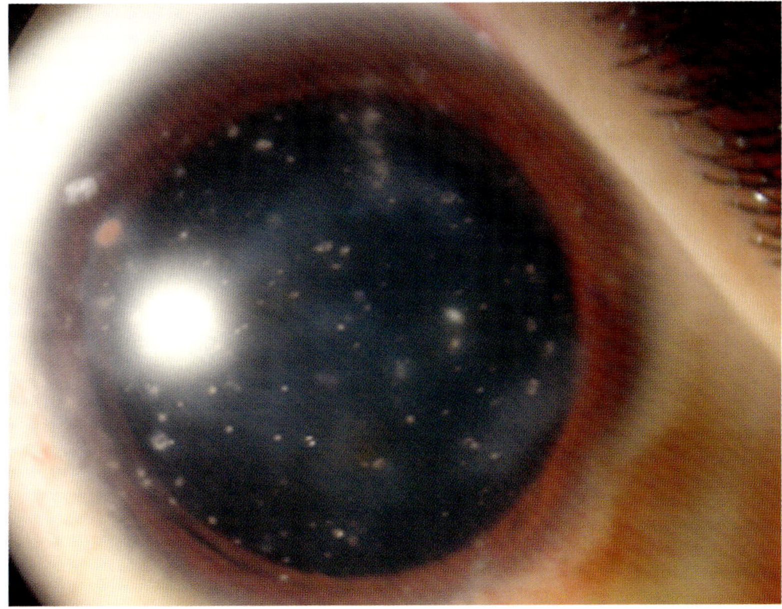

Fig. 66: Corneal opacity with multiple corneal foreign bodies following cracker injury

is created when the collar-button type of formed clot occupies both the anterior and posterior chambers. This produces pupillary block with anterior displacement of the iris-lens diaphragm.

Anterior chamber maintainer: Anterior chamber maintainer has been found useful in the surgical management of traumatic hyphema. With an ACM in place, the fluctuations of intraoperative IOP are minimized and the AC depth is stabilized throughout the operation. The risk of renewed bleeding is reduced because of the continuous positive intraoperative IOP. The ACM is an important tool in the surgical management of traumatic hyphemas because it facilitates AC washout and reduces iatrogenic damage to the iris and corneal endothelium.

Removal of hyphema with vitrectomy: The evacuation of the hyphema can be performed with vitrectomy. The initial clear corneal incision is made with a diamond blade. To avoid the iris and lens, the blade is oriented and pushed into the anterior chamber in such a manner that it is parallel to the plane of the iris. With the vitrectomy cutting port half open and the infusion line in place, it is possible to irrigate and aspirate free blood from the formed clot.

Corneal Blood Staining

Corneal blood staining usually occurs following traumatic hyphema. Hyphema combined with secondary glaucoma are most common risk factors for developing corneal blood staining. Cornea blood staining may rarely occur following non-traumatic hyphema. Coneal blood staining has been reported following hyphema due to proliferative diabetic retinopathy. A case of corneal blood staining due to a hemorrhagic descemet membrane detachment has been reported. Spontaneous resolution of corneal blood staining is known, but may take many months to years.

Iris and angle changes: The classical sign of close globe injury is the ring of pigment clumps over the anterior capsule, known as Vossius ring. The size of the ring is smaller than the size of the pupil. Iridoschisis is lamellar separation of anterior and posterior iris. Sudden increase in the pressure in the anterior chamber puts stress on the iris sphincter, root of the iris circular and longitudinal cilliary muscle fibers, resulting angle recession. Blunt trauma may cause separation of longitudinal fibers from the scleral spur creating a cyclodialysis cleft. Iris is torn at thinnest portion and the thinnest portion of the iris is at root, resulting iridodialysis. A technique for repair of traumatic iridodialysis that avoids the need for iris sutures has been described. Following a limbal peritomy, sclerostomy sites level with the iris base are created at each clock hour of the iridodialysis using a microvitreoretinal blade. Vitreoretinal forceps passed through these ports are used to incarcerate the peripheral iris. No suture material is used to secure the iris.

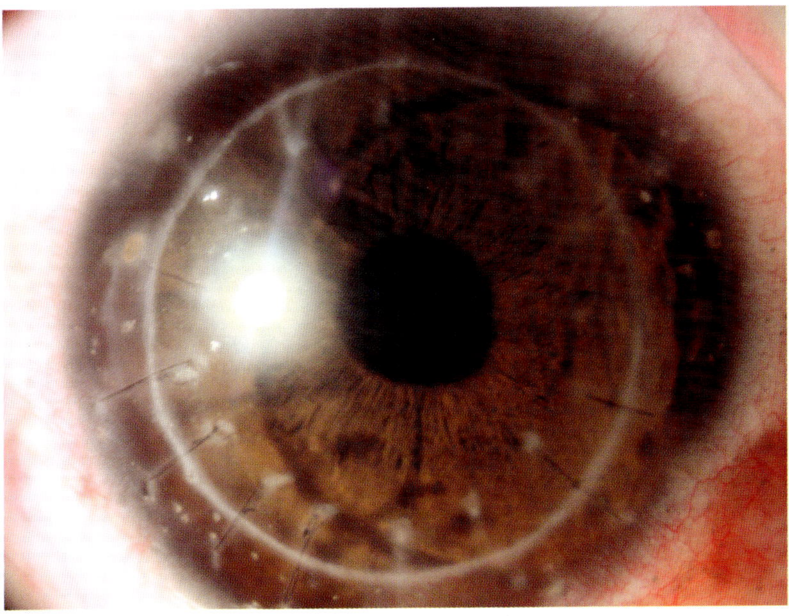

Fig. 67: Deep anterior lamellar keratoplasty

Secondary glaucoma: Glaucoma in hyphema may develop due to variety of mechanisms. These mechanisms include trabecular blockage with erythrocytes, pupillary block due to full chamber clotted blood, angle recession and peripheral anterior synechia Clinically, the presence of increased pigmentation at the angle, elevated baseline IOP, hyphema, lens displacement, and angle recession of more than 180 degrees have been significantly associated with the occurrence of chronic glaucoma after closed globe injury. On UBM findings such as a wider angle and the absence of cyclodialysis were significant predictors for the subsequent development of traumatic glaucoma. Less than 10% of patients having angle recession develop glaucoma. The mechanism of glaucoma is outflow obstruction due to scarring or a hyaline membrane covering the angle. Patients presenting with hyphema and associated vitreous hemorrhage may have raised intraocular pressure 2 weeks to 3 months later. The erythrocytes after losing hemoglobin, become "ghost cells" in the vitreous cavity. The ghost cells may pass forward into the anterior chamber, with resultant elevation of IOP. The condition is described as Ghost cell glaucoma.

Miscellaneous changes: Changes in the refractive status of the eye have been reported following blunt trauma. Blunt trauma can dislocate angle-supported pIOLs. Implantation of these IOLs should be discouraged in patients who perform activities that put them at risk for eye trauma. Tube extension using angiocatheter material is used in glaucoma flitering surgery. Following blunt trauma intrusion of the tube into the anterior chamber has been reported. Ocular blunt trauma activates corneal and lens epithelial cells without apparent corneal ablation or direct injury in the lens epithelium. Eyes with cracker injuries may develop corneal scarring due to multiple foreign bodies and may require deep anterior lamellar keratoplasty. Eyes with scleral rupture after blunt trauma may rarely get complicated by proliferative vitreoretinopathy. In certain cases, retinal detatchment or proliferative vitreoretinopathy may not develop following extensive scleral rupture. Sympathetic ophthalmia has been reported to occur following nonpenetrating ocular trauma.

Prevention of blunt ocular trauma is of paramount importance in decreasing the incidence of these injuries. Use of preventive measures while at work or during high risk sports should be strictly complied. Public education on the use of protective glasses and other protective measures should be given at regular intervals. In case blunt trauma occurs prompt examination and urgent treatment may limit the ocular morbidity.

Acute Chemical Eye Injury

Chemical injury is an important cause of severe limbal stem cell deficiency. Chemical injuries in children and housewives may occur inside the house due to inappropriate handling of the dangerous chemicals. Young adults may get chemical injury while working in labs or in the factories. In most cases of

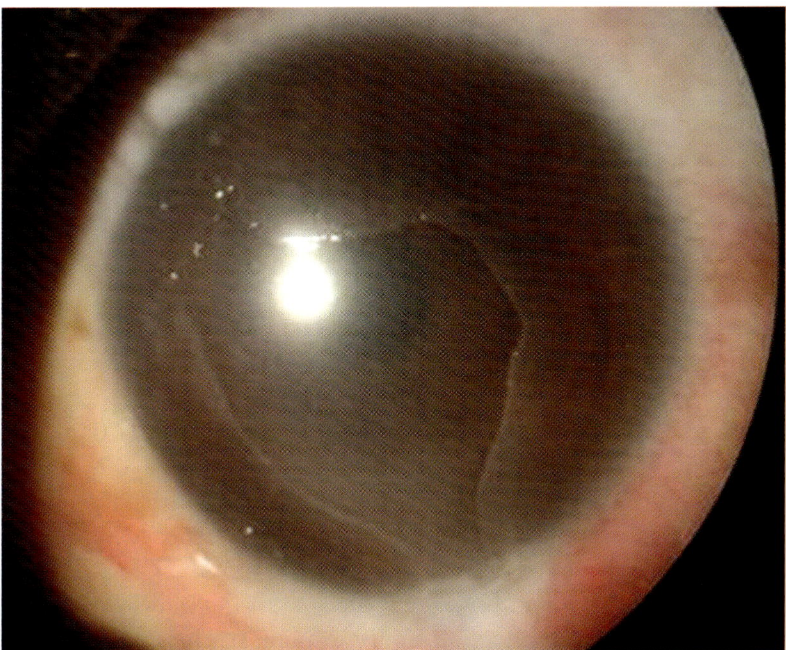

Fig. 68: Epithelial defect and localized limbal stem cell deficiency following severe chemical injury (Acid)

chemical injuries the victim usually had ignored the precautions. Alkalies (Ammonium hydroxide, sodium hydroxide, potassium hydroxide and calcium hydroxide) and acids (Hydrochloric acid and sulphuric acid) are common chemicals implicated in chemical injuries. Alkalies damage cell membrane and penetrate deeper into the tissues in comparison to acids. Of various chemicals, it is ammoium hydroxide which has maximum penetration and causes maximum damage. Acids cause coagulation of proteins and thus form a protective layer on the cornea.

Emergency treatment: To minimize the contact period of the chemical is of paramount importance. This limits the damage by the chemical to the minimum. Thorough irrigation of the conjunctival sac with normal saline decreases the contact time of the chemical and decreases the ocular surface damage. The conjuntival lavage should be continued for at least 45 minutes. We did not find practical estimation and monitoring of pH in chemical injury patients. Patient is put on topical antibiotic, frequent instillation of corticosteroid drops, cycloplegic and anti-glaucoma medication.

In acute chemical injury every effort is made to promote healing of the ocular surface after 48 hours of chemical injury grading of chemical eye injury is done.Modified Roper Hall classification is used. The grading of the chemical injury is performed on the basis of extent of limbal ischemia as degree of limbal ischemia equates with limbal stem cells. Grade 0 and1: No limbal ischemia, Grade 2: Less than 1/3rd limbal ischemia, Grade 3: 1/3rd to 1/2 limbal ischemia, Grade 4: > ½ limbal ischemia. Severe grades (Grade 3 and 4) of chemical injury have poorer prognosis. To promote epithelial healing bandage contact lens or amniotic membrane transplant may be used. Sutureless application of an amniotic membrane patch delivers various factors, which may help preserve and facilitate rapid expansion of remaining limbal stem cells. This may prevent late cicatricial complications in mild and moderate acute alkaline burns.

Limbal stem cell transplant may be required in case the medical measures fail to achieve epithelial healing due to limbal stem cell damage. Patient with persistent epithelial defect should be treated with oral doxycycline 100 mg twice daily. In desperate cases of progressive corneoscleral melt glued on RGP contact lens may be applied. Tectonic penetrating corneal graft is performed for tectonic purpose. The procedure may be combine with amniotic membrane transplants.

Conjunctival epithelium grows onto the cornea. The vascularized pannus formation progress from the area of limbal stem cell deficiency and finally affect the vision. Associated dry eye is due to unstable tear film may worsen the ocular surface. Limbal stem cell deficiency can be total or partial. In partial limbal stem cell deficiency, limbal stem cell hypo-function may result in non-healing epithelial defect.

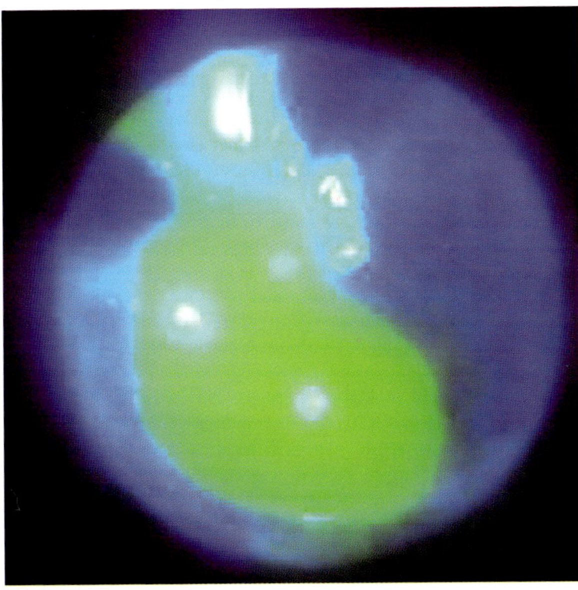

Fig. 69: Fluorescein staining showing localized limbal stem cell deficiency and limbal ulceration

Diagnosis

Conjunctivalization of the cornea, the hallmark of limbal stem cell deficiency, needs to be documented to make diagnosis. A severe form of conjunctivalization is usually obvious to the clinician. The subtle changes in the corneal epithelium texture, permeability, recurrent erosions may be detected on slit lamp biomicroscopy using fluorescein dye. Impression cytology of the cornea and histopathological examination of the excised fibrovascular tissue may show the presence of goblet cells. Impression cytology can be performed by applying nitrocellulose filter paper onto corneal surface. All cytologic specimens are processed and stained with periodic Acid-Schiff reagent and a modified Harris hematoxylin-eosin stain. Under a microscope with a 40× objective, the area with the highest cell density is counted at 5 different areas with each equivalent to 5625 μm^2, while that of goblet cell density is measured in a similar manner but at an area equivalent to 10000 μm^2. These data are then converted to number of cells per millimeter squared and are compared using the Student paired (match) t test.

Visual Rehabilitation

Once acute condition has healed and stable ocular surface has been achieved, ocular surface should be further evaluated. Effect should be made to decrease the corneal vascularization. Limbal stem cell transplants, amniotic membrane transplant may be performed to improve corneal surface and decrease corneal vascularization. Cultured limbal stem cell or corneal epithelial cell transplantation has been need to rehabilitate ocular surface. In a recent report one 60 degrees conjunctival limbal autograft combined with amniotic membrane transplantation as both a permanent graft and a temporary patch was found to resurface the total corneal surface in an eye with total limbal stem cell deficiency. Finally visual rehabilitation in some of the cases occur only after penetrating keratoplasty or deep anterior lamellar keratoplasty.

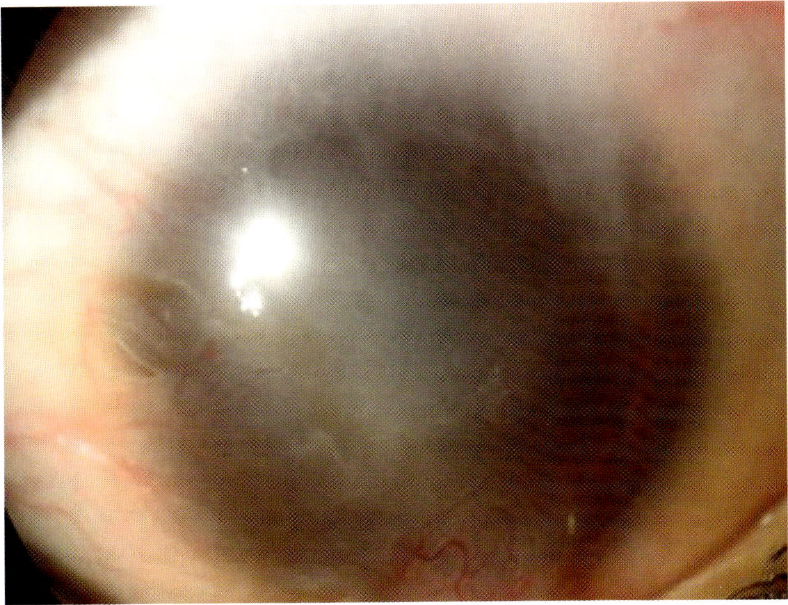

Fig. 70: Healed chemical injury following limbal stem cell transplant

Non-inflammatory Degenerations

Corneal Degenerations

Corneal degenerations are usually unilateral, asymmetrical located either peripherally or eccentrically. These do not have any inheritance or genetic predisposition. The corneal degenerations may occur following trauma, inflammation and due to aging. There is no satisfactory classification for corneal degenerations. Some of the important ones are described as under:

Keratoconus

In this disease the central or paracentral cornea undergoes progressive thinning and ectasia. The cornea assumes the shape of a large cone. Child develops myopia, regular and irregular astigmatism. The hereditary pattern is usually unpredictable. Most of the cases are sporadic in nature. Nearly all cases are bilateral, but one eye may be affected more than the other. The disease is known to occur in chromic vernal conjunctivitis. The management of keratoconus in active vernal disease is extremely difficult. One may have to control vernal conjunctivitis before considering the treatment of keratoconus. The disease tends to progress during the adolescent years and may stabilize later. As the progression occurs, the apical thinning of the central cornea increases, and extreme degrees of irregular astigmatism may develop.

Clinical Presentation

Most of the patients, who are not happy with the initial prescription the should be carefully examined for early keratoconus. Many of the patients are diagnosed during screening or during pre-operation work up as part of laser vision correction. Scissoring of the red reflex on ophthalmoscopy or retinoscopy is considered an early sign of keratoconus. Rizzutti's sign, conical reflection on the nasal cornea as a pen light is show from the temporal side, is another early finding. Iron deposits within the epithelium around the base of the cone described a Fleischer's ring. It is best appreciated with the cobalt-blue filter. Vogt's striae or "stress lines of the stroma" can be observed. Ruptures and scars may occur in Bowman's layer. Higher magnification of slit-lamp may be useful in detecting subtle changes. Currently corneal topography has become the standard procedure to detect early keratoconus and monitor the progress.

Descemet's membrane rupture may results in sudden development of corneal edema, referred to as acute hydrops. The break in the Descemet's membrane may heal in six to eight weeks. The corneal edema disappears and only stromal sign may be left. Hydrops is treated conservatively with topical hypertonic agents and patching or a soft contact lens. A cycloplegic agent may be needed

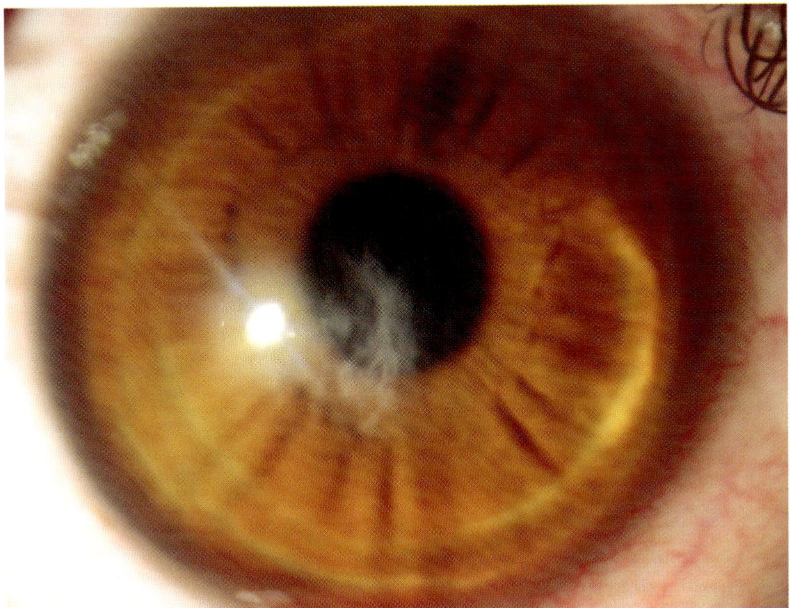

Fig. 71: Advanced keratoconus

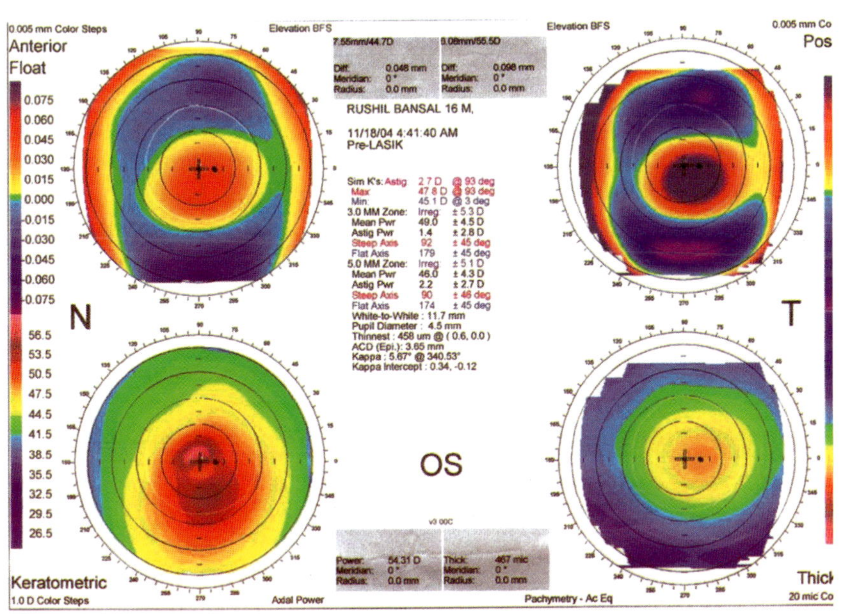

Fig. 72: Keratoconus on corneal topography (orbscan)

for ciliary pain. Air injection into the anterior chamber has been reported to enhance resolution of corneal edema.

Pathogenesis

Recent studies suggest increased expression of lysosomal enzymes and decreased levels of inhibitors of proteolytic enzymes may play an important role in corneal stromal thinning. Several investigators have suggested that abnormality in corneal collagen and its cross-linking may be the cause of keratoconus. Eye rubbing and contact lens wear have bee postulated to play a role.

Treatment

In mild cases of keratoconus vision may be improved with glasses alone. However, RGP contact lenses are helpful in mild to moderate cases. They often cause significant improvement in vision as these are able to neutralize the irregular corneal astigmatism. The majority of patients with keratoconus without central corneal scarring can be fitted contact lenses. When the routine gas permeable contract lenses do not work, one can try speciality contact lenses. Rose K contact lenses and Boston contact lenses are specially designed for keratoconus. These contact lenses provide appropriate fit when the routine contact lenses fail. When contact lenses no longer provide satisfactory vision surgical treatment is considered.

Standard surgical treatment consists of penetrating keratoplasty. Lamellar keratoplasty is also effective, but most surgeons prefer not to use this because of the technical difficulties involved and the slightly reduced visual outcome. Deep anterior lamellar keratoplasty has significantly improved visual results. In patients with advanced keratoconus who have developed corneal hydrops the preferred procedure is penetrating keratoplasty. At the time of keratoplasty, decreasing the donor/ recipient size disparity reduces post keratoplasty myopia. Intracorneal ring's have achieved some success in patients without corneal scarring in reducing the myopia and astigmatism and improving spectacle corrected visual acuity. But these patients can be fitted GP contact lenses as well.

Cross-linking treatment of keratoconus is a new method of treating keratoconus. In this procedure the photosensitizer riboflavin and ultraviolet A-light is used as an effective means for stabilizing the cornea in keratoconus. At the present stage of knowledge, the treatment should only be performed in patients with documented progression of keratoconus. To avoid serious side effects it is mandatory in each patient to perform preoperative pachymetry to exclude cases with less than 400 u m stromal thickness. The UVA irradiance should be checked using a UVA-meter, before every case.

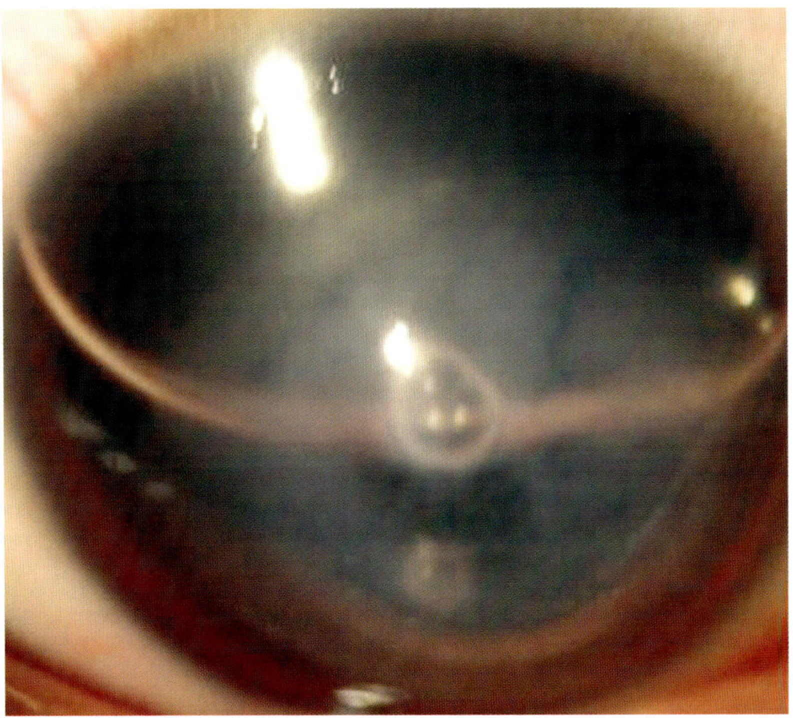

Fig. 73: Air injection for acute hydrops

Pellucid Marginal Corneal Degeneration

Pellucid marginal corneal degeneration is bilateral peripheral corneal ectatic disorder. It is characterized by narrow area of thinning inferiorly extending from 4 to 8 O′ clock. Between the thinned cornea and limbus there is narrow strip of normal cornea. Peripheral corneal thinning, results ectasia of cornea and high astigmatism against the rule. There is inferior corneal steepening and the curvatures may be increased upto 20 D. Unusual case of PMCD with 360° peripheral corneal thinning has been reported. The disease usually occurs in young adults in second to fourth decade. The condition is progressive. Although uncommon cases of corneal hydrops have been reported following Pellucid marginal corneal degeneration. Pellucid marginal degeneration has been reported to cause spontaneous corneal perforation resulting in the need for urgent therapeutic intervention. Pellucid marginal corneal degeneration has potential for severe ocular morbidity in all patients even if the disease appears to be stationary. Patients with unilateral perforation should be observed more closely for development of complications in the fellow eye.

Treatment

In mild disease visual acuity can be improved with glasses. In moderate cases GP contact lenses are ideal. In a recent study, authors could fit GP contact lenses in 23 out of 32 eyes. Calculation of appropriate base curve of the lens by stability factor method is found to be the best method to start with a trial in PMCD. Those patients who are not benefited with GP contact lenses may need lamellar keratoplasty. Wedge resection with relaxing incision have been tried to correct high astigmatism. DALK has been found an useful surgical alternative in the management of PMD. The technique may provide useful visual rehabilitation in patients with PMD even in the presence of previous corneal perforation. Corneal wedge resection combined with paired, opposed clear corneal penetrating relaxing incisions has also been found suitable surgical option for the treatment of PMCD. The procedure provided early adequate and stable astigmatism control.

Terrien's Marginal Degeneration

Terrien's marginal degeneration is a bilateral, ectatic corneal disorder that can occur at any age. It is characterized by localized superior or inferior corneal thinning. The area over the ectatic cornea is flattened and the cornea at 90° to the flatter meridian steepens. Thus these patients present with against the rule astigmatism. Patients to start with have fine, subepithelial opacity and corneal thinning in the superonasal quadrant. As the disease progresses the peripheral opacities as well as corneal thinning increases. Even in the extreme cases of corneal thinning the overlying epithelium remains intact. The peripheral corneal

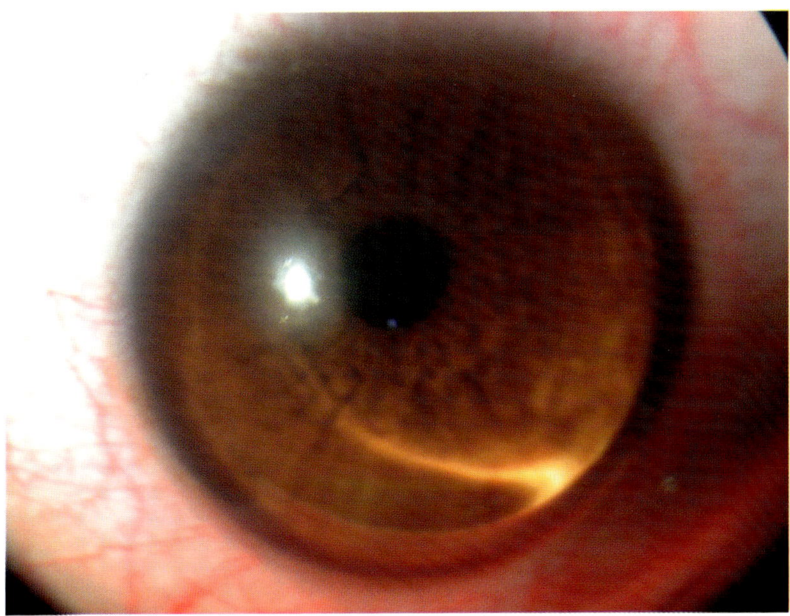

Fig. 74: Pellucid marginal corneal degeneration (Frontal view)

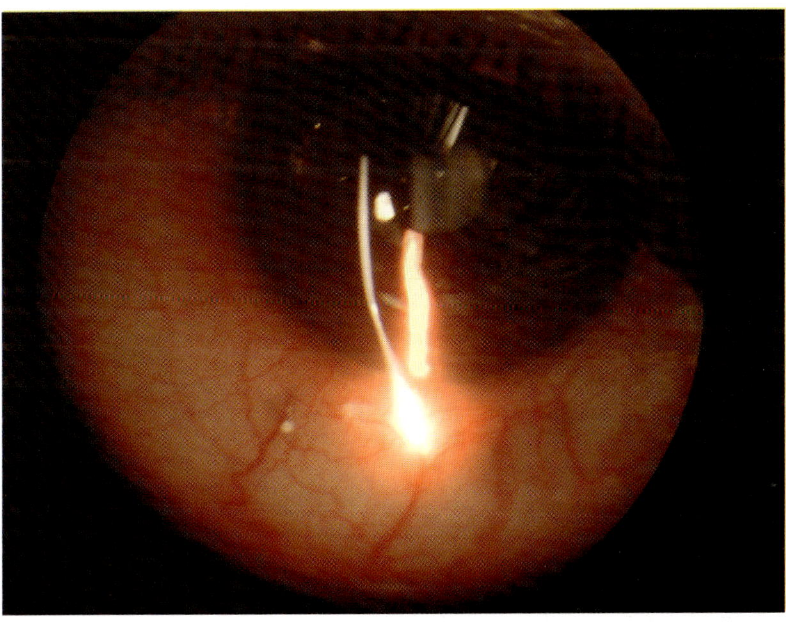

Fig. 75: Pellucid marginal corneal degeneration (Slit photograph)

opacities do not involve the limbus. Hitopathologically the Bowman's membrane and the corneal lamella are fibrillated. The circulating immune complexes in Terrien's marginal degeneration are normal. This signifies that the disease does not have immune mediated inflammation as an etiological factor.

Treatment

In the early cases, glasses or contact lenses may improve the vision. At a stage when the corneal thinning and the corneal ectasia is extreme reconstructive surgery either penetrating or lamellar corneal graft may be necessary. Keratoplasty combined with focal resection has been found effective and safe in the treatment of TMD. This procedure has been reported to preserve and improve the visual activity.

Salzmann's Nodular Degeneration

Salzmann's nodular degeneration has been reported to occur as late sequalae to ocular surface inflammatory conditions. Various diseases following which Salzmann's nodular degeneration has been reported to occur include vernal conjunctivitis, trachoma, phlyctenulosis and various viral diseases. Salzmann's nodules are gray colored, multiple, sub-epithelial and raised above the corneal surface. These nodules tend to occur either in the area of pre-existing corneal scarring or at the junction of transparent and opaque cornea. The cornea in the centre may be lear or opaque. The Salzmann's nodules may be single or multiple. Patients with Salzmann's nodular degeneration may be asymptomatic. Sometimes patients present with irritation watering and redness. Histopathologically these nodules consist of hyaline degeneration of collagen, cellular debris and electron dense hyaline deposits.

Treatment

Patients who are asymptomatic and have normal vision do not require any treatment. Irritation, watering or photophobia or diminution of vision may require excision of the nodules or superficial keratectomy. For superficial keratectomy diamond burr is considered to give better results. In a recent study, diamond burr superficial keratectomy improved visual acuity in patients with visually-significant anterior corneal opacities including Salzmann's nodular degeneration. Amniotic membrane transplant augmented superficial keratectomy helped achieve subjective comfort, visual rehabilitation and clinical regularization of the corneal surface in superficial corneal degenerations.

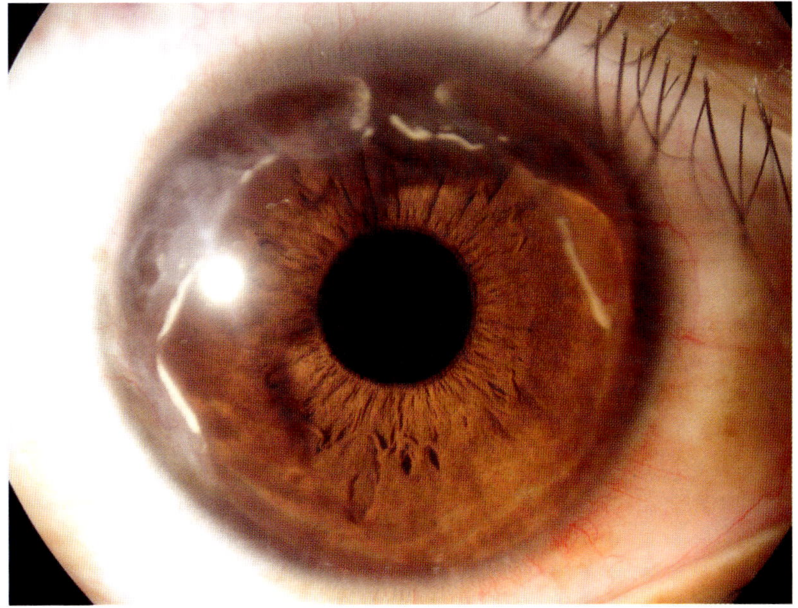

Fig. 76: Terrien's marginal degeneration

Excimer laser PTK provides both symptomatic relief and improvement in the visual acuity. Patients with corneal scarring may require lamellar keratoplasty or deep anterior lamellar keratoplasty. Penetrating keratoplasty is rarely required in some cases with scarring involving the entire thickness of the cornea. Lesion may recur after surgical treatment.

Climatic Droplet Keratopathy

Climatic droplet keratopathy has N number of names. No other medical condition in the literature seem to have such a long list of synonyms as climatic droplet keratopathy. To name a few of them, these include Labrador keratopathy, chronic actinic keratopathy, spheroidal droplet keratopathy, keratinoid degeneration, oil droplet degeneration, elastoid degeneration, hyaline degeneration. Figherman's keratopathy, Nama keratopathy, proteinaceous keratopathy etc. The exact etiopathogenesis of climatic droplet keratopathy is not known. Various factors including aging, microtrauma, UV radiation, welding and pre-existing corneal inflammatory disease have been postulated to be associated with the onset and the progress of the disease. Climatic droplet keratopathy has been categorized into primary and secondary type. Primary type is considered to be age related whereas the secondary variety is associated with pre-existing corneal disease. The disease has high prevalence in the outdoor workers. Slitlamp biomicroscopy reveals sub-epithelial lesions resembling oil droplets, these form yellowish gray band underneath the epithelium. Climatic droplet keratopathy has been assigned three severity grades. Grade 1 has peripheral interpalpebral involvement, Grade 2 lesions involving centre of the cornea (VA >20/100) and Grade 3 with raised lesion in the papillary area (VA <20/200). Climatic droplet keratopathy should be distinguished from lipid and calcific keratopathy.

Histopathology of the lesions reveal elastotic degeneration.

Treatment

Symptomatic patients with Grade 1 disease may treated with topical antibiotics, preservative free artificial tears. The condition can predispose to the development of infective keratitis. Patients with Grade 2 and Grade 3 disease should be treated surgically. Superficial keratectomy should be considered for these patients. Superficial keratectomy using diamond burr has been reported to give better results. In a recent study diamond burr superficial keratectomy improved

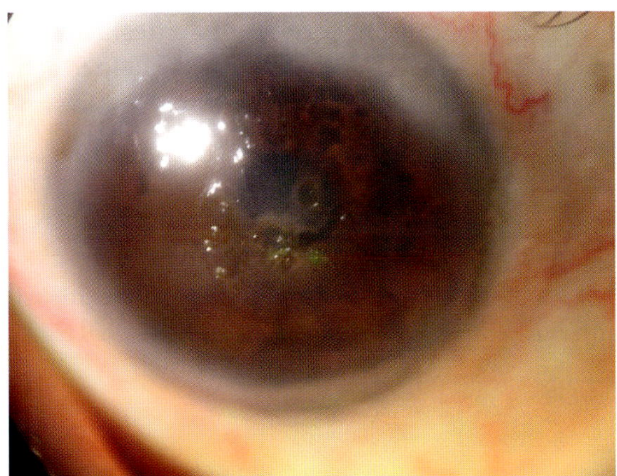

Fig. 77: Climatic droplet keratopathy (Primary)

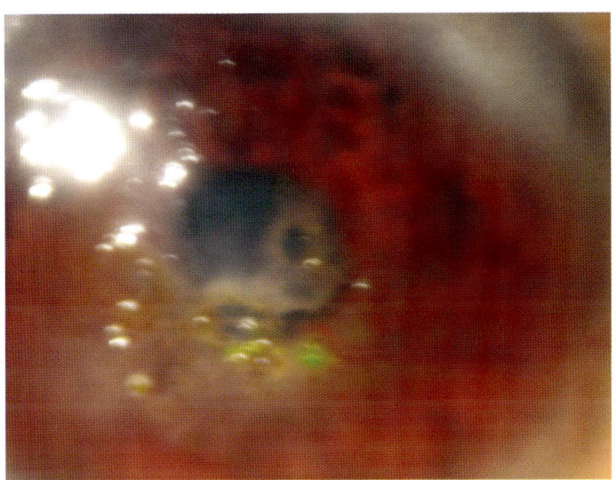

Fig. 78: Climatic droplet keratopathy (Primary, magnified)

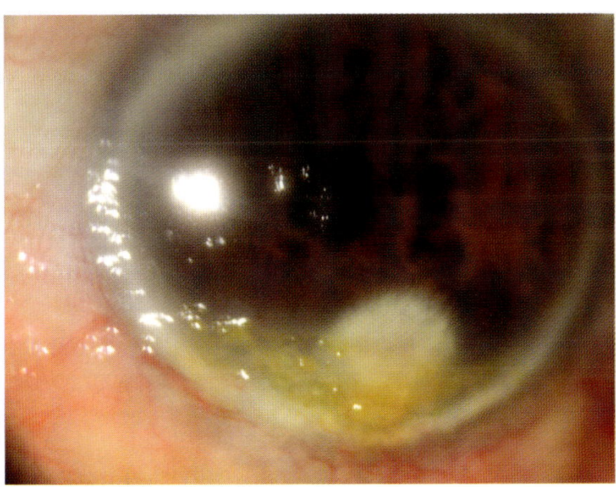

Fig. 79: Climatic droplet keratopathy (Secondary)

Corneal Dystrophies

Recent Advance in Diagnosis and Classification: Corneal dystrophies are a combination of various disorders those cause progressive loss of corneal transparency due to accumulation of deposits within the different corneal layers. Corneal dystrophies were diagnosed based on their classical slitlamp appearance, the characteristic of the deposits and the depth of the corneal involvement. The diagnosis was confirmed on the basis of histopathological features and the staining patterns. The corneal dystrophies were classified on the basis of characteristic clinical appearance and histopathological features. This classification has certain limitations as some of the corneal dystrophies may have similar clinical and histopathological characteristics.

Major advances and developments in molecular genetics have enhanced our understanding of the pathogenesis of corneal dystrophies. In a landmark development in corneal molecular genetics the origin of several corneal dystrophies was traced down to chromosome (5q31). Munier et al reported that the gene transforming growth factor beta-induced (TGFBI) also described as beta-induced gene human cell clone number 3 (BIGH3) located on chromosome 5q31 was responsible for these corneal dystrophies. It was discovered that the four separate mutations resulted a group of these four distinct corneal dystrophies (granular, Avellino, lattice type 1 and Reis Bucklers). The discovery that the different mutations on the same gene can cause four distinct corneal dystrophies has revolutionized our understanding of these conditions (Stone et al, 1994; Munier et al, 1997). This observation also explains the reason for similarities between various corneal dystrophies as they stem from the same gene. Keratoepithelin is an adhesion protein secreted by the epithelium into the stroma. The gene TGFBI encodes for kertoepithelin. A defect in the adhesion process of this protein may be responsible for deposits in the cornea observed in these dystrophies. The presence of keratoepithelin has been confirmed on immunohistochemical studies. The newer discovery has led the researchers to incorporate the responsible gene effect in developing a new classification system.

With the rapidly expanding field of corneal molecular genetics the basic understanding of various corneal dystrophies is becoming more evident. The association of specific gene mutations with specific phenotypes has enabled clinician to use molecular genetic analysis in the diagnosis of corneal dystrophies. Also, identification of the mutations responsible for different types of corneal dystrophies has made it possible to know their genetic and inheritance patterns. The finding of a highly penetrant, dominantly inherited corneal dystrophy in an affected offspring of unaffected parents has confirmed the existence of spontaneous pathogenic mutations. Additionally, molecular analysis for pathogenetic mutations can confirm the diagnosis in cases with atypical presentations of corneal dystrophies. On the other hand, we still know little about how interactions between the environment and the genetic

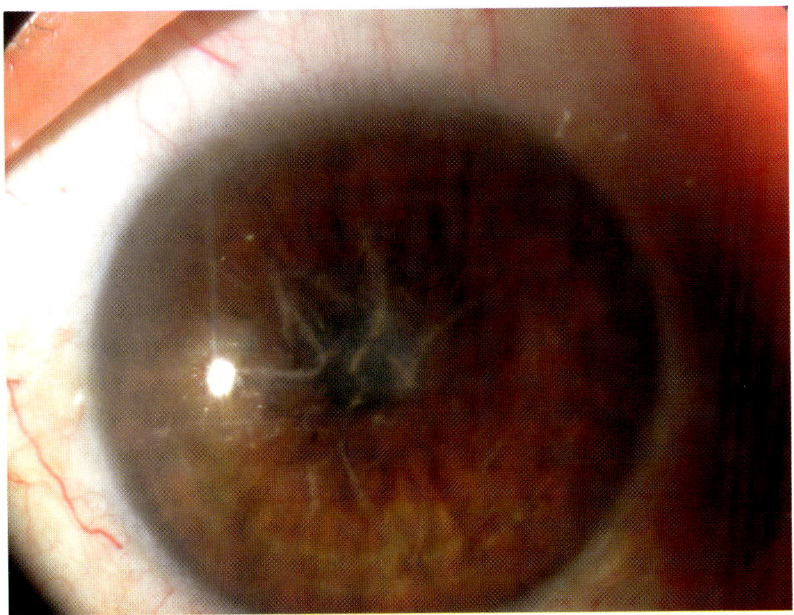

Fig. 81: Lattice dystrophy

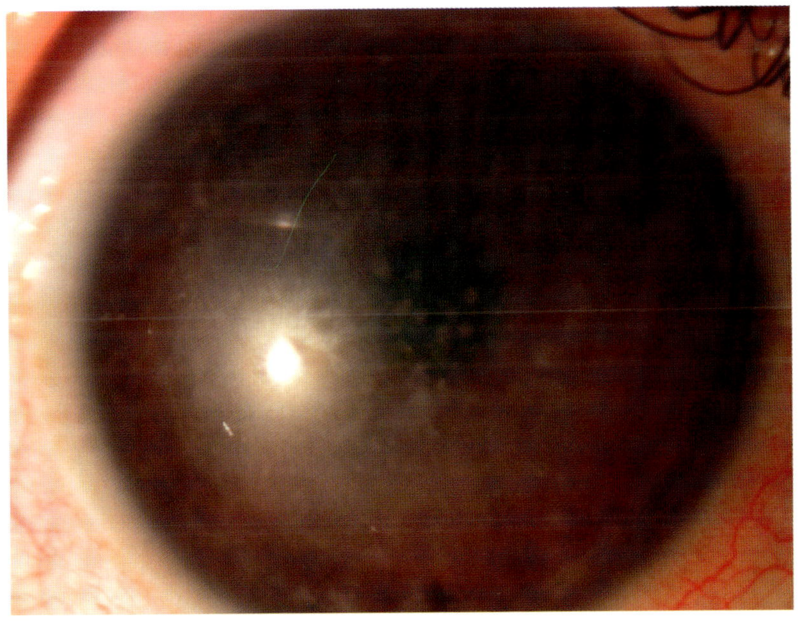

Fig. 82: Macular dystrophy

composition affect the phenotype of these conditions. It is highly likely that even when our understanding of the molecular basis of the corneal dystrophies is complete, this knowledge will be used as an adjunct to clinical findings to make the diagnosis of a corneal dystrophy. In near future the treatment and prevention of corneal dystrophies based on gene therapy may be added to the corneal specialists armamentarium.

Research have already started proposing newer classification based on genetic studies however in the present discussion we have used the conventional classification.

Anterior Corneal Dystrophies

Dystrophies involving the corneal epithelium, epithelium basement membrane and Bowman's layer of the anterior cornea are grouped as anterior corneal dystrophies.

Meesmann's Epithelial Dystrophy

Meesman's dystrophy is the only cornea dystrophy that affects exclusively the corneal epithelium. This is an extremely rare, bilaterally symmetric, autosomal dominant dystrophy with incomplete penetrance. Clinically, this dystrophy presents in the early childhood with minute intraepithelial microcysts or vesicles. The lesions are seen with retroillumination more clearly. These clear cysts consist of cytoplasmic aggregates of keratin in the epithelial cells. Two mutations located on KRT3 (E509K and R503P) and several mutations located on KRT12 (M129T, q130P, R135T, R135G, R135I, L140R, V143L, I426V, Y429C, Y429D, and R430P) are known to cause disease. These mutations are believed to cause dysfunctional keratin formation since this genetic location is essential for keratin filament assembly. These patients usually retain very good vision. Slight diminution may occur the number of cysts increases causing irregularity on the corneal surface. Recurrent corneal erosions are not a feature of this corneal dystrophy unlike many of the other anterior corneal dystrophies. Most patients require no treatment, but lubrication of the corneal surface or soft contact lenses may be warranted for symptomatic patients.

Epithelial Basement Membrane Dystrophy

This dystrophy, also known as map-dot-fingerprint dystrophy, Cogan's microcystic epithelial dystrophy and dystrophic recurrent erosions, is the most common anterior corneal dystrophy. To date, there has been no genetic linkage established and it is more often found sporadically in the population. Epithelial basement membrane dystrophy has, however, been classified as a dystrophy since the changes associated with it occur more commonly in some families. When found with a hereditary component, it is autosomal dominant and often with incomplete penetrance. The primary symptoms in this dystrophy are severe

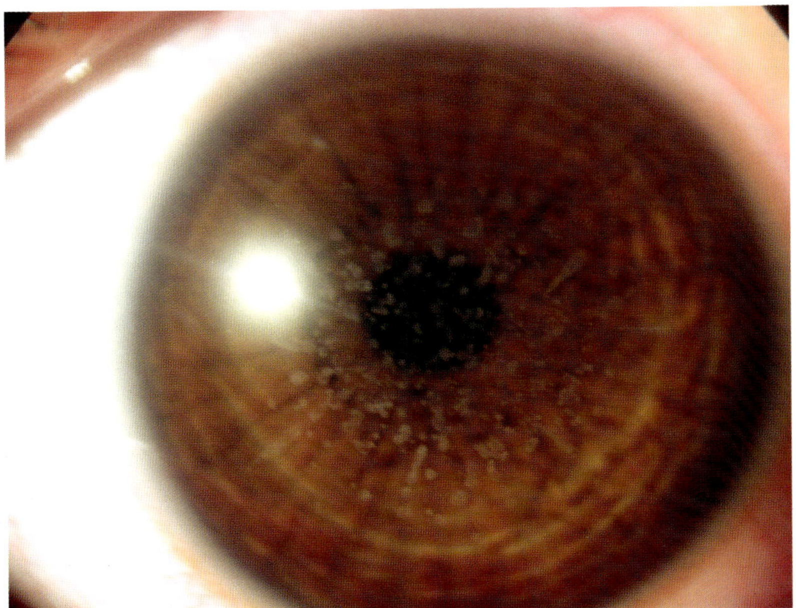

Fig. 83: Granular dystrophy

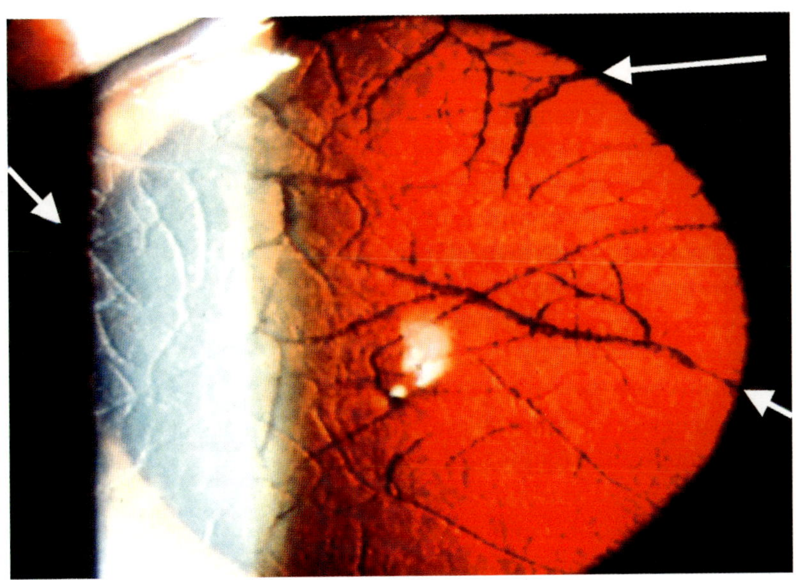

Fig. 84: Lattice dystrophy

pain on waking in the morning, photophobia and blurred vision. These symptoms are due to spontaneous recurrent corneal erosions and irregular astigmatism. On clinical examination the lesions include dots, gray patches resembling maps and fine refractile lines simulating finger prints. The pathogenesis involves synthesis of abnormal epithelial basement membrane. The striking histopathological changes include thickening of the epithelial basement membrane, extension into the epithelium and presence of fibrillar material between basement membrane and Bowman's layer. Recurrent erosions occur due to lack of hemidesmosomes in the epithelial cells overlying the abnormal basement membrane.

Treatment is necessary only when patients are symptomatic. Recurrent corneal erosions can be treated with lubrication, patching, bandage contact lens, mechanical debridement of loose epithelium, stromal puncture, or phototherapeuric keratectomy (PTK) depending on the degree of severity. Irregular astigmatism can be treated with contact lens, mechanical debridement, or more commonly PTK.

Reis-Bucklers Dystrophy

Reis-Bucklers and Thiel-Behnke dystrophies share many similarities as well as some differences, which has caused much debate in categorizing them. Reis-Bucklers dystrophy is autosomal dominant and patients are born with normal appearing corneas. In the first and second decade of life, however, corneal opacification and scarring cause marked visual loss and recurrent corneal crosions lead to significant pain. Thiel- Behnke dystrophy is also an autosomal dominant dystrophy with recurrent corneal erosions developing in the first and second decade of life. Later in life visual acuity decreases due to scarring seen in Reis-Buicklers dystrophy.

In both diseases. Bowman's layer is replaced with fibrocellular scar tissue. Clinically, on slitlamp biomicroscopy, it is often impossible to distinguish one condition from the other. Transmission electron microscopy, however, will differentiate the two dystrophies. In Reis-Bucklers dystrophy, rodlike bodies are seen deposited in Bowman's layer, whereas in Thiel-Behnke dystrophy, curly bodies are seen. Molecular genetic studies have increased our knowledge of these two dystrophies. Both dystrophies are linked to mutations in BIGH3 on chromosome 5q31 (R555Q, R124L and G623D). Thiel-Behnke is also linked to a mutation on chromosome 10q23-24, the gene product is currently unknown. Initial management for both of these dystrophies is aimed at treating recurrent corneal erosions similar for the treatment of recurrent erosions due to epithelial basement membrane dystrophy. If significant corneal scarring or opacification occurs and is superficial, then superficial keratectomy or more commonly PTK can be performed. With deeper opacification and scarring, lamellar or penetrating keratoplasty is necessary. Recurrence rates are high with these dystrophies after penetrating keratoplasty.

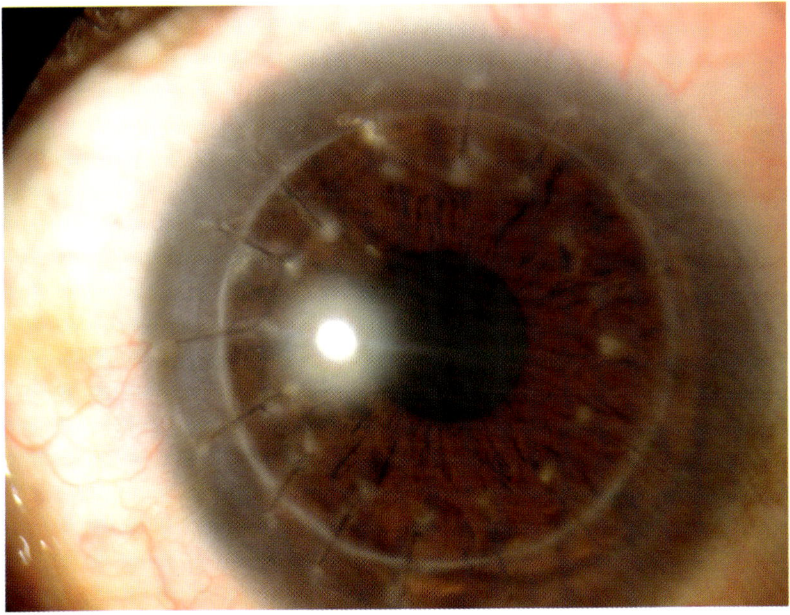

Fig. 85: PKP in macular dystrophy

Stromal Corneal Dystrophies

Dystrophies in this category involve the corneal stroma. As these diseases progress, other cornea layers can become involved.

Granular Dystrophy

Granular dystrophy is an autosomal dominant dystrophy characterized by the deposition of gray-white crumb like opacities in the anterior stroma. These lesions are mainly axial and do not extend to the limbus. In the early stage of the disease the intervening stroma between the opacities remains clear. Due to this reason these patients has good vision. As the disease advances, opacities may increase in number and size, may coalesce, and can involve the deeper stroma. With progression of the disease, the intervening clear stroma gets involved, resulting in decreased vision. Opacities in granular dystrophy are composed of eosinophilic hyaline deposits that stain with Masson trichrome.

Granular dystrophy has been linked to several mutations in BIGH3 on chromosome 5q31; (R124H, R124L, R124S, R555W). R555W mutation in keratoepithelin is found in the classic form granular dystrophy. In the juvenile confluent form of granular dystrophy, the mutation R124H is seen.

Many patients with granular dystrophy retain good vision and will not require treatment. Initial treatment if warranted is aimed at recurrent corneal erosions. Treatment for visually significant superficial corneal disease includes superficial keratectomy, lamellar keratectomy, or more commonly PTK. If the lesions involve deeper layers and vision is severely reduced, then penetrating keratoplasty may be considered. Recurrence in the graft may occur.

Avellino Dystrophy

Avellino dystrophy is a variant of granular dystrophy. Patients affected with Avellino dystrophy have clinical and histological granular dystrophy, as well as the presence of lattice lesions. Lattice lesions always develop after granular deposits are present. The name of the dystrophy comes from Avellino, a city in Italy where three families affected with the disease belonged.

Avellino dystrophy is also autosomal dominant and is linked to the R124H mutation in the TGFβ1 gene. The severity of the corneal deposits is dependent on the heterozygosity or homozygosity of this mutation.

Clinically, patients follow a similar course to granular dystrophy and are treated in the same fashion. Recurrent corneal erosions are seen more commonly in patients with Avellino dystrophy than with classic granular dystrophy.

Lattice Dystrophy

Lattice dystrophy, the most common of the stromal cornea dystrophies. This is an autosomal dominant dystrophy with variable expression. The disease is characterized by refractile lines in the stroma, seen best with retoillumination on slitlamp examination. The spectrum of corneal changes seen with this disease, however, is large. Lattice dystrophy represents a primary localized corneal amyloidosis. These deposits stain orange-red with Congo red, and also demonstrate an apple-green birefringence with a polarizing filter.

Clinically and histologically at least four types of lattice dystrophy have been identified. Type I is characterized by classic branching lattice lines with stromal haze. There is no systemic amylodosis. Type II lattice dystrophy also known as Meretoja syndrome is a systemic amyloidosis associated with corneal dystrophy. Systemic findings include cranial and peripheral neuropathies, mask-like facies and dermatologic changes. Type III b is an autosomal recessive with symptoms occurring much later in life. Type IIIa also has a delayed onset, but is inherited autosomal dominant.

Lattice dystrophy type I and IIIa have been linked to mutations in BIGH3 on chromosome 5q31. Lattice dystrophy type II is associated with mutations in the gelsolin gene on chromosome 9q32-34 (D187N, D187Y, D654Y) Gelsolin is a precursor protein for amyloid.

Treatment for lattice dystrophy depends on the patients symptoms. Recurrent corneal erosions, which often occur due to the predominance of anterior stromal involvement are managed in the usual fashion. If visual acuity is impaired due to superficial opacities, then PTK can be employed. If opacities deepen into stroma, lamellar and penetrating keratoplastry are needed. Recurrence of lattice dystrophy in grafts is more common than in either granular or macular dystrophy.

Macular Dystrophy

Macular dystrophy, inherited in an autosomal recessive fashion, is the least common of the stromal dystrophies but most severe clinically. Patients are born with clear corneas and corneal haze starts between 3 and 9 years of age. The deposits start as central gray-white superficial stromal opacities, which subsequently involve the deeper layers of the peripheral and central corneal stroma. Patients present with progressive decrease in vision and irritation as the diseases worsens. By the third to fourth decade of life the vision is severely affected. In the early stages of the disease macular dystrophy can be mistaken clinically with granular dystrophy. Definite differences involving macular dystrophy, however, make the distinction possible including recessive inheritance, full involvement of the cornea stroma, intervening haze between the opacities, and central corneal thinning. The deposits seen in macular dystrophy are composed of glycosaminoglycans, which stain with Alcian blue, colloidal iron, and periodic acid-Schiff.

Macular dystrophy is divided into two types based on synthesis of keratin sulfate, an important component of corneal proteoglycans. In the more common type I macular dystrophy, there is a lack of keratin sulfate synthesis patients serum. In type II macular dystrophy there is production of keratin sulfate, but it is synthesized at 30% below the normal levels. Both types of macular dystrophy have been linked to chromosome 16q22. Mutations on this chromosome location are found in the carbohydrate sulfotransferase-6 gene (CHST6) which codes for the enzyme catalyzes the sulfatio of keratin sulfate. A comprehensive review of all mutations known to date for macular dystrophy as well as novel mutations found was recently published by Klintworth et at. Treatment for macular dystrophy depends on the patients' symptoms. Recurrent corneal erosions are managed in the usual fashion. Photophobia may be relieved with tinted sunglasses. Vision loss resulting from superficial disease can be treated with PTK and lamellar keratoplasty. Due to the severe nature of this dystrophy and evidence of endothelium involvement, penetrating keratoplasty is considered the treatment of choice. Recurrence of macular dystrophy may occur in the penetrating grafts.

Gelatinous Droplike Dystrophy

Gelatinous droplike dystrophy is rare autosomal recessive dystrophy that presents in the first decade of life and may initially resemble band keratopathy. As the disease progresses, corneal opacification increases as protuberant gelatinous masses accumulate in the subepithelium and anterior stroma. Symptoms include photophobia, lacrimation, foreign-body sensation, and decreased vision. These gelatinous masses are accumulations of amyloid deposits. Gelatinous droplike dystrophy has been linked to mutation so in the MISI gene located on chromosome 1p31. MISI is a cell surface phosphoglycoprotein as well as a substrate for protein kinase C. Mutations in the gene lead to a truncated protein which is thought to initiate amyloid formation in the cornea. Patients with this disease are managed with lamellar and penetrating keratoplasty. Recurrence in the graft is very high.

Endothelial Dystrophies

Fuchs' Endothelial Dystrophy

Fuch's endothelial corneal dystrophy is a common progressive corneal disorder more often affecting women than men. The first signs of this dystrophy are asymptomatic corneal Guttata. As the endothelial cells are further compromised, corneal decompensation occurs. It is rare for patients to have symptomatic Fuchs' dystrophy before age 50 years. As the disease progresses, further marked stromal edema, bullous epithelial edema and finally subepithelial fibrosis occurs.

Fuchs' dystrophy has been reported to have an autosomal dominant mode of inheritance pattern, but also has been sporadic. In some studies this dystrophy has been linked to mutations in the COL8A2 gene on chromosome Ip34. Gottsch et al found a point mutation, L450Q, in COL8A2 responsible for an early onset subtype of Fuchs' corneal dystrophy. COL8A2 encodes a 703 amino acid α2 chain of type VIII collagen, a component of endorhelial basement membrane. In a recent study by Sundin et al. A late onset Fuchs' corneal dystrophy has been linked to new genetic locus 13pTel-13p12. Further molecular gentic studies are needed to elucidate the gene and genetic mutation behind this dystrophy.

Treatment of patients with Fuchs' endothelial dystrophy is aimed at reducing visually significant corneal edema. Medical management may include hypertonic saline solutions and ointments, dehydration of the cornea with a blow dryer, or reduction in intraocular pressure are temporary measures. Lubricating drops and bandage contact lenses are used to treat bullous epithelial keratopathy in advanced cases. Penetrating keratoplasty has been the treatment of choice for patients. Newer lamellar transplant techniques, however are beginning to replae full thickness cornea transplants. These innovative treatments include deep lamellar endothelial keratoplasty and more recent Descemet's stripping endothelial keratoplasty.

Congenital Corneal Dystrophies

Corneal dystrophies are characterized by bilateral, central, symmetrical, non-inflammatory, avascular and progressive corneal lesions. Corneal lesions are morphologically characteristic in different corneal dystrophies and have district features on histopathology. Although the underlying metabolic dysfunction is present congenitally but the disease may manifest later after birth. These features affect biochemical features of cornea. Dystrophies in general are hereditary in origin. Familial patterns may definite in stromal dystrophies but are unpredictable in keratoconus and Fuchs' dystrophy.

Congenital corneal dystrophies include the following disorders:

- Congenital hereditary endothelial dystrophy (CHED)
- Posterior polymorphous dystrophy (PPMD)
- Congenital hereditary stromal dystrophy (CHSD)

Congenital Hereditary Endothelial Dystrophy (CHED)

Congenital hereditary endothelial dystrophy (CHED), resulting bilateral corneal clouding in a full-term infant was first described by Maumenee in 1960. This dystrophy is characterized by bilateral congenital corneal edema normal IOP and normal corneal diameter. Corneal thickness increases two to three times and control corneal thickness may be more than 1.0 mm. Corneal pannus, esotropia, nystagmus and rarely glaucoma have been described in association with CHED. Clinically, two forms of CHED autosomal recessive and autosomal dominatnt have been described.

Autosomal recessive form is characterized by presence of bilateral corneal edema since birth, nystagmus but no photophobia. The corneal edema is non-bullous diffuse. This form of disease remains stationary throughout life. Autosomal dominant form of disease develops in the first or the second year of life. This form of disease is gradually progressive. It is characterized by pain, watering, photophobia but absence of nystagmus. The studies have shown that the locus for autosomal dominant CHED is linked to pericentric region of chromosome. The studies for autosomal recessive form have revealed that the locus for recessive form is distinct from this region of choromosome but it has not been identified.

Clinical Features

CHED is characterized by diffuse epithelial and stromal edema. Examination under anesthesia reveals diffuse ground-glass appearance of corneal stroma. It has slight bluish grey appearance. Corneal diameter (horizontal) and intra-ocular pressure are normal. Rarely CHED may have associated glaucoma. In such a situation IOP should be controlled with medication first. After normalization of IOP if corneal edema still persists it should be labeled as CHED. This condition should be differentiated from congenital glaucoma without buphthalmos. In case of CHED, there are no breaks in the descemet's membrane. Although rare, sensory neural deafness may occur.

Differential Diagnosis

CHED should be differentiated from other conditions resulting bilateral corneal opacification at birth. These conditions include glaucoma without buphthalmos, congenital hereditary stromal dystrophy, posterior polymorphous dystrophy, macular stromal dystrophy, mucopoly saccharidosis, birth trauma due to forceps and intrauterine infections. Of intra-uterine infections congenital rubella syndrome, toxoplasmosis, cytomegalovirus and herpes infection should be considered. The author has performed penetrating keratoplasty on a neonate having central dense leukomatous scar in one eye and the other eye having a healed lesion of congenital toxoplasma retinochoroiditis. Child had in addition central nervous abnormality resulting delayed milestones.

Pathogenesis

The primary abnormality in CHED is considered the degeneration or abnormal formation of endothelial cells during or after fifth month of gestation. CHED has been described as part of anterior segment dysgenesis, resulting from abnormal differentiation of neural crest ectoderm that forms the monolayer of corneal endothelium. Failure to complete the final differentiation lead to the dysfunctional endothelial cells. These abnormal endothelial cells may secrete posterior non-banded (smooth) Descemet's membrane. Histopathology of corneal button shows diffuse epithelial and stromal edema with secondary changes. Spheroidal degeneration in the stroma of CHED patients helps to distinguish it from posterior polymorphous dystrophy.

Treatment

In case patient has mild edema hypertonic drops, ointment or other measures of dehydrating cornea including hair dryer may be effective. Infants and neonates having severe corneal edema require penetrating keratoplasty. However, penetrating keratoplasty is neonates and infants is not only technically difficult but has poorer visual outcome compared to penetrating keratoplasty. Presence of severe amblyopia is another limiting factor even if clear graft following penetrating keratoplasty is achieved.

Posterior Polymorphous Dystrophy

Posterior polymorphous dystrophy (PPMD) was first described in 1916 by Keoppe. This rare dystrophy has a clinical spectrum that ranges from congenital corneal edema to late onset corneal edema in the middle age. Many cases are subclinical and the majority of patients have good vision. Many patients have subtle slitlamp and specular microscopic abnormalities. Posterior polymorphous dystrophy (PPMD) is a bilateral autosomal dominant disorder characterized by polymorphic posterior corneal surface irregularities with variable degrees of corneal decompensation. Characteristic features include, vesicular, curvilinear, and placoid irregularities found on slitlamp examination. On specular microscopy rounded dark areas with central cell detail produce a doughnut-like pattern. Histopathology shows epithelial-like transformation of endothelium. Clinically, these patients had reduced vision due to corneal edema.

Associated features are iridocorneal adhesions, peripheral anterior synechiae and glaucoma. PPMD clinically resembles iridocorneal endothelial (ICE) syndrome, Peters' anomaly, and Axenfeld-Rieger syndrome, suggesting that PPMD may be part of a broader spectrum of disorders resulting from abnormalities of terminal neural crest cell differentiation.

Diagnosis

The majority of patients are diagnosed using the slitlamp by observing vesicular, band-like, or placoid areas on the posterior corneal surface. The diagnosis of PPMD in patients with corneal edema of unknown cause is based on light and electron microscopy of the excised buttons obtained during keratoplasty.

Differential Diagnosis

Differential diagnosis includes tears in Descemet's membrane, interstitial keratitis, Fuchs' dystrophy, and ICE syndrome. As in PPMD, endothelial cells in ICE syndrome may show epithelial characteristics, leading to speculation that they represent a spectrum of the same disease. However, unlike PPMD, ICE syndrome is unilateral, occurs sporadically, is more common in women, and is typically progressive and symptomatic. Glaucoma and iris changes can be found in PPMD but are much more prominent features of ICE syndrome. No systemic associations exist except for rare reports of PPMD associated with Alport's syndrome.

Pathology

Light microscopy of keratoplasty buttons shows pits in the posterior corneal surface, which correspond to the vesicles seen on slitlamp examination. Descemet's membrane in these areas is attenuated, and the endothelium may be multilayered. In other areas, Descemet's membrane appears multilayered, of variable thickness, and with attenuation or loss of endothelium. Discontinuities in Descemet's membrane with anterior migration of cells to form slit-like structures or clefts in pre-Descemet's stroma have been described. Scanning electron microscopy of keratoplasty buttons may show a striking juxtaposition of normal-appearing endothelial cells adjacent to epithelial cell-like areas that show myriad surface microvilli. Transmission electron microscopy of these layers shows the cells to be multilayered and to contain numerous desmosomes and intracytoplasmic filaments. Cell culture studies of these cells demonstrate features similar to cultured epithelial cell lines.

Treatment

The majority of patients require no treatment, but those who have corneal opacification are offered keratoplasty.

Congenital Hereditary Stromal Dystrophy

Congenital hereditary stromal dystrophy (CHSD), an autosomal dominant, rare, stationary dystrophy was first described by Witschel et al (1978). The dystrophy presents at birth with bilateral, symmetrical, non-progressive, central and superficial corneal stromal clouding. The periphery of cornea is clear. The epithelium is uneffected and the anterior stroma gives an ill-defined, flaky or feathery appearance. The child does not have any corneal edema, photophobia or tearing, but stromal opacities can be dense enough to reduce vision. Visual deprivation may lead to nystagmus and congenital esotropia.

In CHSD two types of abnormal collagen lamella constitute the entire stroma. These small collagen fibrils form alternating layers. One layer consists of compact collagen fibrils unformly arranged like normal corneal collagen. The other layer consist of irregularly arranged, loosely packed collegen fibrils.

Early penetrating keratoplasty has been reported to restore good vision. Since Descemet's membrane and endothelium is normal, LK or DALK can also be useful in restoration of vision.

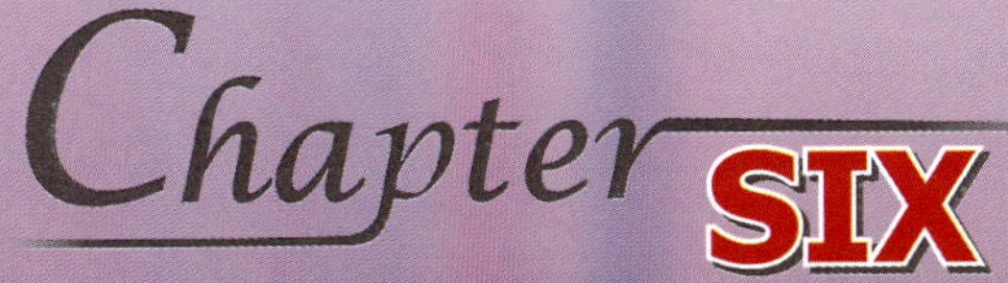

Iris and Ciliary Body

Arturo Perez Arteaga (Mexico)

- **Idiopathic Iritis**
- **Sarcoidosis**
- **Fuchs Heterochromic Iridocyclitis**
- **Juvenile Idiopathic Arthritis**

Idiopathic Iritis

Introduction

Inflammation of the uveal tract has many causes and may involve one or all three portions (iris, ciliary body and choroids) simultaneously. The most frequent form of uveitis is acute anterior uveitis (also termed as iritis). In many cases the cause should remain unknown.

Clinical Signs and Symptoms

Iritis is usually unilateral and characterized by a history of pain, photophobia, blurring of vision, a red eye without purulent discharge, and a small, variably irregular shaped pupil. The presence of keratic precipitates on the posterior surface of the cornea as well as flare and cell in the anterior chamber can be seen with the slit lamp. Slit lamp also shows anterior chamber reaction manifested by inflammatory cells called flare (protein leakage). Shining a light into the normal eye should make the opposite eye hurt if the patient has iritis (because of consensual movement of the inflamed affected contralateral iris).

Investigation

Causes of anterior uveitis can be related to autoimmune disorder (juvenile rheumatoid arthritis, ankylosing spondylitis, Reiter's syndrome, ulcerative colitis, Crohn's, psoriasis), infections (syphilis, TB, herpes zoster, herpes simplex, adenovirus), malignancy (masquerade syndrome-retinoblastoma, leukemia, lymphoma, malignant melanoma), trauma, gout, or after all investigations can become idiopathic.

Differential Diagnosis

It is important to make the diagnosis early, to distinguish for other forms of ocular inflammation and to dilate the pupil to prevent the formation of permanent posterior synechiae related to glaucoma. Signs to improve the differential diagnosis are painful red eye, ciliary flush, decreased visual acuity and marked photophobia. Pupil is constricted secondary to the inflammation. Test with fluorescein stain to rule out corneal abrasion and herpes simplex dendrite.

Treatment

Treatment is with topical steroids nonsteroids and cycloplegic agent meanwhile the cause is determined. If condition is recurrent or persistent, then underlying systemic disorder should be ruled out.

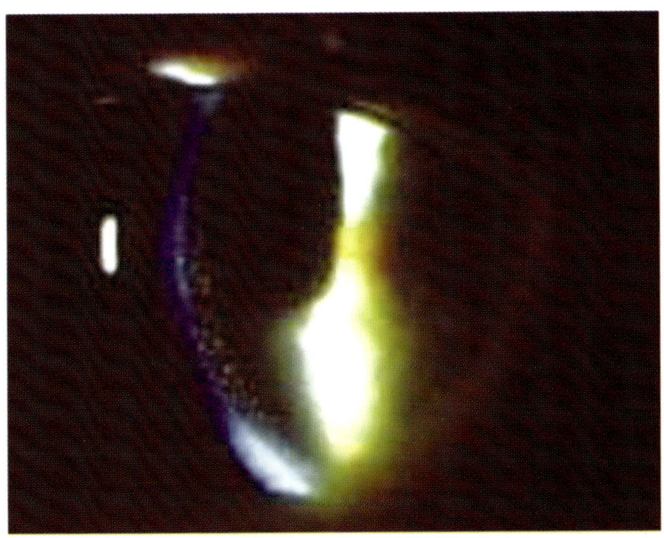

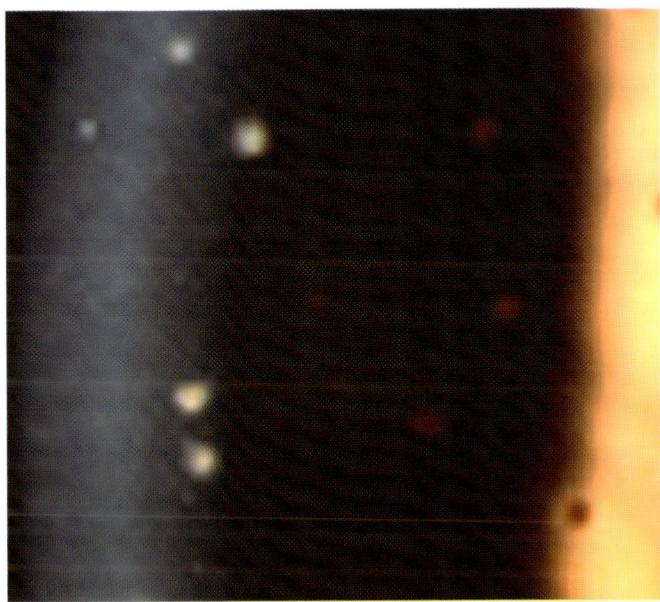

Figs 1 and 2: Idiopathic iritis

Prognosis

It will be variable according the cause of the iritis; if underlying disease is treated with success, ocular inflammation tend to decrease; but in the cases of idiopathic iritis, the control of the inflammation and the advice to possible recurrences, should improve the prognosis if they are made on time.

Sarcoidosis

Introduction

Sarcoidosis is a multisystemic disorder of unknown etiology that most commonly affects adults between 20 and 40 years of age. Patients with sarcoidosis frequently present with bilateral hilar lymphadenopathy and pulmonary infiltration, and often with ocular and skin lesions.

Clinical Signs and Symptoms

Ocular disease affects approximately one quarter of patients with systemic sarcoidosis and may involve any area of the eye in an inflammatory pattern. Uveitis is the most common ocular manifestation of sarcoidosis, affecting almost 25 percent of patients with the disorder, but sarcoidosis is responsible for only 5 to 7 percent of cases of uveitis overall. Ocular disease involves the anterior segment of the eye in about 80 percent of patients and the posterior segment of the eye in about 20 percent of patients, usually in the form of chorioretinitis, but this may experience variations according the stage of the disease. The optic nerve may become involved in patients with neurosarcoidosis. Other ocular manifestations of sarcoidosis include cataracts, blindness, lachrymal gland swelling and inflammation, and retinal periphlebitis. The combination of keratoconjunctivitis and xerostomia, as in Sjögren's syndrome, has also occurred. Uveoparotid fever (also called Heerfordt's syndrome) is also known to affect patients with sarcoidosis. Symptoms include painless swelling of the parotid gland, fever and uveitis. Rarely, cranial nerve involvement (i.e., paralysis of the facial nerve) has been associated with this disease, but it can happen.

Investigation

Sarcoidosis is also characterized by distinctive laboratory abnormalities, including hyperglobulinemia, an elevated serum angiotensin converting enzyme level, evidence of depressed cellular immunity manifested by cutaneous anergy and, occasionally, hypercalcemia and hypercalciuria.

Differential Diagnosis

The diagnosis is established when clinical and radiographic findings are supported by histological evidence of non-caseating epithelioid cell granulomas found on tissue biopsy; tissue biopsy is mandatory for the confirmation of the

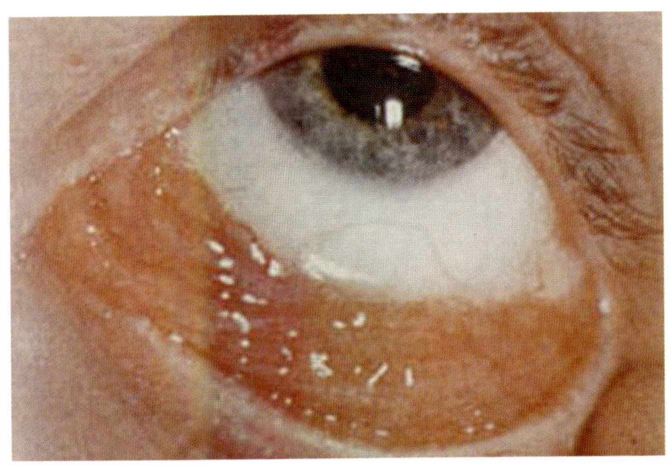

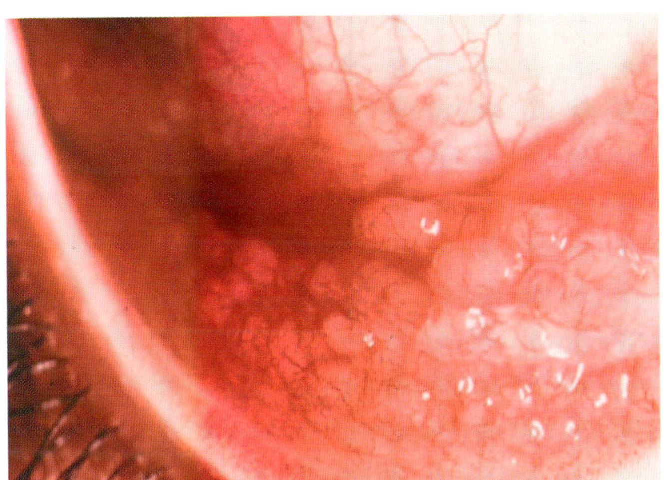

Figs 3 and 4: Sarcoidosis

a posterior subcapsular cataract, which matured rapidly. No laboratory studies are useful to the clinician in making the diagnosis; it is based on both the clinical history and the physical examination.

Investigations

The trigger for inflammation of the iris and the ciliary body is unknown. Several unsubstantiated theories have been proposed, including infection from *Toxoplasma gondii*, an immune dysfunction, infiltration of sensitized lymphocytes, and chronic herpetic infection. Additionally, because iris heterochromia occurs in congenital Horner syndrome, a neurogenic factor contributing to inflammation and structural changes has been proposed. Degenerative changes of the trabecular meshwork are the most common cause of secondary glaucoma. Other factors leading to the development of secondary glaucoma include inflammation of the trabecular meshwork, chronic corticosteroid therapy, inhibition of uveoscleral outflow mechanisms, presence of peripheral anterior synechiae, and neovascularization of the trabecular meshwork. The presence of glaucoma is of particular importance when planning a cataract surgery.

Differential Diagnosis

Glaucoma pigmentary, herpex simplex, herpes zoster, HIV, HLA-B27 syndromes, horner syndrome, Posner-Schlossman syndrome, retinitis, CMV, sarcoidosis, toxoplasmosis, tuberculosis.

Treatment

In general, treatment is not necessary for patients with the typical low-grade inflammation, unless some investigators are planning the role of topical nonsteroidal anti-inflammatory agents. Symptomatic flare-ups may require short-term topical corticosteroids; however, chronic therapy is not indicated. Unlike other uveitides, topical steroids should not be used to eliminate cells from the anterior chamber as part of the cells and flare is contributed by the breakdown of the blood-aqueous barrier and leakage of inflammatory infiltrate. Overall, the surgical outcome of patients with this disease is equivalent to patients with age-related cataracts; these patients tend to have better outcomes following cataract extraction than patients with other forms of uveitis. The incidence of glaucoma ranges from 15-59% according to different series. Fortunately, most secondary glaucoma can be controlled with traditional antiglaucoma medications; because it is an inflammatory disease prostaglandin analogs tend to be avoided. Argon laser trabeculoplasty does not appear effective in improving the outflow where trabecular sclerosis and peripheral anterior synechiae are present. Glaucoma filtering procedures are less successful compared with that for patients with primary open-angle glaucoma.

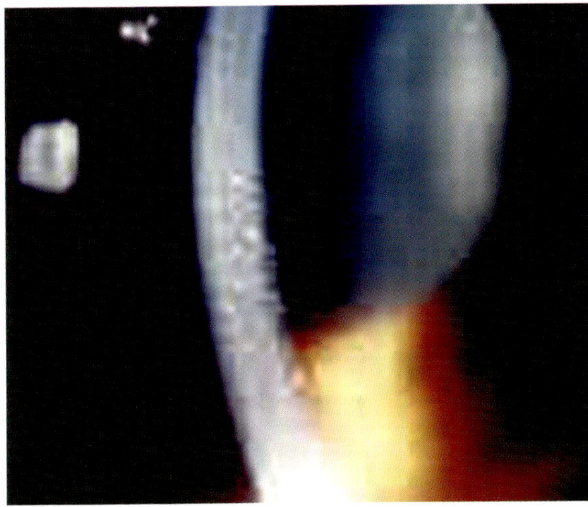

Fig. 7: Juvenile idiopathic arthritis

Prognosis

The low-grade inflammation smolders over decades. Initially, vision is not significantly impaired. All patients eventually develop cataracts that require surgical removal with good prognosis.

Juvenile Idiopathic Arthritis

Introduction

Juvenile idiopathic arthritis (JIA) is a chronic disease present in children that can lead to serious ophthalmic complications. The cause is genetic with some associated environmental factors under research; recently with new therapies, a decrease in chronic consequences of inflammation have been seen, even so, it can be a terrible disease causing chronic systemic disability.

Clinical Signs and Symptoms

Despite the systemic manifestations, we will focus at the ophthalmic manifestations. Chronic uveitis is a serious complication; 6% of the cases occur in children. From all the cases 12% of them associated with the pauciarticular form of the disease, still develop permanent blindness as a result of low-grade chronic intraocular inflammation. The vision-robbing consequences of low-grade uveitis occur extremely slowly, typically over a period of 4 to 8 years, and the end result is clear: even low-grade uveitis may lead eventually to ocular damage, including band keratopathy, maculopathy (macular edema, macular cysts, and epiretinal membrane), glaucomatous optic neuropathy, and cataract formation from chronic inflammation and corticosteroid therapy.

Investigation

Although remarkable progress has been made in the care of these patients since the development of corticosteroids for systemic and ophthalmic use, up to 12% of children with uveitis develop severe visual impairment. Ironically, these children are often under careful observation by ophthalmologists who may opt to tolerate low-grade ocular inflammation, hoping to avoid the development of corticosteroid-induced ocular adverse effects such as cataracts and glaucoma. New chronic therapies with nonsteroidal topical agents are under investigation because of their low side effects.

Differential Diagnosis

Some other diseases of the autoimmune system like lupus and some types of tumors like lymphoma. All the uveitis protocol must be performed in these patients.

Treatment

Although surgical treatment of cataract and glaucoma is remarkably successful in the general population, it is consistently less so in patients with JIA-associated uveitis. Corticosteroids are still the treatment of choice, making a good judge between beneficial and side effects. New chronic therapies with nonsteroidal topical agents are under investigation because of their low side effects and the possibility of long term use for control of ocular inflammation.

Prognosis

Not always good, taking in count that inflammatory intraocular process is chronic and due to the systemic disease; prognosis is better if systemic treatment is performed early in the disease and with good results. Surgery should be the final approach.

Chapter SEVEN

Tear Film Disorders

Pathophysiology of Tear Film

Ashok Garg (India)

Introduction

The exposed part of the ocular globe—the cornea and the bulbar conjunctiva is covered by a thin fluid film known as preocular tear film. **Tear film is that surface of the eye, which remains most directly in contact with the environment.** It is critically important for protecting the eye from external influences and for maintaining the health of the underlying cornea and conjunctiva. The optical stability and normal function of the eye depend on an adequate supply of fluid covering its surface.

The tear film is a highly specialized and well-organized moist film which covers the bulbar and palpebral conjunctiva and cornea. It is formed and maintained by an elaborate system—the lacrimal apparatus consisting of secretory, distributive and excretory parts. The secretory part includes the lacrimal gland, accessory lacrimal gland tissue, sebaceous glands of the eyelids, goblet cells and other mucin-secreting elements of the conjunctiva. The elimination of the lacrimal secretions is based on the movement of tears across the eye aided by the act of blinking and a drainage system consisting of lacrimal puncta, canaliculi, sac and nasolacrimal duct.

By definition, a film is a thin layer that can stand vertically without appreciable gravitational flow and the tear film meets this criteria very well. The presence of continuous tear film over the exposed ocular surface is imperative for good visual acuity and wellbeing of the epithelium and facilitates blinking. Tear film serves:

- An optical function by maintaining an optically uniform corneal surface
- A mechanical function by flushing cellular debris, foreign matter from the cornea and conjunctival sac and by lubricating the surface
- A corneal nutritional function
- An antibacterial function.

The composition of the tear film must be kept within rather narrow quantitative and qualitative limits in order to maintain the wellbeing and proper functioning of the visual system. Abnormalities of the tear film affecting its constituents or volume lead to serious dysfunction of the eyelids and the conjunctiva with the concomitant loss of corneal transparency. A thin tear film is uniformally spread over the cornea by blinking and ocular movements. The tear film can be arbitrarily divided into four main parts:

- The marginal tear film along the moist portions of the eyelid which lie posterior to the lipid strip secreted by the tarsal glands

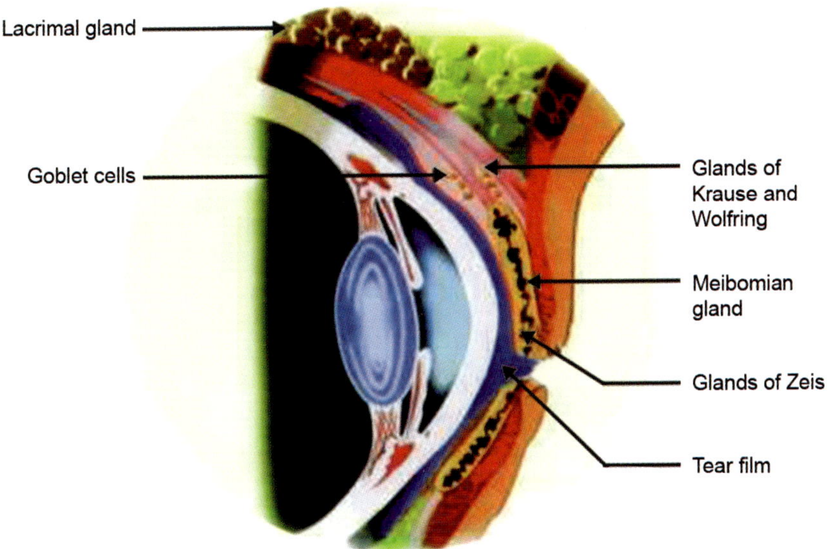

Fig. 1: Cross-section of eye showing tear film (blue) in its natural distribution along with tear producing glands (*Courtesy:* Allergan India Limited)

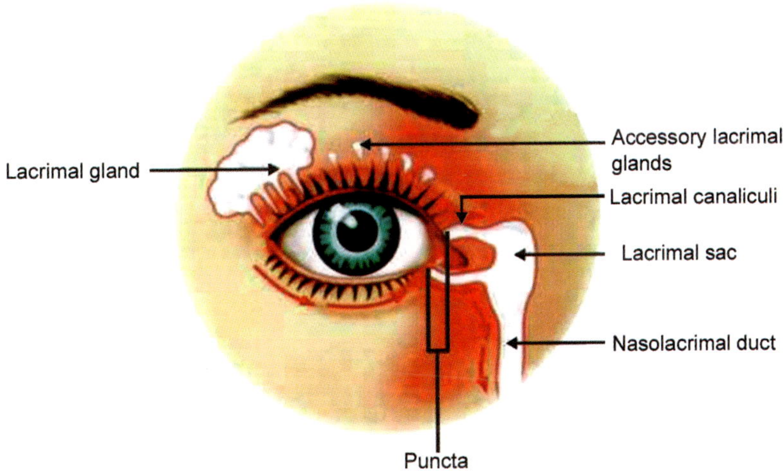

Fig. 2: Tear drainage system (*Courtesy:* Allergan India Limited)

- Portion covering the palpebral conjunctiva
- Portion covering the bulbar conjunctiva
- Precorneal tear film which covers the cornea.

The marginal, palpebral and conjunctival portions are regarded as making the preocular tear film.

Tears refers to the fluid present as the precorneal film and in the conjunctival sac. The volume of tear fluid is about 5 to 10 ml with normal rate of secretion about 1 to 2 ml/minute. About 95 percent of it is produced by the lacrimal gland and lesser amounts are produced by goblet cells and the accessory lacrimal glands of the conjunctiva. The total mass of the latter is about one-tenth of the mass of the main lacrimal gland.

The secretory part of the lacrimal apparatus provides the aqueous tear, lipids and mucus all the important components of the tear film and its boundary.

The tear film is composed of three layers.

Superficial Lipid Layer

The superficial layer at the air-tear interface is formed over the aqueous part of the tear film from the oily secretions of meibomian glands and the accessory sebaceous glands of Zeis and Moll. The meibomian gland openings are distributed along the eyelid margin immediately behind the lash follicles.

The chemical nature of the lipid layer is essentially waxy and consists of cholesterol esters and some polar lipids. The thickness of this layer varies with the width of the palpebral fissure and is between 0.1 and 0.2 μm. Being oily in nature it forms a barrier along the lid margins that retains the lid margin tear strip and prevents its overflow on to skin. This layer is so thin that there are no interference color patterns such as one normally sees on an oily surface. However, if one squints, the oily layer thickness and distinct interference colors may be seen.

While the bulk of tarsal gland secretions are nonpolar lipid compounds which do not spread over an aqueous surface alone, many surface active components are also present. It appears that the tarsal gland secretions which are transported to the cornea in the tear film are massaged into the outermost layer of corneal epithelial cells by eyelid action and then possibly are changed by local metabolic processes in the epithelium combining with conjunctival mucus to form a stable hydrophilic base for the precorneal tear film.

This outer lipid layer has the following main functions:

- It reduces the rate of evaporations of the underlying aqueous tear layer.
- It increases surface tension and assists in the vertical stability of the tear film so that tears do not overflow the lower lid margin.
- It lubricates the eyelids as they pass over the surface of the globe.

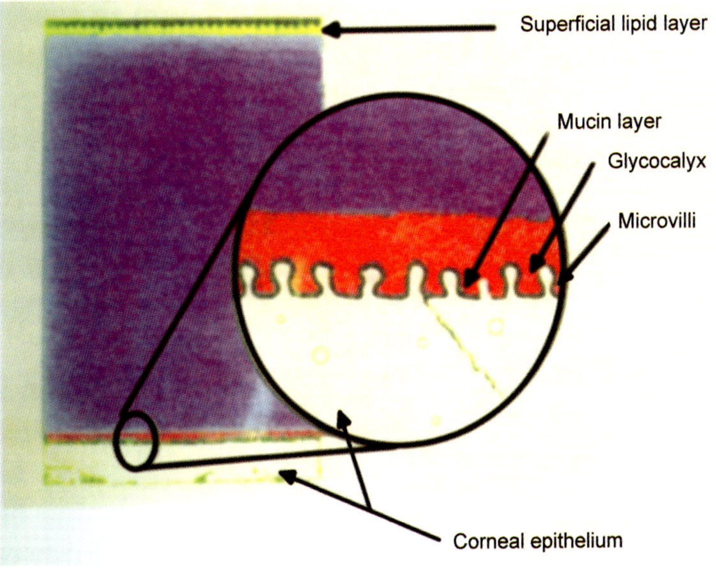

Fig. 3: Tear film layers (*Courtesy:* Allergan India Limited)

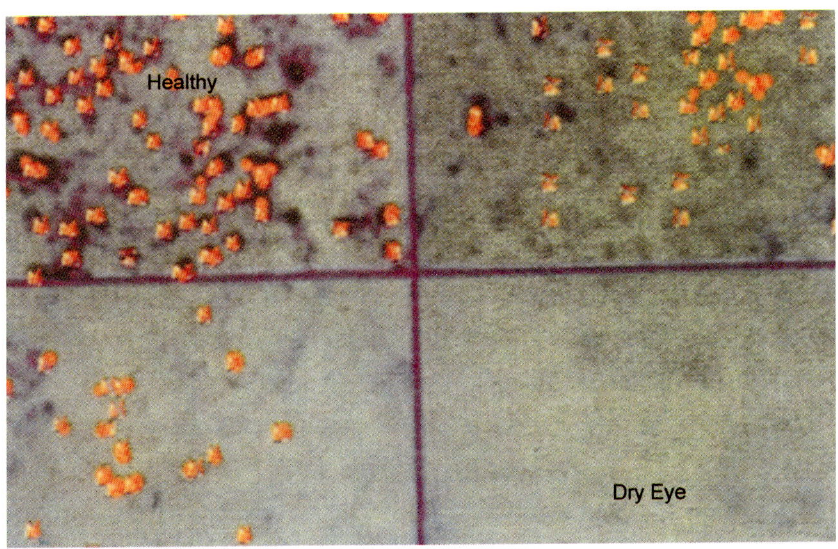

Fig. 4: Impression cytology mapping (*Courtesy:* Allergan India Limited)

Middle Aqueous Layer

The intermediate layer of tear film is the aqueous phase which is secreted by the main lacrimal gland and the accessory glands of Krause and Wolfring.

This layer constitutes almost the total thickness of the tear film 6.5 to 10 um, many times thicker than the fine superficial oily layer. This layer contains two phases—a more concentrated and a highly dilute one. The interfacial tension at the adsorbed mucin-aqueous layer is apt to be rather small due to the intensive hydrogen bond formation across the interface. This layer contains inorganic salts, water proteins, enzymes, glucose, urea, metabolites, electrolytes, glycoproteins and surface active biopolymers. Uptake of oxygen through the tear film is essential to normal corneal metabolism. This layer has four main functions:

- Most importantly it supplies atmospheric oxygen to the corneal epithelium.
- It has antibacterial substances like lactoferrin and lysozyme. Therefore, dry eye patients are more susceptible to infection than a normal eye.
- It provides smooth optical surface by removing any minute irregularities of the cornea.
- It washes away debris from the cornea and conjunctiva.

Posterior Mucin Layer

The innermost layer of tear film is a thin mucoid layer elaborated by goblet cells of the conjunctiva and also by the crypts of Henle and glands of Manz. It is the deepest stratum of the precorneal tear film. This layer is even thinner than the lipid layer and is 0.02 to 0.04 μm thick. This adsorbs on the epithelial surface of the cornea and conjunctiva rendering them hydrophilic. It assumes the ridged appearance of the microvilli of superficial epithelial cells which it covers. The preocular tear film is dependent upon a constant supply of mucus which must be of proper chemical and physical nature to maintain corneal and conjunctival surfaces in the proper state of hydration. The mucous threads present in the tear film provides lubrication allowing the eyelid margin and palpebral conjunctiva to slide smoothly over one another with minimal energy lost as friction during blinking and ocular rotation movements. They also cover foreign bodies with a slippery coating thereby protecting the cornea and conjunctiva against the abrasive effects of such particles as they are moved about by the constant blinking movements of eyelids. The mucus contributes stability to the preocular tear film as well as furnishing an attachment for the tear film to the conjunctiva but not to the corneal surface. The corneal surface is covered with a myriad of fine microvilli which provides some support for the tear film. The mucus dissolved in the aqueous phase facilitates spreading of the tear film by smoothening the film over the corneal surface to form a perfect, regular refracting surface.

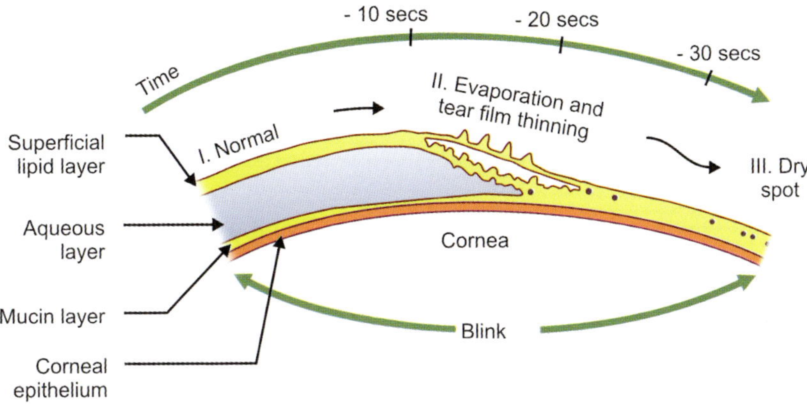

Fig. 5: Mechanism of tear film break up (*Courtesy:* Allergan India Limited)

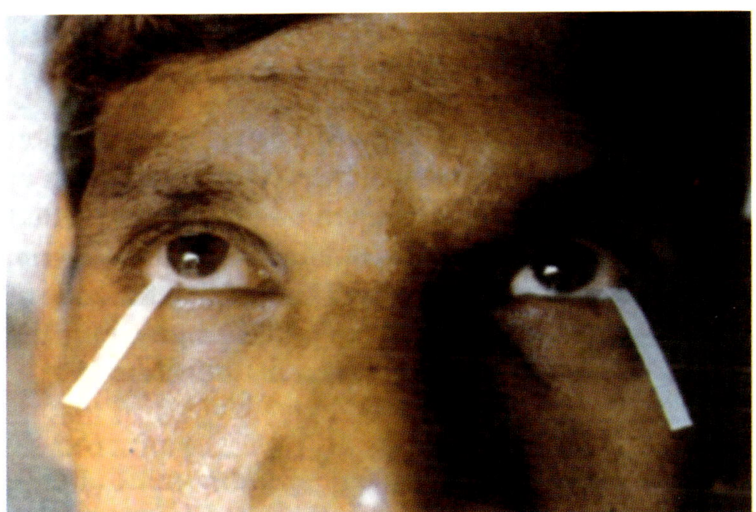

Fig. 6: Modified Schirmer's test

So the mucin layer which is a glycoprotein converts a hydrophobic surface into a hydrophilic surface and enables the corneal epithelium to be adequately wetted.

In addition to sufficient amounts of aqueous tears and mucin three other important factors are necessary for effective resurfacing of the cornea by the precorneal tear film.

- A normal blink reflex is essential to ensure that the mucin is brought from the inferior conjunctiva and rubbed into the corneal epithelium. Patients suffering from facial palsy and lagophthalmos therefore develop corneal drying.
- Congruity between external ocular surface and the eyelids ensures that the precorneal tear film shall spread evenly over the entire cornea. Patients suffering from limbal lesions like dermoids face the problem of apposition of the eyelids to the globe leading to local selective areas of drying.
- Normal epithelium is necessary for the adsorption of mucin on to its surface cells. Patients suffering from corneal scars and keratinizations have problem of interference with the corneal wetting.

The tear film is not visible apparently on the surface of the eye but at the upper and lower lid margins a 1 mm strip of tear fluid with concave outer surface can be seen. It is here that the oily surface prevents spillage of the tear fluid over the lid margin. Tears forming the upper tear strip are conducted nasally from the upper temporal fornix. At the lateral canthus the tears fall by gravity to form the lower strip, spreading medially the upper and lower strips reach the plica and caruncle where they join together. The tear fluid does not flow over the eye by gravity but a thin film is spread over the cornea by blinking and eye movements.

Tear Film Formation Dynamics

It is interesting to know the tear film formation. Generally during the closure of the eyelids the superficial lipid layer of the tear film is compressed by the eyelid edges because it is energetically unfavorable for the lipid to penetrate under the lids into the fornix. The thickness of lipid layer therefore increases by a factor of 1000 resulting in thickness of 0.1 mm which is easily contained between the adjacent eyelid edges. The aqueous tear layer remains uniform under the lids and acts as a lubricant between the eyelids and the globe. In a complete blink phenomenon, the two tear minisci join and most of their bulk is held at their junction to fill the slight bridge formed by the meeting eyelids and at the canthus.

When the eyelids open, first they form an aqueous tear surface on which the compressed lipid rapidly spread. Monomolecular lipid layer is the first to spread at speeds limited only by the moving eyelid. Following the spread of lipid monolayer, the excess lipid and associated macromolecules shall distribute

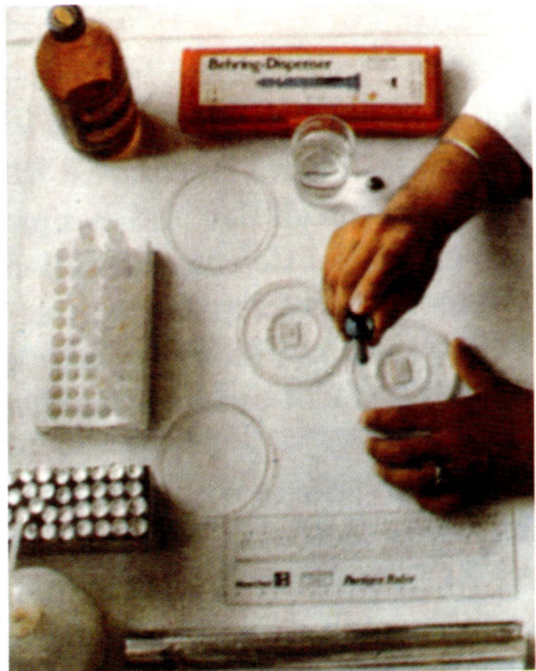

Fig. 7: Tear globulin assay (diagnostic test)

themselves over the tear film surface at a lower speed, usually the lipid layer ceases within 1 second after the opening of the eye.

Under normal conditions a person blinks on an average 15 times per minute. Some of these blinks may not be complete (the upper eyelid descends only half way towards the lower eyelid). Normally the tear film break up time (BUT) is longer than the interval between blinks and no corneal drying occurs.

A deficiency in the conjunctival secretions can lead to dry eye symptoms even in the presence of an adequate aqueous tear component.

BUT (Break up Time) is generally determined after the instillation of a drop of fluorescein solution in the eye or after staining the tear miniscus and the tear film by a wetted paper strip containing fluorescein. Normal BUT value ranges from 10 to 40 seconds for normal eyes when the BUT is determined by a non-invasive method (e.g. by the toposcope). BUT values of as long as 3 to 5 minutes can be recorded.

If the BUT is shorter than the average time interval between two consecutive blinks, tear film rupture can cause pathological changes in the underlying epithelium. The tear film breaks up prematurely over the damaged epithelial surface thereby exacerbating the injury.

Generally there is balance between the secretion and excretion of tears and the rate of tear drainage increases with increased tear volume.

Normal Tear Drainage

In the normal tear film between 10 and 25% of the total tears secreted are lost by evaporation. Evaporation rate is low because of the protective oily surface.

In the absence of the protective oily layer the rate of evaporation is increased 10 to 20 times. Normally tear flows along the upper and lower marginal strips and enters the upper and lower canaliculi by capillarity and possibly by suction also. About 70% of tear drainage is via the lower canaliculus and the remaining through the upper canaliculus. With each blink the superficial and deep heads of pretarsal orbicularis muscle compress the ampullae, shorten the horizontal canaliculi and move the puncta medially. Simultaneously the deep heads of preseptal orbicularis muscle which are attached to the fascia of the lacrimal sac contract and expand the sac. This creates a negative pressure which sucks the tears from the canaliculi into the sac. When the eyes are opened the muscles relax, the sac collapses and a positive pressure is created which forces the tear down the duct into the nose. Gravity also plays an important role in the sac emptying. The puncta move laterally, the canaliculi lengthen and become filled with tears.

Tear Composition

Tears contain 98.2% water and 1.8% solids. The high percentage of water in tears is a natural consequence of the need for lubrication of the conjunctiva and

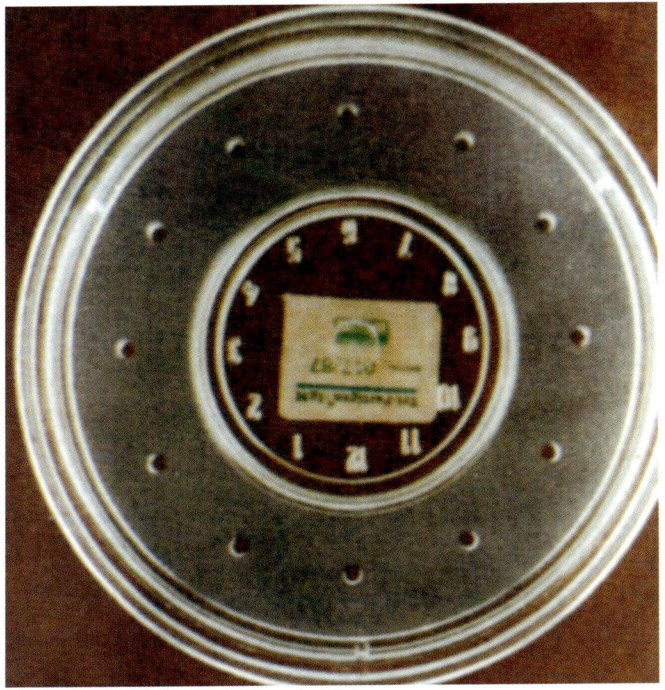

Fig. 8: Tripartigen immunodiffusion plates
(diffusion of rings around agar wells is measured up to 0.1 mm)

corneal surface. The evaporation of water between blinks may influence the concentration of the tear film. The evaporation rate of water from the intact precorneal tear film through the superficial lipid layer has been shown to be 8×10^{-7} cm^{-2} sec^{-1}. In a time interval of 10 seconds (between two consecutive blinks) the thickness of the tear film decreases about 0.1 mm resulting in nearly 1 to 2% decrease in water concentration. The solute concentration, however, increases about 20%.

Table 1: Relative water contents of tears and other body fluids

Fluid	*Percentage water*
Tear	98.2
Aqueous humor	98.9
Vitreous humor	99.0
Blood	79.5
Serum	91.0
Urine	96.5

Physical Properties of Tears

Tear pH

The pH of unstimulated tears is about 7.4 and it approximates that of blood plasma. Although wide variations are found in normal individuals (between 5.0-8.35) the usual range is from 7.3 to 7.7. **A more acidic pH of about 7.25 is found following prolonged lid closure possibly due to carbon dioxide produced by the cornea and trapped in the tear pool under the eyelids.** Tear pH is characteristic for each individual and the normal buffering mechanism maintain the pH at a relatively constant level during waking hours. The permeability of the corneal epithelium does not seem to be affected by wide variations in the pH of tear fluid.

Osmotic Pressure

The osmotic pressure in tears mainly caused by the presence of electrolytes is about 305 mOsm/kg equivalent to 0.95% sodium chloride. Individual values over the waking day may range from 0.90 to 1.02% NaCl equivalents. A decrease to an average of 285 mOsm/kg equivalent to 0.89% NaCl has been reported following prolonged lid closure which accounts for the reduced evaporation. When the aqueous component of tears decreases, the tears become markedly hypertonic (0.97% NaCl solution or more) and corneal dehydration results. When the eyes are closed, there is no evaporation of tears and the precorneal tear film is in osmotic equilibrium with the cornea. When the eyes are open evaporation takes place, increasing the tonicity of the tear film and producing an osmotic gradient from the aqueous through the cornea to the tear film. This direction of flow will continue as long

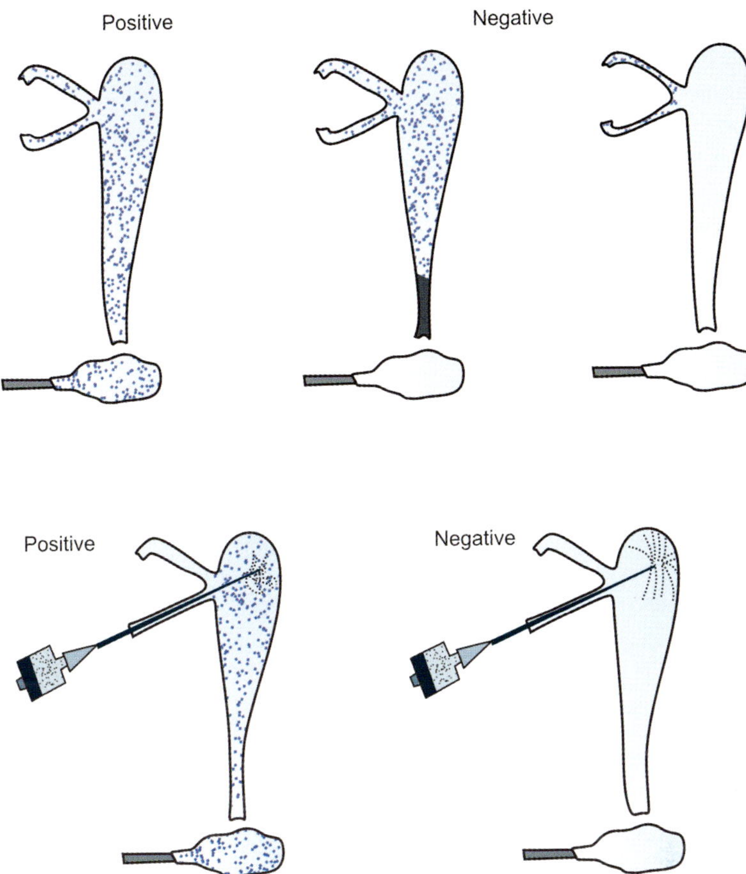

Fig. 9: Dye testing: Jones primary test (top) and Jones secondary test (bottom) (*Courtesy: Kanski Clinical Ophthalmology Butterworth International*)

as evaporation maintains the hypertonicity of the tear film. Osmotic pressure is sensitive to changes in tear flow. Reflex stimulation of tears in early adaptation to contact lenses results in a decrease in electrolytes and in total protein leading to hypotonicity. This relative hypotonicity may account for the corneal edema often seen in early stages of contact lens wearing.

Other Physical Properties of Tear

- Refractive index—1.357
- Tear volume—0.50-0.67 g/16 hr (waking).

Chemical Composition of Tear Fluid

The chemical composition of tear fluid is quite complex. The first chemical analysis of tears was studied in 1791 by Fourcroy and Van Que Lin Fleming (1922) and Ridley (1934) demonstrated the detailed chemical composition of normal tears.

Immunoelectrophoretic studies have shown that tears contain lipids, proteins, enzymes, metabolites, electrolytes and hydrogen ions, etc.

Lipids

Lipids are present in small amount in tears as they are contained only in the very thin superficial lipid layer of the tear film. Chromatographic studies of meibomian lipids reveal the presence of all possible lipid classes mainly waxy esters, hydrocarbons, triglycerides, cholesterol esters and in lesser amount diglycerides, monoglycerides, free fatty acids, free cholesterol and phospholipid. However, great individual variations occur in lipid composition.

Cholesterol

Cholesterol has been reported to be present in tear fluid in concentrations of about 200 mg% which is same as in the blood. Like all lipids in biological fluids cholesterol has to be transported by α and β lipoproteins. In normal tears the very low protein content and the absence of lipoproteins is incompatible with a cholesterol concentration of 20 mg%.

Proteins

About 60 components to tear protein fraction have been reported which form the first line of defense against an external infection and seen to be more effective than systemically produced antibodies. The protein content of tears differ from that of blood plasma in several respects. Proteins can be divided in two groups.

Table 2: Composition of human tears and plasma

Tears		*Plasma*
Physical properties		
pH	7.4 (7.2-7.7)	7.39
Osmotic pressure	305 mOsm/kg Equiv. 0.95% NaCl	6.64 atm
Refractive index	1.357	1.35
Volume	0.50-0.67 g/16 hour (waking)	
Chemical properties		
1. General tear composition		
Water	98.2 g/100 ml	98 g/100 ml
Solids (total)	1.8 g/100 ml	8.6 g/100 ml
Ash	1.05 g/100 ml	0.6-1.0 g/100 ml
2. Electrolytes		
Sodium	120-170 mmol/l	140 mmol/l
Potassium	26-42 mmol/l	4.5 mmol/l
Calcium	0.3-2.0 mmol/l	2.5 mmol/l
Magnesium	0.5-1.1 mmol/l	0.9 mmol/l
Chloride	120-135 mmol/l	100 mmol/l
Bicarbonate	26 mmol/l	30 mmol/l
3. Antiproteinasis		
α_1-Anti trypsin(α_1-at)	0.1-3.0 mg%	280 mg%
α_1-Anti Chymotrypsin	1.4 mg%	24 mg%
Inter-α trypsin inhibitor	0.5 mg%	20 mg%
α_2 Macroglobulin	3-6 mg%	—
4. Nitrogenous substances		
Total protein	0.668-0.800 g/100 ml	6.7 g/100 ml
Albumin	0.392 g/100 ml	4.0-4.8 g/100 ml
Globulin	0.2758 g/100 ml	2.3 g/100 ml
Ammonia	0.005 g/100 ml	0.047 g/100 ml
Uric acid		
Urea	0.04 mg/100 ml	26.8 mg/100 ml
Total nitrogen	158 mg/100 ml	1140 mg/100 ml
Nonprotein nitrogen	51 mg/100 ml	15-42 mg/100 ml
5. Carbohydrates		
Glucose	2.5 (0-5.0) mg/100 ml	80-90 mg/100 ml
6. Sterols		
Cholesterol and cholesterol esters	8-32 mg/100 ml	200-300 mg/100 ml
7. Miscellaneous		
Citric acid	0.6 mg/100 ml	2.2-2.8 mg/100 ml
Ascorbic acid	0.14 mg/100 ml	0.1-0.7 mg/100 ml
Lysozyme	1-2 mg/ml	—
Amino acid	7.58 mg/100 ml	—
Lactate	1-5 mmol/l	0.5-0.8 mmol/l
Prostaglandin	75 pg PF/ml 300 pg PF/ml	80-90 pg PF/ml
Catecholamine	0.5-1.5 µg/ml	
Complement	1:4 dilution (Hemolytic assay)	1.32 dilution (Hemolytic assay)

Group A: Proteins which are similar to serum proteins with a low concentration representing less than 15% of all tear proteins. Some of them are always present in tears. Albumin, IgG, α-L antitrypsin, transferrin, α-L antichymotrypsin and β-2 microglobulin others which appears sporadically are ceruloplasmin, haptoglobin and Zinc α-2 glycoprotein.

Group B: Specific proteins synthesized by tear gland are RMP (rapid migration protein) and some other proteins which are also present in other external secretions (lysozyme, lactoferrin and IgA).

Tear Albumin

Albumin represents about 60% of the total protein in tears as it does in plasma. Tear albumin is a unique protein fraction. It is electrophoretically a prealbumin and migrates to a position similar to serum prealbumin. Genetic polymorphism has been reported of the tear albumin.

Electrophoresis of tears shows several peaks of migration. These peaks are main which correspond to proteins synthesized by the lacrimal gland—rapid migrant proteins and lactoferrin migrating to the anode and lysozyme migrating to the cathode.

The total tear proteins content strongly depends upon the method of collection of tears. Small unstimulated tears show levels of about 20 mg/ml while stimulated tears show much lower values in the range of 3 to 7 mg/ml reflecting the level of lacrimal gland fluid.

Lysozyme

Fleming first discovered an antibacterial substance and showed that this substance is an enzyme which he named lysozyme because of its capacity to lyze bacteria. In normal tears concentration of lysozyme is much higher than in any other body fluid. The normal level for human tear lysozyme (HTL) is 1 to 2 mg/ml. The enzymic activity of lysozyme is optimal at pH 5.2 and decreases above and below this pH value.

Lysozyme is a long chain, high molecular weight proteolytic enzyme produced by lysosomes—a known cellular ultra structure. Lysozyme acts upon certain bacteria and dissolves them by cleaning the polysaccharide component of their cell walls. As the function of cell wall in bacteria is to confer mechanical support a bacterium devoid of its cell wall usually bursts because of the high osmotic pressure inside the cell.

Lysozyme level in tears can be measured with a diffusion method or with a spectrophotometric assay.

In addition to lysozyme, presence of other antibacterial factors in human tears have been shown. The nonlysozymal bactericidal protein beta lysin has been reported to be derived chiefly from platelets but it exists in higher

Table 3: Amino acid composition of human tear lysozyme

Amino acids	*Residues (gm/100 g protein)*
Aspartic acid	13.23
Arginine	13.05
Glutamic acid	8.55
Tryptophane	6.89
Alanine	6.36
Leucine	6.11
Trypsin	5.65
Glycine	4.94
Lysine	4.92
Valine	4.62
Serine	4.02
Half-cysteine	4.01
Threonine	3.67
Isoleucine	3.59
Phenylalanine	1.97
Proline	1.72
Methionine	1.50
Histidine	1.01

Table 4: Relative quantity of various protein fractions in tears

Fractions	*Normal tears (Percentage)*	*Stimulated flow (Tears) Percentage*
Albumin	58.2	20.2
Globulin	23.9	56.9
Lysozyme	17.9	22.9

Table 5: Origin of various tear protein fractions

Protein fraction	*Lacrimal gland proper*	*Accessory lacrimal gland*	*Goblet cells*
Lysozyme	+	—	—
Component-I	—	+	±
Component-II	+	±	±
Component-III	+	±	±
Serum albumin	—	—	+
Tear albumin	+	—	—
Mucin	—	—	+

+means fraction is present
— means fraction is absent
±Means fraction is indifferently present

concentration in tears than in blood plasma. The lysozyme and beta lysin protein fractions can be separated by filtering the tears. The antibacterial activity of the filtrate results from lysozyme but in whole tears beta lysin is responsible for three-fourth of the bactericidal effect. Beta lysin acts primarily on cellular membrane while lysozyme dissolves bacterial cell walls.

The action of lysozyme depends on the pH. The optimum pH for lysis varies with the solubility of the bacterial proteins but in general it ranges between 6.0 and 7.4. Low salt concentrations favor lysis by increasing solubility.

Human tear lysozyme (HTL) levels have been shown to be greatly decreased in tears of patients suffering from Sjögren's syndrome and ocular toxicity from long-term use of practolol therapy thus making it a useful diagnostic aid. Other disease states where HTL level is lowered include herpes simplex virus infection and malnutrition in children.

Lactoferrin

It is an iron carrying protein and appears to be a major tear protein in the intermediate fraction. Its property of iron binding (Fe III) is 300 times stronger than the other iron binding protein (transferrin). This is probably significant for its bacteriostatic activity in tears making essential metal ions unavailable for microbial metabolism.

Transferrin

Transferrin has been shown to be present in tears. Transferrin along with serum albumin and IgG can be detected only after mild trauma to the mucosal surface of the conjunctiva or in tears.

Ceruloplasmin

Ceruloplasmin, a copper carrying protein is regularly found in tears. In electrophoresis the migration rate of tear ceruloplasmin varies from its serum counter part.

Immunoglobulins

Tiselius (1939) for the first time separated the plasma proteins by electrophoresis and isolated three types of globulins—alpha, beta and gamma. Antibody property of the immune serum resides in the gamma globulin fraction. Immunoglobulins are elaborated by plasma cells following transformation of antigen stimulated B-lymphocytes. This elaboration constitutes the humoral immune system.

Five major classes of immunoglobulins have been recognized. These are:

Immunoglobulin A (IgA)

Immunoglobulin G (IgG)

Table 6: Immunoglobulin levels in tear and serum

Ig class	*Tears*	*Serum*
Total proteins	800 mg/100 ml	6500 mg/100 ml
IgA	14-24 mg/100 ml	170-200 mg/100 ml
IgG	17 mg/100 ml	1000 mg/100 ml
IgM	5-7 mg/100 ml	100 mg/100 ml
IgE	26-250 µg/ml	2000 µg/ml

Immunoglobulin M (IgM)
Immunoglobulin E (IgE)
Immunoglobulin D (IgD)

Immunoglobulin A (IgA): It is the major immunoglobulin present in tears, saliva and colostrum. Almost all of the IgA have a secretory component attached to them when they occur in external secretions. It participates in the functioning of IgA as antibody in the external environment. The possible functions of secretory IgA include prevention of viral and bacterial infections that may have an access to the external secretions, e.g. tears and participate as opsonins in the phagocytosis process.

The average levels of IgA—the predominant immunoglobulin in normal human tear is 14 mg/dl.

In the human lacrimal gland, IgA appears to be synthesized by interstitial plasma cells and after entry into the intercellular spaces it is coupled to SC and secreted as secretory IgA (IgA-SC) through the blood-tear barrier involving intracellular transport by acinar epithelial cells into the lumens. In the conjunctiva IgA and plasma cells are located in the substantia propria. Only in the acinar epithelium of the accessory lacrimal glands can SC material be present indicating that these are the sites of synthesis of secretory IgA of the conjunctival secretions. Depending upon the method of tear collection IgA values can vary from 10 to 100 mg%.

Immunoglobulin G (IgG): It is present in very low concentrations in normal tears. However, after mild trauma to the mucosal surface of the conjunctiva it can be easily detected.

IgG is the most prominent circulating (serum) immunoglobulin present in concentrations five times that of IgA. The average level of IgG in normal human tears range from 17 to 20 mg/100 ml.

The serum level of IgG is about 1000 mg/dl. IgG molecule has a molecular weight of about 150,000. Each molecule of IgG consists of 2 L chains and 2 H chains linked by 20-25-S-S bonds. The antigenic analysis of IgG myelomas show four subclasses now termed as IgG_1, IgG_2, IgG_3, and IgG_4,. IgG_1 is the predominant variant and together with IgG_3 possesses the ability to combine with complement to bind to macrophages and to cross the placenta. IgG synthesis in humans is about 35 mg/kg/d and its half-life is about 23 days. IgG molecules are Y-shaped with a hinge region near the middle of the heavy chain connecting the 2 Fab segments to the Fc segment.

During the secondary response, IgG is the major immunoglobulin to be synthesized probably because of its small size, IgG diffuses more readily than other immunoglobulins into the tears, therefore as the predominating immunoglobulin it carries the major burden of neutralizing bacterial toxins and of binding to microorganisms (specially streptococci, pneumococci and staphylococci) to enhance their phagocytosis. IgG is most efficient in killing and stopping the progress of microorganism's invasion.

Immunoglobulin M (IgM): It is present in very low concentrations in normal tears. The average level of IgM in normal tears range from 5 to 7 mg%. Barnett (1968) reported first the presence of IgM in normal tears.

The serum level of IgM is about 100 mg/dl. The IgM molecule with a molecular weight 900,000 is the largest of the immunoglobulins. Often referred to as macroglobulin because of its size, the IgM molecule are pentamers with a high valency or anticombining capacity. Due to its high valency IgM is extremely efficient agglutinating and cytolytic agent and is the first type of antibody which is formed after the initial encounter with antigen. It appears early in response to infection and is confined mainly to the bloodstream.

Even minimum trauma to conjunctiva would cause serum proteins to leak into the tears. There is increased concentrations of IgA, IgG and IgE in tears. Either these immunoglobulins are selectively excreted into the tears or they are locally synthesized. Increased concentrations of IgA, IgG and IgM are reported in cases of blepharoconjunctivitis, herpes keratitis, vernal conjunctivitis, acute follicular conjunctivitis, phlyctenular conjunctivitis, keratomalacia, corneal ulcer and acute endogenous uveitis.

Immunoglobulin E (IgE): It is mostly extravascular in distribution. IgE values ranges from 26 to 144 µg/ml in normal tears. Normal serum contains only traces of IgE but greatly elevated levels are seen in atopic conditions.

Immunoglobulin D (IgD): IgD levels are quite low in tears as well as in serum. It is mostly intravascular.

Complement

Complement in tears has been shown in hemolytic assays up to dilution of 1.4 whereas serum is active in this system up to 1:32.

Glycoproteins

Glycoproteins are present in the mucoid layer as well as in the tear fluid since they are highly soluble in water. Glycoproteins contribute significantly to the stickiness of the material forming the mucoid layer. N-acetyleneuraminic acid (a sialic acid) has been indentified in normal tears. Glycoproteins may play a critical role in the lubrication of the corneal surface by rendering its hydrophobic surface more hydrophilic permitting spreading and stabilization of the tear film. The mucus is secreted by the conjunctival goblet cells as a solution of glycoproteins (mucoids) and this sticky mixture adheres to the surface of the epithelium even though the glycoproteins are water soluble.

The glycoproteins are carbohydrate-protein complexes characterized by the presence of hexosamines, hexoses and sialic acid. In normal tears relative hexosamine content of the protein which is used as indicator for glycoproteins varies from 0.5 to 17%, the hexosamine concentration from 0.05 to 3 g/l. Sialic acid concentration of human tears has been reported to be 114 μmol/100 ml.

Antiproteinases

Antiproteinases, inhibitors of proteinases are present in tears at levels much lower than in plasma.

These includes α_1-antitrypsin, α_1-antichymotrypsin, inter-α-trypsin inhibitor and α_2-macroglobulin. The source of-α_1 antitrypsin is the lacrimal gland while other antiproteinases originate from corneal and conjunctival surfaces. In various inflammatory conditions of the eye the levels of α_1-at and α_2-m in tear fluid are increased.

In bacterial and viral infections of the eye and in corneal ulceration the levels of α_1-at and α_2-m in tear fluids are increased. Using albumin as a marker protein there is evidence suggesting that these two collagenase inhibitors are derived either from plasma by a general increase in vascular permeability to proteins or they are produced locally.

Metabolites

A number of metabolites have been reported to be present in normal human tears. These include organic constituents of low molecular weight like glucose, urea, amino acids and other metabolites like lactate, histamine, prostaglandins and catecholamines.

Table 7: Antiproteinasis concentration in tears and plasma

Antiproteinasis	*Plasma*	*mg percentage* *Tears*
α_1-antitrypsin ($\alpha_1$at)	280	0.1-0.4
α_1-antichymotrypsin		1.5
		3.0
α_1-antichymotrypsin	24	1.4
Inter-α-trypsin inhibitor	20	0.5
α_2-macroglobulin		3
		6

Table 8: Antimicrobial factors in tears

Compound	*Evidence*
Lysozyme	+
IgA	+
IgG	±
IgE	+
IgM	±
Complement	+
Lactoferrin	+
Transferrin	±
Betalysin	+
Antibiotic producing Commensal organism	+

+Present in normal tears.
± Present in tears after stimulation (mild trauma to the conjunctiva).

Glucose

Glucose is present in minimal amounts of about 0.2 mmol/liter in tear fluids of normal glycemic persons. This low concentration of glucose appear to be insufficient for corneal nutrition. There is no definitive evidence that cornea metabolizes glucose emanating from the tears.

It has been shown that some glucose in tears originates from the goblet cells of the conjunctiva. There is corresponding rise in tear glucose level with elevation of plasma glucose level above 100 mg%. However, there is no significant rise in tear glucose levels in diabetics with blood glucose level of more than 20 mmol/liter which demonstrates the barrier function of the corneal and conjunctival epithelium against loss of glucose from the tissues into the tear fluid. It is the tissue fluid which contributes to the tear glucose after mechanically stimulated methods of tear collection.

Urea

Urea concentration in tear fluid and plasma have been found to be equivalent suggesting an unrestricted passage through the blood-tear barrier in the lacrimal gland. Urea concentration in tears decreases with increasing secretion rate.

Amino Acids

Free amino acid concentration in tears is reported to be 7.58 mg/100 ml. This value is 3 to 4 times higher than the free amino acid concentration in serum.

Lactate

Lactate levels of 1 to 5 mmol/l in tears are far higher than the normal blood levels of 0.5 to 0.8 mmol/l. Pyruvate from 0.05 to 0.35 mmol/l is about the same as is normal for blood (0.1-0.2 mmol/l). These levels do not show significant alterations after mechanical irritation. The epithelium does not possess a barrier function for lactate and pyruvate.

Histamine

Histamine is present in normal tears collected from the conjunctival sac at a level of about 10 mg/ml. In vernal conjunctivitis specifically a variable increase up to 125 mg/ml has been observed.

Prostaglandins

Prostaglandins are present in normal tears at the level of 75 pg prostaglandin F/ml and it is little lower than in serum. In inflammatory conditions of the eye significant higher values are found up to 300 pg/ml of tears.

Catecholamines, Dopamine, Noradrenaline and Dopa

Catecholamines, dopamine, noradrenaline and dopa have been found in the tear fluid. The levels vary from 0.5 to 1.5 mg/ml. Dopamine has values as high as 280 mg/ml.

In glaucoma patients lower values have been reported for these compounds which reflect the diminished activity of the sympathetic innervation of the eye. The determination of catecholamines in tears has been advocated as a test in glaucoma diagnosis.

Electrolytes and Hydrogen Ions

The predominant positively charged electrolytes (cation) in tears are mainly sodium and potassium while the negative ions (anions) are chloride and bicarbonate.

Sodium

Sodium concentration in tears 120 to 170 mmol/liter is about equal to that in plasma suggesting a passive secretion into the tears. While potassium

Table 9: Human tear electrolytes

	Concentration in mmol/l					
	Na^+	K^+	Ca^{++}	Mg^{++}	Cl^-	HCO_3^-
Tears	120-170	6-26	0.5-1.1	0.3-0.6	118-138	26
	145	24	0.4-1.1	0.5-1.1	106-130	
	134-170	26-42	0.3-2.0		120-135	
Serum	140	4.5	2.5	0.9	100	30

with an average value of about 20 mmol/l is much higher than the corresponding plasma concentration of about 5 mmol/l. This indicates an active secretion of potassium into the tears. It is interesting to observe that while the main cationic constituent of the aqueous and vitreous humor is sodium while cornea (mainly corneal epithelium) contains a much higher concentration of potassium than sodium. These two cations play an essential role in the osmotic regulation of the extracellular and intracellular spaces and in general changes in sodium level are the reverse of changes in potassium level.

Calcium

Calcium is independent of the tear production and is lower than the free fraction of plasma. In cystic fibrosis patients have much higher calcium values. An average of 2.5 mmol/l have been shown only at slow rates concomitant with lower tear sodium values.

Magnesium

Magnesium in tears is little lower than corresponding serum value possibly reflecting the free fraction of magnesium. Both calcium and magnesium play a role in controlling membrane permeability.

Chloride

Chloride, an anion essential to all tissues also plays an important role in osmotic regulation much like sodium and potassium. The chloride concentration is slightly higher in tears than in serum.

Bicarbonate

The bicarbonate together with the carbonate ions in tears may be involved in the regulation of pH. This buffer system maintains the near neutral pH of the tear film, the surface of which is exposed to atmospheric changes.

Enzymes

Enzymes of Energy Producing Metabolisms

Glycolytic enzymes and enzymes of tricarboxylic acid cycle can be detected in high values only in human tear samples. These enzymes form a blood-tear barrier against penetration from the blood. The source of these enzymes is in the conjunctiva where they are secreted in small amounts. The lacrimal gland apparently does not secrete these enzymes. These enzymes can be obtained during mechanical irritation.

Lactate Dehydrogenase

Lactate dehydrogenase (LDH) is the enzyme in the highest concentration in tears. It can be separated electrophoretically into its five isoenzymes showing a pattern with more of the slower migrating muscle type isoenzymes. This is closely related to the distribution pattern of corneal tissue in contrast to serum LDH where the faster migrating heart type isoenzymes prevail.

These findings indicate that tear LDH originates from the corneal epithelium. Therefore, in patients suffering from corneal disease, the distribution of LDH isoenzymes in tears differs from those found in healthy individuals. LDH isoenzymes bound to immunoglobulin have been found in blood and it is probable that here an analogous binding takes place in tears.

Lysosomal Enzymes

Lysosomal enzymes include a number of lysosomal acid hydrolases which are present in tears in concentration of 2 to 10 times than those in serum. **The lacrimal gland is the main source of the lysosomal enzymes but conjunctiva may act as a second source for lysosomal enzymes after mild trauma.** The relative high values are found in tear fluid collection where the epithelial cells of conjunctiva remain intact and contain very low levels of lactate dehydrogenase or other cytoplasmic enzymes. Lysosomal enzyme activities in tears are used for diagnosis and identification of carriers of several inborn errors of metabolism.

The concentration of β-hexosaminidase in tears collected on filter paper strips is an index for the development and prognosis of diabetic retinopathy. The tears would reflect the decreased enzyme activity of β-hexosaminidase and of other lysosomal glycosidases in the retina showing a negative correlation with the increased plasma levels of these enzymes.

Amylase

Amylase is the enzyme present in tear fluid in relatively moderate levels. The origin of this enzyme is in lacrimal gland. The reported presence of amylase in the cornea might be due to contamination by tear fluid.

Peroxidase

Peroxidase (POD) is present in human tears originating from the lacrimal gland and not from the conjunctiva. The level of tear POD in human tears is $10^3 \mu/l$. POD activity found in the conjunctiva is probably derived from the tears.

Plasminogen Activator

Plasminogen activator has been demonstrated in tear fluid and corneal epithelium is suggested to be the source of this urokinase-like fibrinolytic activity.

Collagenase

Collagenase has been shown to be present in tear fluid in the presence of corneal ulceration, due to infection, chemical burn, trauma and desiccation. Corneal collagenase is present as an inactive precursor "latent collagenase" which can be activated with trypsin and *in vivo* possibly by plasmin resulting from plasminogen activator activity in tears.

Drugs Excreted in Tears

Tears represent a potentially more stable body fluid of low protein content and with modest variations of pH. Passage of drugs from the plasma to the tears apparently takes place by diffusion of the non-protein bound fraction. However, presence of tight junctions between the acinar epithelial cells in the lacrimal gland forming a blood-tear barrier, the lipid solubility is expected to play a major role. The blood-tear barrier shows the same characteristics as that of cell membrane. Phenobarbital and carbamazepine are excreted in tears in about 0.5% of corresponding plasma concentration.

Methotrexate, an antimetabolite reaches tear levels of 5% of the corresponding plasma concentrations and is in equilibrium with the unbound fraction in plasma. Ampicillin is present in tears in concentration of about 0.02 of the corresponding serum level.

Applied Physiology

Basic secretion of tear fluid is made up of the secretions of the lacrimal gland and accessory lacrimal gland tissue together with the secretions of meibomian glands and the mucous glands of the conjunctiva. Reflex secretions of tears is hundreds time greater than basal or resting secretion. The stimulus to reflex secretions appears to be derived from the superficial corneal and conjunctival sensory stimulation as a result of tear break up and dry spot formation. The secretory stimulus to the lacrimal glands is parasympathetic with reflex secretions occurring in both eyes following superficial stimulation of one eye. The whole mass of lacrimal tissue responds as one unit to reflex tearing. Reflex secretion is reduced by topical corneal and conjunctival anesthesia.

Hyposecretion of Tears

Hyposecretion means decreased formation of tears.

Lacrimal hyposecretion may be congenital although not very common.

Acquired lacrimal hyposecretion may be due to:

- Atrophy and fibrosis of lacrimal tissue due to a destructive infiltration by mononuclear cells as in keratoconjunctivitis sicca and Sjögren's syndrome.
- Local inflammatory diseases of the conjunctival commonly conjunctival scarring secondary to bacterial or viral infection.
- Chronic inflammatory disease of the salivary and lacrimal glands (Mikulicz's syndrome).
- Damage or destruction of lacrimal tissue by granulomatous (sarcoidosis), pseudotumor or neoplastic lesions.
- Absence of lacrimal gland.
- Blockage of excretory ducts of the lacrimal gland.
- Neurogenic lesions.
- Meibomian gland dysfunction.

Diagnostic Tests for Tear Hyposecretions

Tear Film Break-up Time (BUT)

The tear film break-up time is a simple physiological test to assess the stability of the precorneal tear film. This test is performed by instilling fluorescein into the lower fornix, taking precaution not to touch cornea. The patient is asked to blink several times and then to refrain from blinking. The tear film is scanned with a broad beam and cobalt blue filter. After an interval of time black spots or line indicating dry spots appear in the tear film. **BUT is the interval between the last blink and appearance of the first randomly distributed dry spot.** Ideally average of three measurements is taken. A normal BUT is more than 10 seconds and a BUT of less than 10 seconds is considered abnormal. This test may also be abnormal in eyes with mucin or lipid deficiency.

Table 10: Diagnostic tests and drug assays in tears

Compound	*Diagnosis*	*Usefulness*
Lysozyme	Sjögren's disease	+
	Practolol induced toxicity	+
	Traumatic inflammation of eye	+
Lysosomal enzymes	Lysosomal storage disease	+
Collagenase	Corneal ulceration	+
α_1-Antitrypsin	Bacterial infections	±
Glucose	Diabetes mellitus	±
Tear albumin	Genetic marker	+
Immunoglobulins (IgA, IgG and IgM)	Iatrogenic inflammation of anterior-segment	+

+ Useful
± Comparatively useful

Schirmer's Test

The rate of tear formation is estimated by measuring the amount of wetting on a special filter paper which is 5 mm wide and 35 mm long.

Previously Schirmer's test 1 and 2 were used in diagnostic practice but nowadays modified Schirmer-I test is employed. This test is performed as follows.

Schirmer strips are prepared by cutting out Whatman filter paper No. 41 into the strips of 5 mm × 35 mm dimensions. A 5 mm tab is folded over at one end. Before use, these strips are autoclaved.

The bent end is placed into lower conjunctival sac at the junction of lateral one-third and medial two-third of the lower eyelid so that a 5 mm bent end rests on the palpebral conjunctiva and the folding crease lies over the eyelid margin. This test is usually performed in sitting posture in dim light.

The patient is asked to keep the eyelid open and look slightly upwards at a fixation point. Blinking is allowed while the patient gazes at the fixation point.

After one minute, the strips are carefully removed and moistening of the exposed portion of the strip is measured in millimeters with the help of a millimeter ruler.

The measurements are made from the notch at the bend of the Schirmer strip to the distal end of the wetting on the strip (excluding the folded over tab). The amount of wetting of the Schirmer strip in one minute is multiplied by three to correspond roughly to the amount of wetting that would have occurred in five minutes (Jones, 1972). It is a measure of the rate of tear secretion in a five-minute period.

A normal eye will wet between 10 and 25 mm during that period. Measurements between 5 and 10 mm are considered borderline and values less than 5 mm is indicative of impaired secretion.

Vital Dye Staining

- Rose Bengal 1% has an affinity for devitalized epithelial cells and mucus in contrast to fluorescein which remains extracellular and is more useful in showing up epithelial defects. Rose Bengal is very useful in detecting even mild cases of keratoconjunctivitis sicca (KCS) by staining the interpalpebral conjunctiva in the form of two triangles with their base at the limbus.

  The only disadvantage with Rose Bengal staining is that it may cause ocular irritation specially in eyes with severe KCS. In order to reduce that amount of irritation only a small drop should be instilled into the eye. A topical anesthetic should not be used prior to the instillation of Rose Bengal as it may produce a false-positive result.

- Alcian blue has similar properties as Rose Bengal and is less irritant but it is not generally available.

Lysozyme Assay

Lysozyme assay is based on the fact that in hyposecretion of tears, there may be reduction in the concentration of lysozyme. This test is performed by placing the wetted filter strip into an agar plate containing specific bacteria. The plate is then incubated for 24 hours and the zone of the lysis is measured. The zone will be reduced if the concentration of lysozyme in the tears is decreased.

Tear Globulin Assay

Tear IgA levels are measured in this test. This test is also based on the principle that decreased tear formation will lead to decreased IgA (immunoglobulin A) levels in tears. This test is performed on a specific tripartigan immunodiffusion plates containing specific agar gel in wells. 20 μl of tear samples is put into these wells and plates are incubated for 48 hours. The diffusion of rings around wells are measured to the nearest 0.1 mm with a partigen ruler. The ring will be reduced if the concentration of IgA in tears is decreased. This is a reliable test for measuring tear globulins.

Tear Osmolarity

Tear osmolarity is increased in cases of hyposecretion.

Biopsy of the Conjunctiva

Biopsy of the conjunctiva and an estimation of the number of goblet cells are other tests which can be done. In mucin deficiency states the number of goblet cells shall be decreased.

Hypersecretion of Tears

In practice when patient complains of a wet eye there are two possibilities of excessive watering of the eye.

- Lacrimation from reflex hypersecretion due to irritation of cornea and conjunctiva.
- Obstructive epiphora as a result of failure of tear drainage or evacuation system. The main causes are lacrimal pump failure due to lower lid laxity or weakness of the orbicularis muscle and more commonly due to mechanical obstructions of the drainage system.

If the wet eye is caused by hypersecretion the Schirmer's test values (technique already mentioned) will be increased and the Jones Fluorescein dye test will reveal normal outflow function.

Physiological Diagnostic Test for Hypersecretions

Jones I (Primary) Test

This is a physiological test which differentiates an excessive watering due to a partial obstruction of the lacrimal passages from primary hypersecretion of tears.

In this test 1 drop of 2% fluorescein solution is instilled into the conjunctival sac. After about 5 minutes a cotton-tipped bud or applicator (moistened in cocaine 4% or proparacaine 0.75%) is inserted under the inferior turbinate at the nasolacrimal duct opening. This is situated about 3 cm from the external nares.

The results are interpreted as follows.

- If the fluorescein is recovered from the nose on the applicator and aqueous solution passes from the conjunctival sac to the nose in 1 minute then the excretory system is patent and cause of watering is primary hypersecretion. No further tests are required then and the test is inferred as positive.
- If no dye is recovered from the nose a partial obstruction is present or there is failure of the lacrimal pump mechanism. In this situation secondary dye test or Jones II test is required.

Jones II (Secondary Irrigation) Test

This test helps to identify the probable site of partial obstruction.

In this procedure topical anesthesia (4% Xylocaine or 0.5% proparacaine) is instilled into the conjunctival sac and any residual fluorescein is washed out. The nasolacrimal system is then irrigated with normal saline. The patient is positioned with his or her head down by about 45° so that the saline runs out of the nose into white paper tissues and not into the pharynx.

This test is interpreted as follows.

- Positive—If fluorescein-stained saline is recovered from the nose, the dye must have reached the lacrimal sac during the primary dye test but was stopped from entering the nose by a partial obstruction in the nasolacrimal duct. However, syringing of the lacrimal system had pushed the dye past the obstruction into the nose. A positive secondary dye test indicates a partial obstruction to the nasolacrimal duct which can be treated by a dacryocystorhinostomy (DCR) procedure.
- Negative—If unstained saline is recovered from the nose it means that no dye has entered the lacrimal sac during the primary dye test. This means a partial obstruction in the upper drainage system (punctum, canaliculi or common canaliculus) or a defective lacrimal pump mechanism. In such a situation DCR would fail and some other operative procedure will be required.

Fluorescein Dye Disappearance Test

An accurate status of the excretory capability of the lacrimal system can be obtained by observing the behavior of a single drop of 2% fluorescein solution instilled into the inferior conjunctival cul-de-sac. The color intensity after 5 minutes is measured and graded on a scale of 0 to 4+. The normal excretion of the retained fluorescein shall be 0-1+. Any greater residual then is indicative of impaired outflow. However, by this test one cannot distinguish between impairment of the upper and lower segments of the system, but it may complement the Jones tests.

- Nasal examination should be performed in order to determine the position of normal nasal structures specially the position of the anterior end of the middle turbinate when surgery is contemplated. It will also detect the presence of polyps or tumors, etc.

Special Tests

Intubation Dacryocystography

The conventional method of dacryocystography consists of injecting contrast medium into one of the canaliculi followed by the taking of posteroanterior (PA) and lateral views, radiographs. However, far superior status of the canalicular system can be obtained by using a technique that combines injection of lipoidol ultra fluid through a catheter with macrography. In common canalicular lesions, subtraction macrodacryocystography may provide more sophisticated details.

These specific investigations are not only extremely valuable in depicting the exact location of the obstruction but they are also of help in the diagnosis of diverticula, fistulae, filling defects due to tumors, stones and infections by streptothrix species.

Scintillography (Radionuclide Testing)

This test involves the labeling of tears with gamma-emitting substances such as technetium-99m and monitoring their progress through the drainage system. This is a sophisticated and reliable test for better understanding of excretory physiology.

Color Doppler Scanography

Color Doppler scanography is the latest technique for evaluating the status of the drainage system. It is a recently introduced test with accurate results.

Diagnostic Tests and Principles in Dry Eye Syndrome

David Meyer (South Africa)

Any practicing comprehensive ophthalmologist will confirm that dry eye is the most common complaint of patients presenting to their offices, albeit most frequently in a mild form. The National Eye Institute/Industry Workshop on Clinical Trials in Dry Eyes, have formulated a "global definition" of Dry Eye Syndrome (DES) or Keratoconjunctivitis Sicca (KCS). They suggest that dry eye is a disorder of the tear film due to tear deficiency or excessive tear evaporation that causes damage to the interpalpebral ocular surface and is associated with symptoms of ocular discomfort. DES is a chronic condition and currently has no real cure. It is an apparently benign condition but with an intractable course. This is often frustrating for the sufferer and unrewarding for the ophthalmologist. However, timely therapy after early recognition usually helps to avert late complications. Traditional therapy has included the long-term use of topical lubricants, but for want of a definitive causative treatment, efficacy is usually only partial. With the increasing recognition of ocular surface inflammation as a contributory component of DES and the availability of new specific therapies for this condition, it has become prudent that clinicians diagnose and objectively monitor this condition intelligently.

Classification

Despite the high prevalence of this condition, it still remains remarkably under diagnosed. This is due in part to the lack of understanding of its classification and partly because of a lack of a single universal diagnostic test. There are two clear categories of DES as proposed by the National Eye Institute, one related to *insufficient production* and the other to *increased evaporation* of tears. There are several subgroups in each of the two categories. Sjögren's and non- Sjögren's Syndrome are the two main subgroups in the *insufficient production* arm whilst meibomian gland disease (MGD), exposure, blink abnormality and contact lens wear form the essential subgroups of the *increased evaporation* arm. Tests for one category may be positive and for another category negative; yet, both may lead to DES. Additionally, there is often a crossover of conditions between the two groups e.g. (MGD), which is the leading cause of evaporative DES, may also occur in a significant number of cases with aqueous deficiency.

OCULAR SURFACE DISEASE INDEX (OSDI)

Patient Number	Patient Initials	Physician's Name	Date of Visit
______	___ ___ ___	______	___/___/___ Month Day Year

Have you experienced any of the following during the last week:	ALL of the time	MOST of the time	HALF of the time	SOME of the time	NONE of the time
1. Eyes that are sensitive to light?	☐	☐	☐	☐	☐
2. Eyes that feel gritty?	☐	☐	☐	☐	☐
3. Painful or sore eyes?	☐	☐	☐	☐	☐
4. Blurred vision?	☐	☐	☐	☐	☐
5. Poor vision?	☐	☐	☐	☐	☐

Have problems with your eyes limited you in performing any of the following during the last week:	ALL of the time	MOST of the time	HALF of the time	SOME of the time	NONE of the time	NOT applicable
6. Reading?	☐	☐	☐	☐	☐	☐
7. Driving at night?	☐	☐	☐	☐	☐	☐
8. Working with a computer or bank machine (ATM)?	☐	☐	☐	☐	☐	☐
9. Watching TV?	☐	☐	☐	☐	☐	☐

Have your eyes felt uncomfortable in any of the following situations during the last week:	ALL of the time	MOST of the time	HALF of the time	SOME of the time	NONE of the time	NOT applicable
10. Windy conditions:	☐	☐	☐	☐	☐	☐
11. Places or areas with low humidity (very dry)?	☐	☐	☐	☐	☐	☐
12. Areas that are air conditioned?	☐	☐	☐	☐	☐	☐

Calculation of OSDI: OSDI= Sum of severity for all questions answered / 4 x (total number of questions answered)

ALL of the time = 4 SOME of the time = 1
MOST of the time = 3 NONE of the time = 0
HALF of the time = 2

NOTE: question answered N/A for the calculation = a NON answered question

Fig. 1: OSDI questionnaire designed to assess DES symptoms and severity

Diagnosis

Not only is there a plethora of symptoms in DES, but also numerous diagnostic tests are available. Diagnosing the DES starts with a good clinical history and proceeds to an applicable systemic physical examination, a complete ocular and slit lamp examination followed by one or more of several specific clinical diagnostic tests. Depending on the availability, laboratory supported tests like tear film osmolarity, tear lysozyme and lactoferrin concentrations as well as conjunctival impression cytology may also be added to the diagnostic routine. The average clinician generally relies on the history in conjunction with Schirmer testing, supravital conjunctival staining, tear film break up time, tear fluorescein clearance, tear meniscus height, and the presence or absence of tear film debris.

Patient History

Diagnosing DES begins with the patient history, where a host of symptoms have been ascribed to the condition. Symptoms are a hallmark of the disease, and the most frequently encountered symptoms are dryness, foreign-body or gritty sensation, burning and photophobia. Additional complaints may include itching, mucus secretions, heaviness of the eyelids, inability to produce emotional tears, pain and redness. Patients would often use the term "dryness"; buy will have difficulty defining exactly what it means. The term "discomfort" may be a more accurate summation of all the patient's symptoms. Various questionnaires have been developed to assess symptoms in DES patients. The Ocular Surface Disease Index (OSDI) in lists 12 common symptoms of dry eye patients and scores each from 1 to 4 in terms of severity. This permits quantification of symptoms and provides a reasonably objective approach to the evaluation of symptoms over time. These questionnaires are valuable tools in clinical treatment trials.

A series of further specific questions during the interview may be of extreme importance.

How do winds or drafts affect your eyes?

DES patients are extremely sensitive to drafts and winds, e.g. driving with the windows down and intolerance in air conditioned surroundings. They feel worse in a dry, cold environment with conditions of increased evaporation.

Does reading affect your eyes?

Reading also often elicits symptoms and many suffer because of the reduced blink rate during periods of concentration.

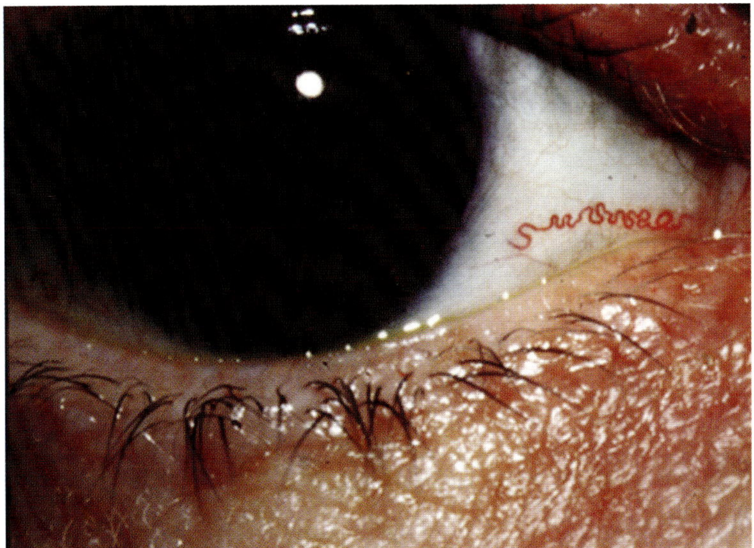

Fig. 2: Thin and irregular tear meniscus supporting suspicion of DES
(Courtesy: Dr Samir Al-Manouri)

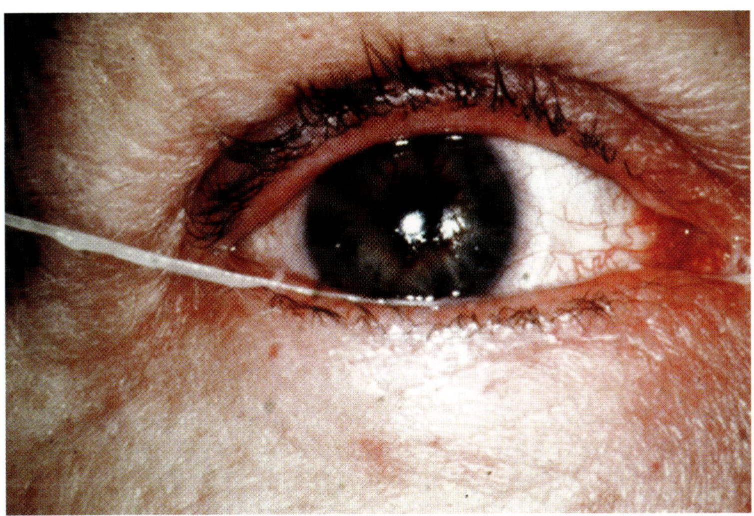

Fig. 3: Mucin strand significant in mucin deficient states

Any problems when you awake at night?

Patients often complain that night-time awaking is the worst part of their lives. Sleep decreases tear production just like general anesthesia. Further reduction in tear flow during sleep in an already compromised eye, will produce nocturnal symptoms. Smoke produces discomfort because smoke is in reality only a suspension of solids in air. It is valuable to determine whether symptoms are better or worse, indoors or outdoors, at home or at work in order to identify high risk environments that may need modification to improve the patient's symptoms.

Do your eyes tear when you peel onions? Can you cry when you feel sad or hurt?

Questioning patients as to their ability to produce irritant and/or emotional tears is important. Affirmative responses suggest that at least some lacrimal function remains, whereas negative responses would suggest the lacrimal gland's inability to secrete tears in response to stimuli. In patients with DES/KCS, the ability to generate irritant tears is lost before the ability to generate emotional tears.

What medications do you take?

Systemic antihistamines, antidepressants, anticholinergics, and diuretics are notorious for reducing tear production. The use of systemic steroids, and other immunosuppressants which may be used for the treatment of Sjögren's syndrome and other collagen vascular diseases should be noted. A history of any collagen vascular disease, thyroid eye disease, lymphoma or AIDS should be sought.

Can you feel saliva in your mouth? Can you swallow bread without additional fluids?

Determining whether the patient has any associated systemic symptoms or conditions is important. Dry mouth and dental gum disease may be pointers to DES. Women should be asked as to noticeable decrease of vaginal secretions.

Do you have any skin problems?

Looking for dermatological conditions may provided useful clues for example scleroderma, facial rash in lupus, pemphigoid, old scars of Stevens-Johnson syndrome and acne rosacea. Family history should be elicited as there may be blood relatives with associated diseases.

What topical lubricants do you use? Are they preserved or unpreserved? How long and how often do you use them?

Information on drops and ointments should be obtained concentrating on type and frequency of use. Most patients will not consider topical treatment when

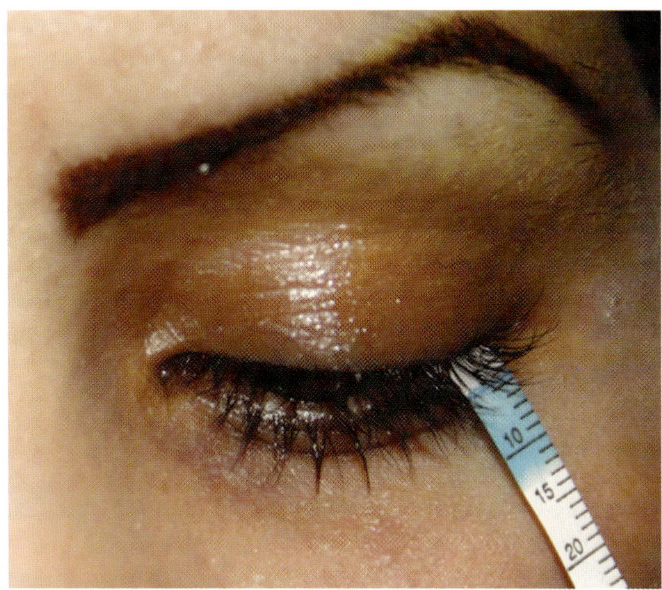

Fig. 4: Schirmer/Jones strip placed at the junction of the middle and lateral one third of the lower eyelid. When performed with local anesthetic the test is called Schirmer 1 and without local anesthetic Jones' test

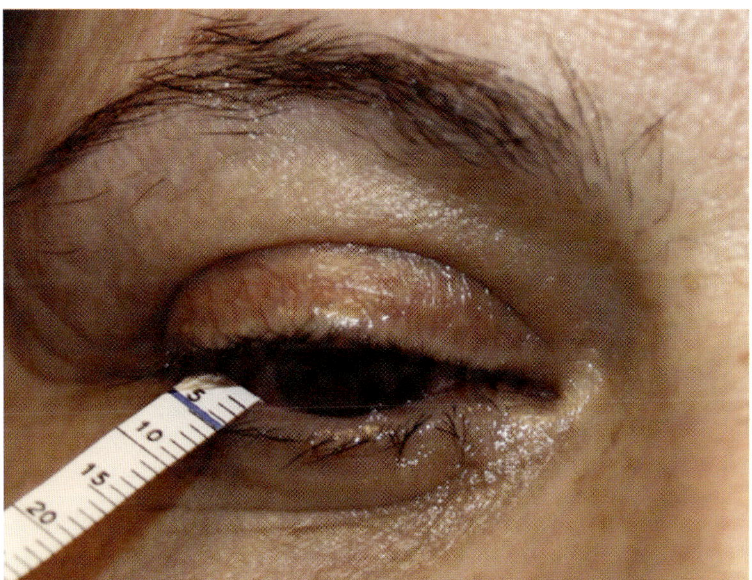

Fig. 5: A Schirmer 1 test value of $\leq$ 6 mm of strip wetting in 5 minutes is accepted as diagnostic for aqueous tear deficiency

generally asked about medications. Most DES sufferers improve on topical lubricant therapy. Valid deductions as to the severity of the condition may often be made from how frequently topical lubricants are used. Patients with severe DES will use the lubricants more often than those with mild DES. Mild cases may be made worse when using preserved lubricants. Other non-lubricant topical medications may be important because of the active drug or the preservative's (most notably benzalconium chloride) effect on the ocular surface. Furthermore, any topical medication is potentially toxic because of the dry eye's inability to dilute the drug. Information about previous temporary or permanent occlusive punctal plugs is essential. If so, was there any improvement in symptoms or did epiphora occur?

Physical Examination

A limited physical examination before focusing on the ophthalmic examination is advised.

Systemic Examination

The facial skin must be examined for evidence of acne rosacea or signs of SLE. The parotid, and submandibular glands should be palpated for presence of enlargement or masses. Thyroid gland palpation is important in patients with thyroid eye disease (TED). Superior limbic keratitis and Sjögren's syndrome are both frequently seen in TED. Lid retraction, exophthalmos and decreased blinking which occur in TED can cause symptoms of dry eye due to increased evaporation. The mouth and tongue are examined for the presence or absence of saliva and oral candidiasis. The hands are assessed for joint disease. Rashes and eczema is looked for on the extremities.

Ocular Examination

A perfectly noncontributory and normal ocular examination may be found in cases of early or mild DES.

External Eyelid Examination

Note the presence or absence of dermatochalasis, the function of the eyelids, completeness of the blink response as well as the blink rate should be noted. The size of the lacrimal gland is assessed by requesting that the patient looks down while the upper eyelid is retracted. Presence of eyelid abnormalities like entropion, ectropion, ptosis, trichiasis, lagophthalmos, and cicatricial conditions should be noted.

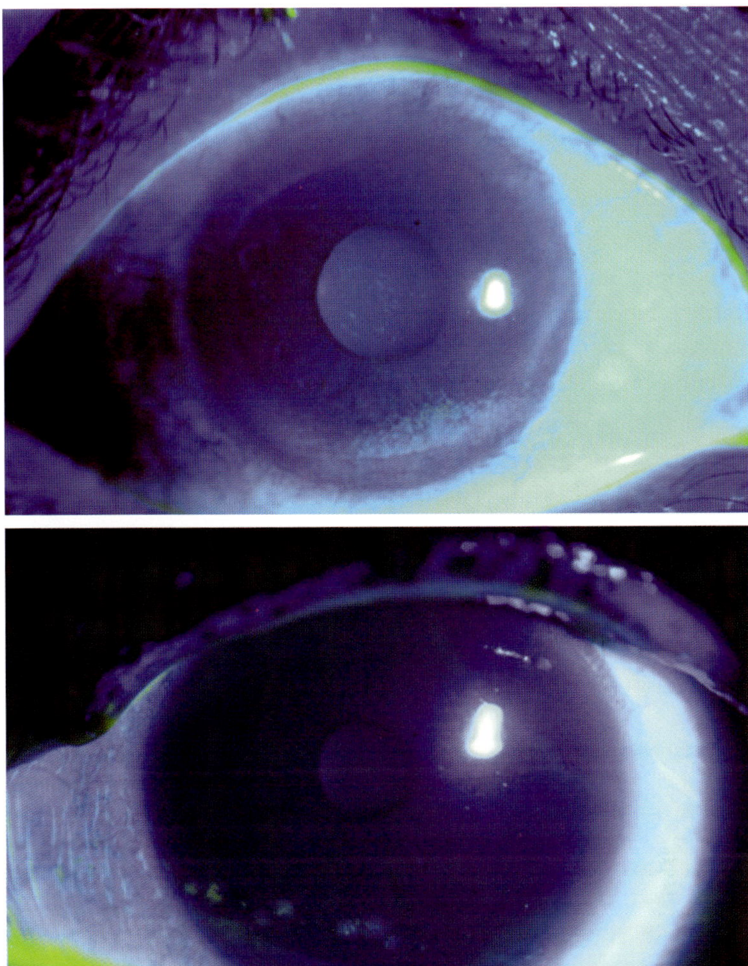

Figs 6 and 7: Fluorescein staining patterns in dry eye syndrome

Slit-lamp Biomicroscopy (SLB)

The most characteristic finding on SLB is an abnormality of the inferior *tear meniscus*. In 85% of normal subjects the height will be 0.2-0.3 mm. In DES, tear meniscus volume is reduced, as indicated by reduced height and radius of curvature. Radius of curvature can be measured by slit lamp photography. Note *meniscus "floaters"* in dry eye cases. They are common and are seen as tiny bits of debris suspended in the tear meniscus. Some are dead epithelial cells that have come off the corneal surface and some are small fibrils of lipid-contaminated mucin. Although extremely common, these floaters are not pathognomonic for DES, as eyes with conjunctivitis and blepharitis may also display them.

Mucous strands may be seen in the more severe cases of DES. They are in reality strings of lipid-contaminated mucus that have been rolled up and pushed into the cul-de-sac by the shearing action of the lids. They are common in the aqueous-deficient states, but become extremely significant in the mucin-deficient conditions. If mucin and excess lipid become intermingled, mucous strands form.

Corneal filaments are commonly seen in dry eye corneas. These filaments are < 2 mm in length and look like short "tails" that are suspended from the surface of the cornea. The exact pathogenesis of filament formation is not known, but these filaments are anchored to epithelial cells and pulling on them can be very painful. This is what happens during blinking, with the resultant symptoms mimicking those of a foreign body.

Eyelid margins are be examined for irregularity, telangiectasia, thickening, and broken or missing eyelashes all of which suggest chronic blepharitis. The condition of the meibomian glands is assessed. Meibomian gland disease (MGD) is suggested by the following: The presence of oil or foam, pouting, plugged or missing meibomian gland orifices, and toothpaste-like thick turbid secretions expressible from the orifices. The percentage of meibomian gland acinar dropout can be quantified by transilluminating the inferior tarsus with a halogen Finhoff transilluminator (Welch Allyn) as suggested by Pflugfelder et al. They quantify the percentage of dropout in the nasal and temporal halves of the lower lid by using a standardized 4-point scale (0, no dropout; 1 ≤ 33%; 234-66%; 3, 67-100%). They also quantify the expressibility of meibomian gland secretions by digitally both the upper and lower lids just above and below the lash line against the globe over an area of five visible meibomian gland orifices. The number of meibomian glands from which meibum can be expressed is quantified on a four point scale as well: (0, all five glands; 1, three to four glands; 2, one to two glands; 3, zero glands).

The *bulbar conjunctiva* may lose its normal luster and may become thickened, hyperemic and edematous. Papillary conjunctivitis especially visible on the

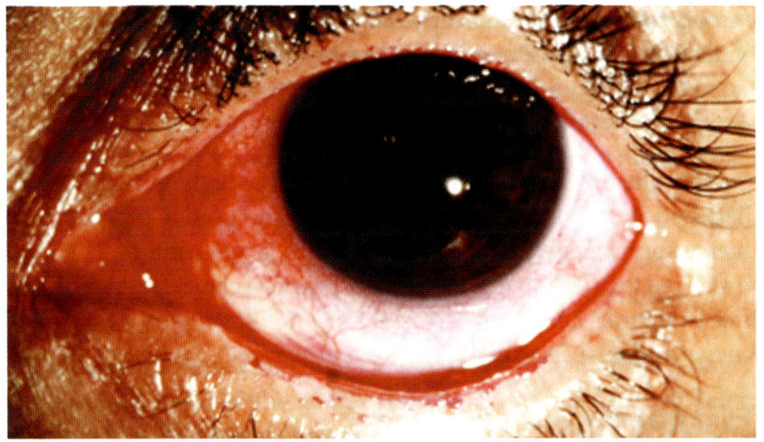

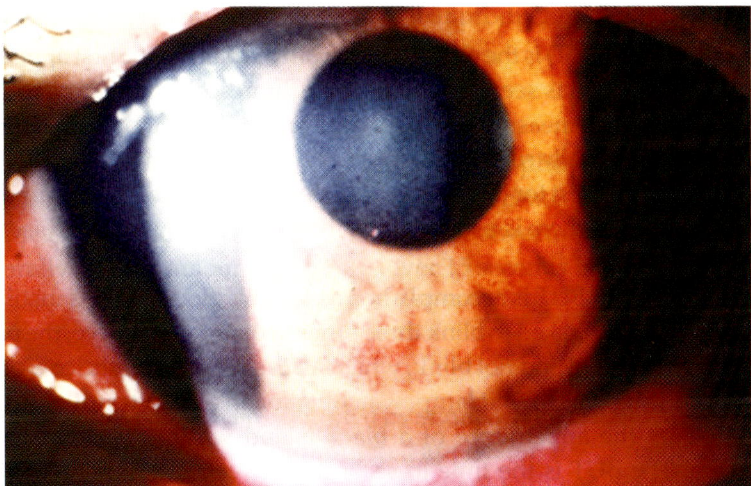

Figs 8 and 9: Staining patterns with rose bengal vital stain

Blepharitis and Meibomianitis

Henry D Perry, Eric D Donnenfeld (USA)

Blepharitis is an acute or chronic inflammatory process involving the eyelids that is frequently associated with conjunctivitis. There are many forms of blepharitis, including bacterial, parasitic, seborrheic, eczematoid, and neoplastic. Generally speaking, blepharitis may be divided into anterior and posterior forms. Anterior blepharitis may be associated with staphylococcal infection and seborrheic dermatitis. Posterior blepharitis is associated with various disorders of the meibomian glands, known collectively as meibomian gland dysfunction.

Meibomian gland dysfunction, a condition associated with obstruction and inflammation of the meibomian glands, is a widespread and chronic problem.

Table 1. Mean total ocular symptoms scores at each visit for the tCSA and Refresh groups. t-test on means was utilized

Visit	*tCSA*	*Refresh*	*P Value*
Baseline	17.7 (n=16)	18.4 (n=17)	0.68
1 month	8.9 (n=15)	9.9 (n=16)	0.63
2 months	6.3 (n=13)	8.1 (n=15)	0.42
3 months	5.8 (n=12)	9.3 (n=14)	0.21

Table 2. Meibomian gland inclusions, fluorescein staining, tear breakup time, and Schirmer scores at each visit for the tCSA and Refresh groups. t-test on means was utilized. Data used is from the worse eye

Visit	*tCSA*	*Refresh*	*P Value*
Mean number of meibomian gland inclusions			
Baseline	26.0	23.8	0.54
1 month	19.3	22.0	0.38
2 months	14.3	21.5	0.02
3 months	12.2	23.9	0.001
Mean fluorescein staining scores			
Baseline	3.3	4.4	0.23
3 months	1.3	3.9	0.01
Mean tear breakup time (in seconds)			
Baseline	9.9	7.4	0.40
1 month	11.2	5.3	0.24
2 months	10.3	6.4	0.19
3 months	10.8	6.1	0.08
Mean Schirmer scores (in millimeters of wetting at 5 minutes)			
Baseline	14.2	11.6	0.31
3 months	11.5	11.2	0.92

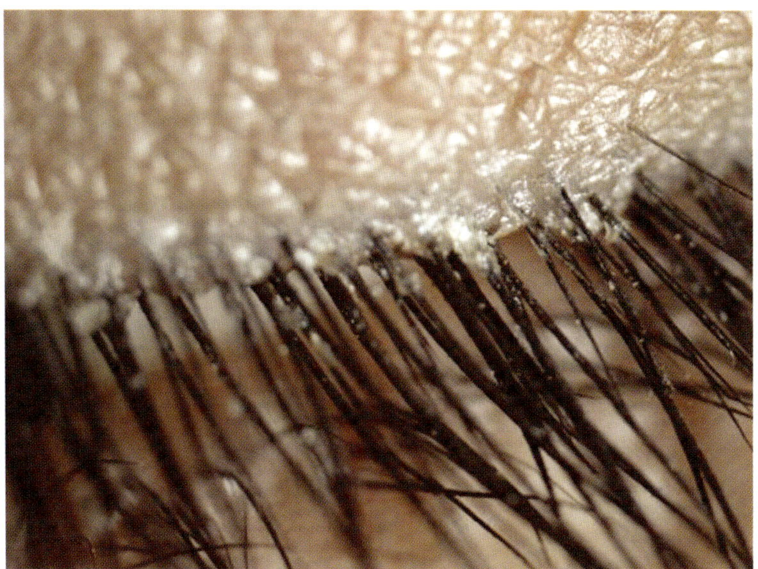

Fig. 1: Seborrheic blepharitis

Table 3. Number of patients in each lid margin vascular injection category at each visit for the tCSA and Refresh groups. Fisher' exact test was utilized after the table was collapsed for analysis. Data used is from the worse eye

	tCSA				*Refresh*				
Visit	*None*	*Mild*	*Moderate*	*Severe*	*None*	*Mild*	*Moderate*	*Severe*	*P value*
Baseline	0	2	8	6	0	3	2	12	0.34
1 month	1	4	3	7	0	2	5	9	0.14
2 months	0	4	4	5	0	2	4	9	0.20
3 months	3	4	2	3	0	0	5	9	0.001

Table 4. Number of patients with presence or absence of tarsal telangiectasis at each visit in the tCSA and Refresh groups. Fisher's exact test was utilized. Data used considers both eyes

	tCSA		*Refresh*		*P value*
Visit	*Present*	*Absent*	*Present*	*Absent*	
Baseline	16	0	16	1	0.52
1 month	15	0	16	0	—
2 months	13	0	13	2	0.28
3 months	8	4	14	0	0.03

It may be the most common cause of dry eye. Other sequelae which confront the ophthalmologist include chalazia, punctuate keratopathy, pannus, phlyctenules, recurrent conjunctivitis, and in severe cases, even corneal ulceration and endophthalmitis. Although blepharitis, in its many clinical forms, is one of the most common diseases seen by ophthalmologists, it remains a diagnostic and therapeutic challenge. The management of blepharitis is time consuming and frequently ineffective in part because little is known about the underlying pathophysiology of the condition, and in part because of the difficulty in categorizing an entity that frequently coexists with other ocular conditions, including ocular rosacea and keratoconjunctivitis sicca. Current treatment for meibomian gland dysfunction includes lid hygiene, oral tetracycline, doxycycline or minocycline, topical erthromycin or bacitracin, and topical corticosteroids.

Dietary supplementation with omega-3 fatty acids and their metabolites can play a significant therapeutic role in dry eye and meibomian gland dysfunction.

Underlying the pathophysiology of posterior blepharitis is meibomian gland dysfunction. The signs and symptoms of this disease are exacerbated by abnormalities in the lipid layer of the tear film, which is produced by the meibomian glands. Obstruction of the meibomian ducts causes accumulation of meibomian gland secretions, known as meibum. Accumulation of meibum within the meibomian gland can lead to inflammation of the gland and bacterial colonization. The colonizing bacteria have lipases that break the nonpolar wax and sterol esters into triglycerides and free fatty acids (polar lipids), thus altering the normal composition of the meibum. The polar lipids diffuse more easily through the aqueous layer and contaminate the mucin layer, making it hydrophobic. This causes the tear film to become unstable, and the surface of the eye becomes unwettable. The abnormal meibum has a melting point above the ocular surface temperature, in contrast to normal meibum, which has a melting point equal to or lower than the ocular surface temperature. The abnormal meibum therefore solidifies and obstructs the ducts, leading to further inflammation and perpetuating the vicious cycle.

Blepharitis and meibomianitis are two of the most common forms of ocular surface dysfunction. Their sequelae may lead to breakdown of the ocular surface including dry eye symptoms which are usually worse in the morning than in the evening. In addition these entities may be associated with staphylococcal immune disease such as cattarhal ulcers, phlyctenules, and inferior corneal staining. The lid manifestations include chalazia and hordeolum. Meibomianits and blepharitis are chronic diseases which often require long term therapy. A comprehensive approach in conjunction with a dermatologist may be necessary.

Dry Eye after Refractive Surgery

Belquiz A Nassaralla, João J Nassaralla (Brazil)

INTRODUCTION

The past two decades have seen changing trends in refractive surgery, with the evolution of several different procedures. Reshaping the anterior corneal surface by excimer laser photorefractive keratectomy (PRK), laser *in situ* keratomileusis (LASIK) or laser subepithelial keratomileusis (LASEK) has shown considerable promise for the surgical correction of refractive errors. In PRK, the refractive surgical ablation is performed on the corneal surface after epithelial debridement. During LASIK, a hinged lamellar corneal flap is raised with a mikrokeratome followed by ablation in the stromal bed and repositioning of the flap. A LASEK procedure involves preserving the extremely thin epithelial layer by lifting it from the eye's surface before laser energy is applied for reshaping. After LASEK, the epithelium is replaced on the eye's surface. Injuries to the ocular surface, occur with all three procedures.

Investigations

Corneal sensitivity is mediated by stromal nerves originating from the long ciliary nerves that penetrate the cornea in the middle and anterior stromal layers and run forward in a radial fashion toward the center of the cornea. These nerves form a network called the subepithelial plexus, beneath Bowman's layer, with free nerve endings in the corneal epithelium.

Ordinarily, the production of tears is monitored by the long ciliary nerves, which create a feedback loop that links the lacrimal glands to sensory receptors on the ocular surface. During flap creation and laser ablation, corneal nerves are transected, resulting in decreased corneal sensitivity and a transient neurotrophic cornea. As a result, it derails the reflex arc of lubrication. Clinical and experimental evidence shows that decreased afferent input from the corneal surface results in decreased tear secretion, decreased mucin production, decreased blink rate, and loss of trophic effects on surface cells, leading to dry eyes.

Dry eyes are a common complaint after refractive surgery, with an incidence ranging from 3% to 60%. Over the course of weeks to months to years, the nerves regenerate, and tear dynamics can return to normal.

Clinical Signs and Symptoms

Dry eye signs and symptoms after refractive surgery are usually transient but can cause significant discomfort for many patients; in rare cases, they persist

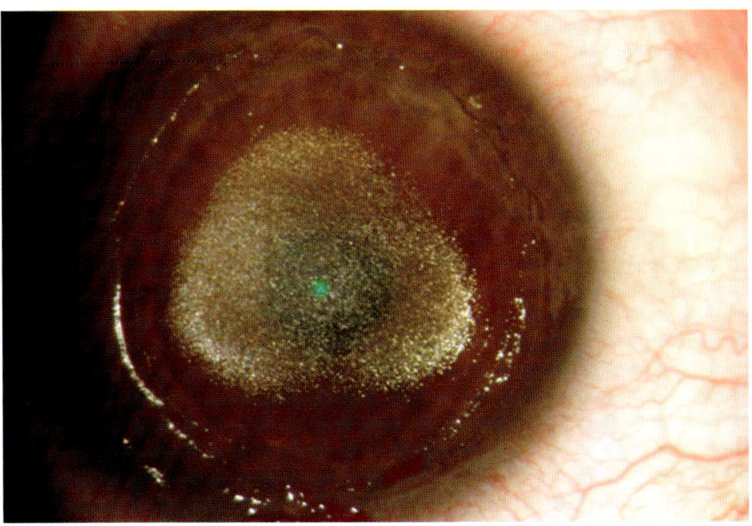

Fig. 1: Photorefractive keratectomy for myopia (PRK)

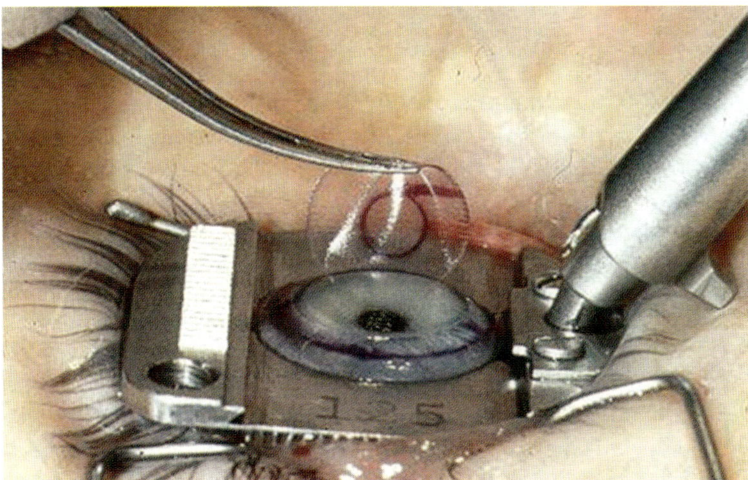

Fig. 2: Flap creation during LASIK. The superficial corneal flap is attached to the underlying cornea by hinge

for more than a year postoperatively. Several mechanisms for dry eye symptoms after refractive surgery have been proposed; these include damage to the goblet cells by suction-ring-induced pressure in LASIK, decreased corneal sensation and blink reflex, altered tear-film stability caused by changes in corneal curvature, inflammation caused by surgical trauma and medication-induced effects. Patients should be prepared for some postrefractive surgery dry eye symptoms, including pain, itchiness, redness, and bouts of blurred vision. Some patients with dry eye after refractive surgery will suffer more severe symptoms than others.

Chronic Dry Eye after LASIK

If postrefractive surgery dry eye symptoms persist, they can develop into chronic dry eye syndrome. In a certain percentage of patients, dry eye after refractive surgery may last for a prolonged period of time and can even become permanent. It is crucial that patients consider the potential for chronic dry eye after LASIK among the risks associated with refractive surgery.

Risk Factors for Dry Eye after Refractive Surgery

The risk factors for developing dry eye after refractive surgery include the preoperative level of myopia, the ablation depth, and the LASIK flap thickness. The increased risk of dry eye accompanying these factors may be explained by their effects on the corneal sensory nerves. The greater the amount of myopia that is treated, the greater the ablation depth that is required, and the greater the distance the surgically amputated nerve trunks will have to regenerate to reinervate the corneal epithelium following surgery.

Some patients with preexisting dry eyes are at risk for prolonged dry eyes that can cause significant symptoms and persist for many years following surgery. For this reason, it is important to screen for dry eye prior to refractive surgery and decide whether patients should be treated for dry eyes in advance.

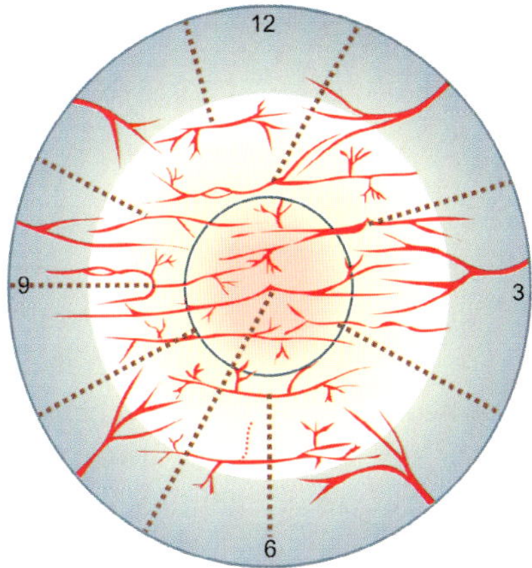

Fig. 3: Nerve fibers distribution in the cornea (Müller et al)

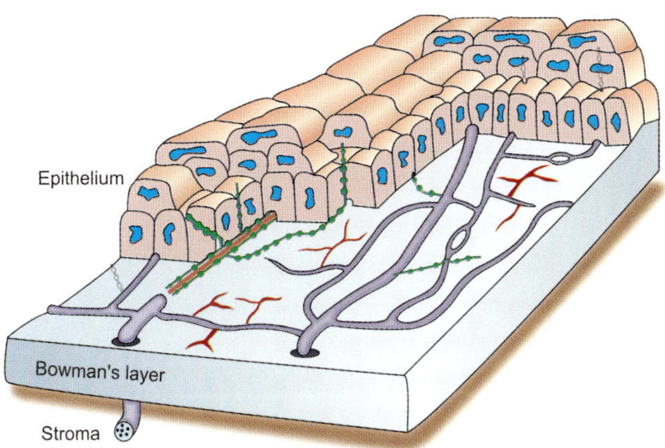

Fig. 4: Subepithelial plexus, beneath Bowman's layer, with free nerve endings in the corneal epithelium (Müller et al)

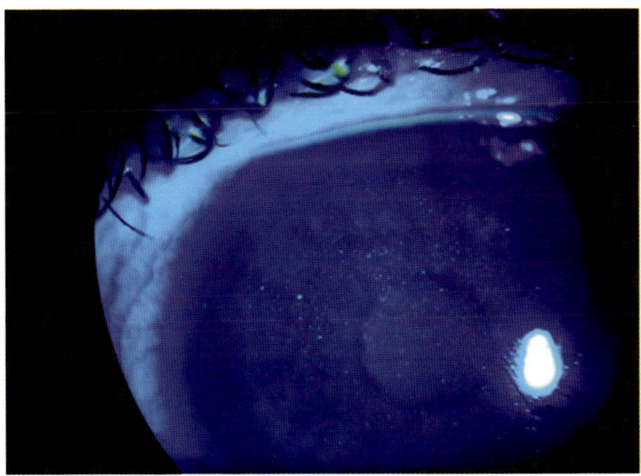

Fig. 5: Slight superficial punctate keratopathy 18 months after PRK for high myopia (-7.5 D)

Treatment

The selection of treatment modalities for patients with dry eye after refractive surgery depends largely on the severity of their disease. Mild cases may require no more than the use of artificial tear solutions. If the condition is not sufficiently managed with artificial tears, the use of sustained-release ocular lubricants may be considered. It may also be appropriate to modify the patient's environment in an effort to reduce evaporation of the tear film. Severe dry eye after refractive surgery is rare; however, in this case, therapy includes all of the above measures as well as punctal occlusion. The mainstay of treatment for dry eye is the use of topical tear substitutes (eye drops, gels, and ointments). Preservative-free tear substitutes are recommended to avoid toxicity in patients who use these agents frequently. Topical cyclosporine A has been proposed as a treatment for the inflammatory component of dry eye after refractive surgery. Although there are several dry eye treatment options available for postrefractive surgery dry eye, prevention should always be a top priority.

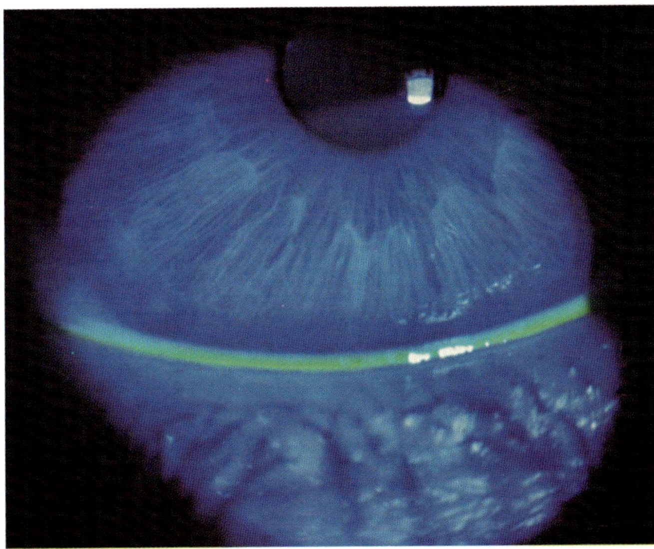

Fig. 6: Normal tear film. Notice an adequate tear lake between the lower lid and the cornea. The cornea is clear and there are no staining irregularities of the corneal epithelium

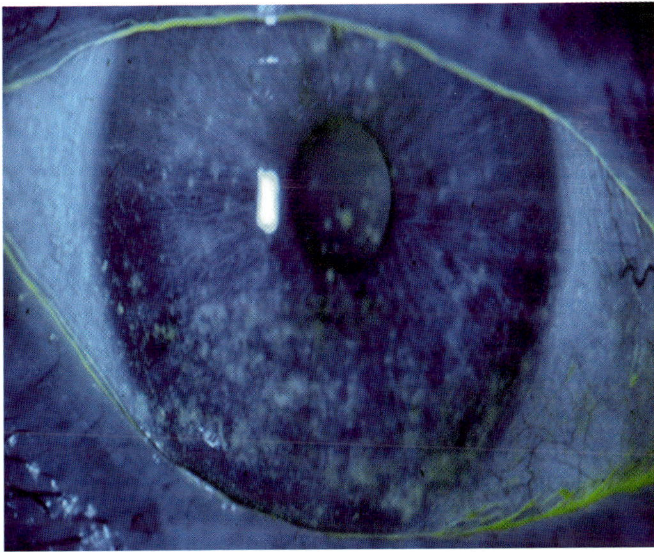

Fig. 7: Dry eye syndrome. Dry eyes can occur as both quantitative and qualitative disorder of tear production. In this example, there is a moderate superficial punctate keratopathy. This is a common finding in patients with dry eye syndrome

Computer Vision Syndrome and Dry Eye

Ashok Garg (India)

Introduction

Computer vision syndrome (CVS) is a condition affecting people working on the computer monitor. Considering the undisputable invasion of technology into our lives, this is a problem to reckon with.

Factors responsible for the development of CVS includes improper positioning like sitting too close to the computer monitor, poor room lighting and increased glare from the screen and infrequent blinking.

Computer Vision Syndrome (CVS) is a temporary condition resulting from focusing the eyes on a computer display for protracted, uninterrupted periods of time.

Pathophysiology

CVS is caused by decreased blinking reflex while working long hours focusing on computer screens. The normal blink rate in human eyes is 16-20 per minute. Studies have shown the blink rate to decrease to as low as 6-8 blinks/minute for persons working on the computer screen. This leads to dry eyes. Additionally, the near focusing effort required for such long hours puts strain on ciliary muscles of the eye. This induces symptoms of asthenopia and leads to a feeling of tiredness in the eyes after long hours of work. Some patients present with inability to properly focus on near objects after a short duration. This can be seen in people aged around 30-40 years of age, leading to a decrease in the accommodative focusing mechanisms of the eye. This can be a setting for early presbyopia.

The prints on a computer monitor, unlike in paper in made up of pixels which are small dots. Their edges are fuzzy giving rise to poor contrast and indistinct margins. The eye has to constantly refocus to keep the images sharp. This leads to strain of the eye muscles. Further, when sealed to close to the computer monitor, a lag of accommodation develops which the subject tries to adjust for and therefore it results in eye strain. Also, letters on computer monitors may be of variable light intensify thereby adding to the poor contrast levels. As already mentioned, poor room lighting and glare from the monitor also adds to the problem.

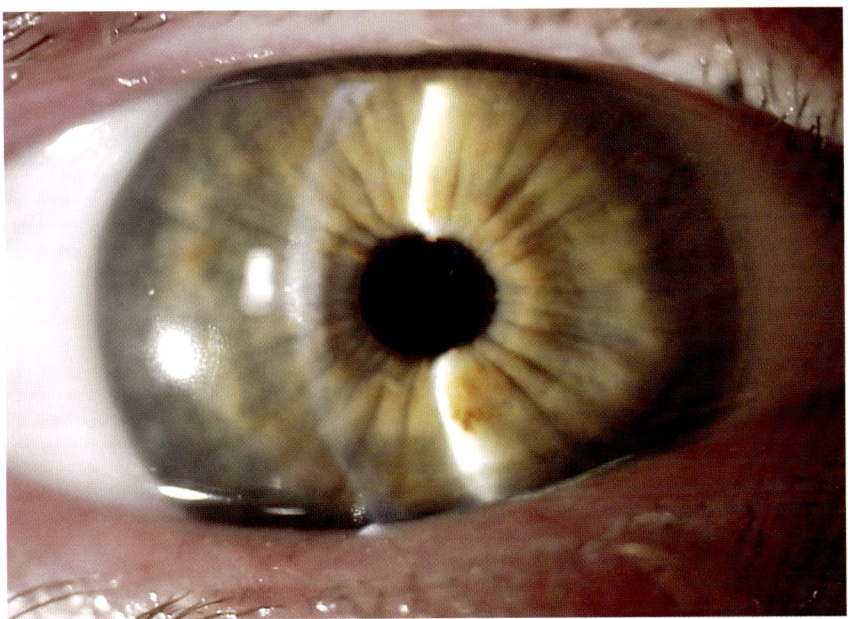

Fig. 1: Clinical photograph of marginal tear strip in dry eye patient due to computer vision syndrome

Clinical Signs and Symptoms

People who suffer from comptuer vision syndrome may experience the following symptoms:

- Dry eyes.
- Headache.
- Eye irritation.
- Foreign body sensation.
- Blurred vision.
- Light sensitivity.
- Double vision.
- Temporary inability to focus on a distant object (Pseudomyopia).
- Squint.
- Neck and shoulder pain.
- Halos appear around objects on the screen.
- Body Fatigue and tiredness.
- Driving/night vision difficulty.

It is characterized by symptoms of like burning, tearing, heaviness of lids, eye pain, headache etc.

Investigations

Investigations recommended for CVS patients are as follows :-

- Ocular examination.
- Direct ophthalmoscopy.
- Visual acuity
- Tonometry.

Differential Diagnosis

Dry eye symptoms in computer vision syndrome are usually confused with Dry eye post refractive surgery. In early grades symptoms may be similar. A thorough history of refractive surgery and ocular examination is mandatory in every case of dry eye to differentiate between the two clinical conditions.

Treatment

Dry eye is a major symptoms targeted in the therapy CVS. The use of over-the counter artificial tear solutions can reduce the effects of dry eye in CVS.

Asthenopic symtoms in the eye are responsible much of the morbidity in CVS. Proper rest to the eye and its muscles is recommended to relieve the associated eye strain. Various catch-phrases have been propagated for spreading awareness about giving rest while working on computers. A routinely recommended approach is a tonsciously blink the eyes every now and then (this helps replenish the tear film), and look out of the window into a distance object or the sky—(this provides rest to the ciliary muscles). One of the catch

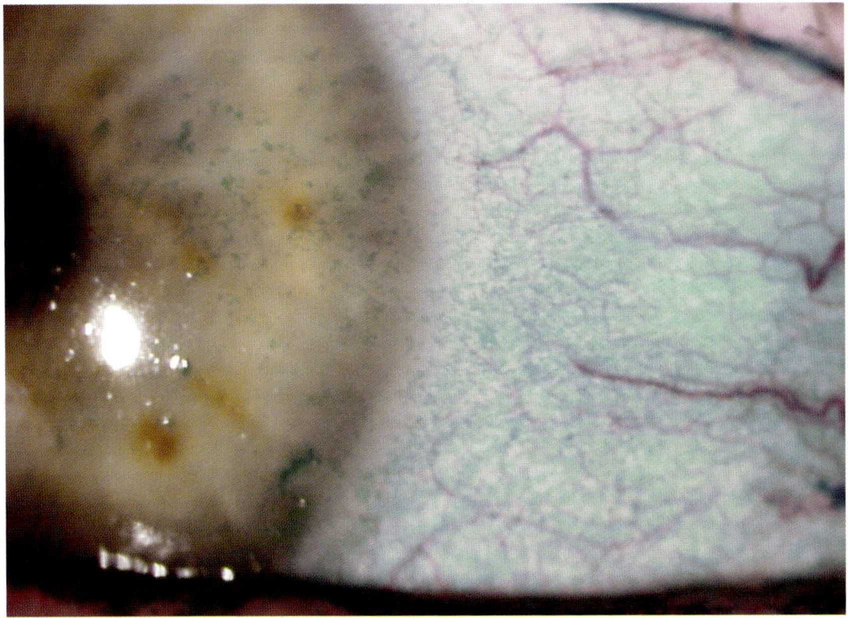

Fig. 2. Clinical photograph demonstrating lissamine green staining pattern of the interpalpebral conjunctiva and cornea in a patient with dry eye due to computer vision syndrome

phrases is the "20-20-20 rule" : every 20 minutes, focus the eyes on an object 20 feet (6 meters) away for 20 seconds. This basically gives a convenient distance and time frame for a person to follow the advice from the ophthalmologist. Otherwise, the patient is advised to close his/her eyes (which has a similar effect) for 20 seconds, at least half hour or even more frequently.

Decreased focusing capability is mitigated by wearing a small plus powered over-the-counter glasses (+1 to +1.50). It helps such patients regain their ability to focus on near objects. Other occupations such as tailors engaged in embroidery can experience similar symptoms and can be helped by the these glasses.

Preventive Measures

1. Maintain a distance of 20-26 inches from the computer monitor.
2. Computer monitor should be placed 10-15 degrees below eye level on straight gaze.
3. Use of antiglare screen.
4. Glarefree room lighting.
5. Position computer to avoid falling of direct sunlight and therefore minimize glare.
6. Take breaks from the computer screen.
7. Remember of blink at regular intervals.
8. Computer monitor may be placed horizontally on the table which will help the subject to read with his presbyopic correction.

Computer Glasses

Computer glasses here actually means glasses for the intermediate working distance where the monitor is placed. This has to be carefully determined according to the working distance of the patient after determining the distance and near corrections. One option would be to use a single vision lens which can be used only while working at the computer. However, this will cause difficulty to the subjects when he looks around. Therefore, the other option would be to use progressive lenses which will have corrections, for distance, near as well as for the intermediate working distance. These include lenses like the interview lenses, desktop lenses, access lenses and technical lenses.

Coating the computer glasses could also help in improving the visual quality. Antireflective coating is beneficial in individuals working in an environment where the amount of lighting can be controlled. For individuals working in offices with bright fluorescent lighting, 400 nm UV coating helps is absorbing blue light component of fluorescent light. Tinted glassed also may be of use in reducing the brightness of harsh fluorescent light.

Prognosis

With proper preventive care and precautions computer vision syndrome symptoms can be controlled to a greater extent. A proper counseling regarding pros and cons of computer is required in each patient. Prognosis is good.

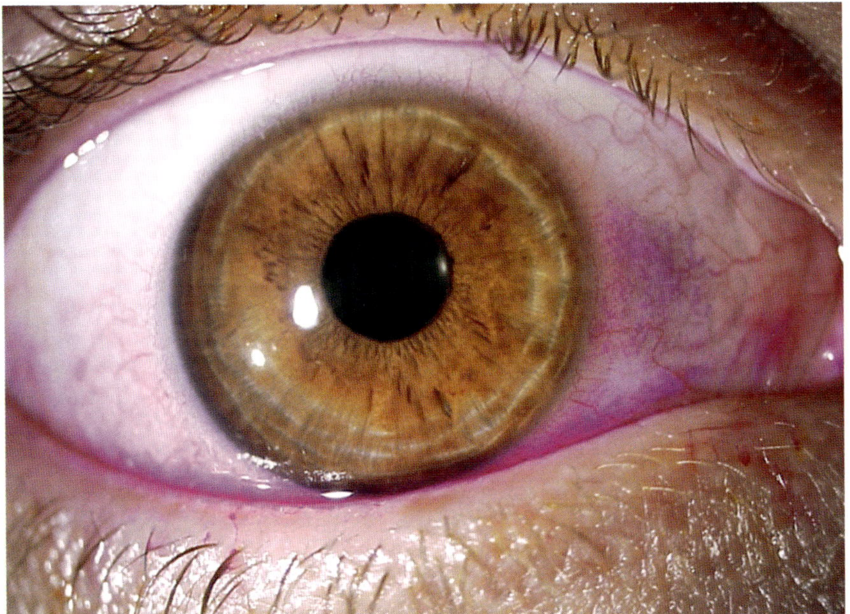

Fig. 3: Clinical photograph demonstrating rose bengal staining pattern of the nasal interpalpebral conjunctiva and cornea in a patient with dry eye due to computer vision syndrome

Pediatric Dry Eye

John D Sheppard (USA)

Dry eye is classically related to aging, androgen deficit, ocular surface inflammation, or systemic medication use. Thus, pediatric dry eye is exceedingly rare because these classic causes are by nature age related. The etiologic factors involved in pediatric dry eye differ significantly from adult disease, yet the principles of diagnosis and treatment remain the same. While the typical adult dry eye patient is a postmenopausal female with arthritis, the typical pediatric dry eye patient suffers from a congenital syndrome or a significant systemic disease requiring powerful sustained systemic medications. So many different classification systems exist for dry eye disease that determining a treatment regimen can almost become intimidating. It is important to analyze patients' potential for improvement and interventions that will actually be meaningful, and thereby determine the etiology of their dry eye.

Dry eye is an extremely common and often unrecognized disease. Due to a wide variety of presentations and symptoms, dry eye syndrome frustrates doctors as well as patients. The etiology is both elusive and multivariate. Because it is difficult to successfully identify a cause, it is also challenging to find efficacious therapy. New therapeutic options beyond the customary aqueous tear replacement so long the standard for ophthalmologists, optometrists, and rheumatologists has rendered the field of dry eye more exciting for clinicians. Since not all dry eye results from a lack of tears, but rather from instabilities in the tear film, even more therapeutic options excite pharmaceutical development teams.

Classification and Treatments

As a pediatric ophthalmologist attempts to classify dry eye patients, they must determine whether the condition is associated with a systemic disease such as arthritis, a congenital condition such as a cranial nerve disorder or Riley-Day syndrome, or with oral medications that may cause or exacerbate preexisting dry the eyes. Directed interventions regarding systemic factors may prove highly beneficial with relatively rapid ocular results, particularly in the context of anticipated elective eye surgery. These interventions may will have other benefits for the patients, including tightened supervision by their pediatricians, improvements in their oral regimens, or even.

Alternately, a young patient's dry eye may be due to either an aqueous or a mucin deficiency or, surprisingly commonly, a problem with the lipid layer in the eye related to blepharitis. In a patient with aqueous deficiency, the treatment strategy may often involve significant environmental manipulation and tear conservation efforts (such as punctal occlusion). To replace the tears in a beneficial way, I always use preservative-free tears or a vanishing preservative such as the refresh line with sodium chlorite (Purite), because the cost differential is minimal and patients respond well to these treatments. Many patients develop sensitivities to preserved tears, and many over-the-counter products available contain vasoconstrictors that are deleterious in both the short- and long-term.

Many cases of pediatric dry eye have a combined mechanism problem, such as a lid and neurologic deficiency coupled with an aqueous deficiency. Another example might be an evaporative dry eye due to a dysfunction of the lipid layer in their tears coupled with a structural lid dysfunction. Therefore, a multi-faceted interventional strategy may be beneficial. This approach would involve changing the diet or adding omega-3 fatty acids to the diet, treating the underlying lid disease with warm compresses or lid scrubs, adding nonaqueous components to the tear film that may be beneficial such as the oil emulsion found in refresh endura tears, Soothe tears, or Systane tears, and conserving any evaporative tear loss. In addition, structural changes in the lid architecture may require oculoplastic surgical intervention.

Diagnosis of Pediatric Dry Eye

First and foremost, obtaining a good patient history will provide useful clues for the diagnosis of dry eye. Though a child suffering from dry eye may not complain of dryness, the child will probably describe the presence of other ocular irritation symptoms such as burning, scratchiness, itching and, rarely, photophobia. Parents may have noted an irritable and/or moderately red eye and that the child's symptoms change with different environmental conditions.

For example, symptoms may worsen during a vacation in a place with dry weather or during an airplane trip. Question parents whether the child sleeps with his eyes partially open at night. Also inquire about the presence of diseases involving the joints, skin, guts and respiratory system. Note the child's current systemic or topical medication schedule. Finally, note any form of radiation therapy or chemotherapy, as these can damage many of the glands involved in tear secretion.

Diagnosis of dry eye usually necessitates a wide variety of tests, many of which are difficult in children. Thus, first implement the least invasive tests in the shortest possible time and then progress to other tests. The most useful information comes from external inspection and from a basic biomicroscopic exam:

- Assess blink rates
- Assess lid architecture
- Determine whether the blink completely covers the ocular surface
- Examine the child for lid/orbital abnormalities, skin lesions and scars
- Slit lamp biomicroscopy
- Check for blepharitis, meibomitis, tear film debris, mucus filaments, superficial punctuate keratitis
- Assess the tear meniscus
- Tear film break-up time
- Vital stains: fluorescein, rose bengal and lissamine green staining
- Schirmer

- Tear osmolarity in experimental settings (>312 mOsm/Kg diagnostic)
- Epiphora
- Rule out nasolacrimal duct obstruction
- Rule out subtarsal or corneal foreign bodies
- Rule out conjunctivitis
- Rule out glaucoma
- Rule out crocodile tears
- Rule out contact lens-associated epiphora

Both historical and examination based data will produce valuable information, which is beneficial because a number of conditions can affect one or more layers of the tear film and can cause dry eye in infants, children or young adults.

Keratic sensitivity, or corneal sensation should be assessed when trigeminal nerve dysfunction is suspected (Heigle 1996). A laboratory and clinical evaluation for autoimmune disorders should be considered for patients with significant dry eyes, other signs and symptoms of an autoimmune disorder such as dry mouth, rash, arthritis, colitis, renal dysfunction, or a family history of an autoimmune disorder.

Etiology of Pediatric Dry Eye

Pediatric dry eye parallels to some extent the more unusual causes of dry eye in adults. This includes deficiencies in each of the three tear film layers, as well as other components of the ocular surface. The tear film, which consists of the lipid, aqueous, and mucin layers, performs a specific role in protecting the ocular surface. If one component is deficient, then the tear film destabilizes more rapidly than normal, resulting in exposed ocular surface epithelium or basement membrane. Prolonged or repeated exposure creates the uncomfortable symptoms of dry eye as well as damaged conjunctival and corneal epithelium. The entire therapeutic strategy revolves around preservation of the intact ocular surface unit, important interactive system, with every component collaborating to produce central corneal clarity for clear vision:

1. Tri-layer tear film and its many constituents
2. Lids, meibomian glands, and cilia
3. Lacrimal gland, minor lacrimal glands, and accessory secretory apparatus
4. Nasolacrimal drainage system, including puntae, canaliculi, lacrimal sac, and duct
5. 5th Cranial nerve (Trigeminal)
6. 7th Cranial nerve (Facial)
7. Conjunctival epithelium (17 fold greater surface area than the corneal epithelium)
8. Corneal epithelium

Tear secreting glands and the ocular surface function as an integrated unit to refresh the tear supply and to clear used tears (Stern 1998). Disease or dysfunction of this unit results in ocular irritation and dry eye syndrome. Decreased tear secretion and clearance initiate an inflammatory response on the ocular surface, and research suggests that this inflammation plays a role in the pathogenesis of dry eye (Pflugfelder 2000).

Significant ocular surface dysfunction may develop from aging, a decrease in supportive factors (such as androgen hormones), systemic inflammatory diseases (such as rheumatoid arthritis), ocular surface diseases (such as herpes zoster ophthalmicus), surgery that disrupts the trigeminal afferent sensory nerves, including laser *in situ* keratomileusis, extracapsular cataract extraction, or penetrating keratoplasty, and systemic diseases or medications that disrupt the efferent cholinergic nerves that stimulate tear secretion (Bacman 2001).

The causes of pediatric dry eye are many, and require a high index of suspicion in less than obvious cases. These causes include mucin, lipid, aqueous, lid, and neurologic deficiencies.

- *Mucin deficiency.* Goblet cells are the primary producers of tear mucin. Ocular surface epithelial cells also secrete certain types of mucins. Deficiency of tear mucin destabilizes the tear film. Stevens-Johnson syndrome, acid and alkali chemical burns, pemphigoid or linear IgA deficiency in older children are the common causes of mucin deficiency. In the developing world, vitamin A deficiency or xerophthalmia and trachoma are the most important conditions that affect ocular surface mucin.

- *Lipid deficiency.* The tarsal meibomian glands produce the anterior oily layer of the tear film. A decrease in tear lipid layer promotes a faster evaporation of the tear film. The most common causes of tear lipid deficiency include blepharitis and meibomitis. Radiation therapy can cause meibomian gland loss, leading to a serious deficiency in the tear lipid layer.

- *Aqueous tear deficiency.* The aqueous layer of the tear film lies in between the lipid and mucin layers forming most of the tear film. The aqueous layer also dissolves tear mucins, making it more of a gel-like layer. The main lacrimal gland produces 90% of the aqueous layer, with essential input from the corneal nerve plexus and cranial nerve V. Classic aqueous tear deficiency, also known as keratoconjunctivitis sicca or chronic dry eye disease (CDED), is more a disease of the middle age, or in the rare case of progeria. Sjögren's syndrome occurs when CDED is associated with systemic autoimmune disease. Rarely seen in children, polyarteritis nodosa, Wegener's granulomatosis, acquired immunodeficiency syndrome (AIDS) and iatrogenic immunodeficiency following bone marrow transplantation create CDED.
- Lid deformity may result from previous injury, surgery, or congenital malformations. Patients with multiple cranial nerve abnormalities, Crouzon's syndrome, Alport syndrome, or Goldenhar's syndrome may have exposure keratopathy from the secondary evaporative dry eye. Localized drying of the exposed palpebral surface can occur because of lagophthalmos, proptosis or facial palsy and even following ocular surgeries such as those for strabismus.
- Neurotrophic disease occurs with cranial facial malformations, cranial nerve abnormalities, and a number of other congenital syndromes including

congenital alacrima (or hypolacrima), corneal hypesthesia associated with decreased reflex tearing, familial glucocorticoid deficiency (Allgrove syndrome), ectopic lacrimal gland development, lacrimal fistulas, lacrimal tissue with dermoid cysts, and familial dysautonomia (Riley-Day syndrome).

CDED symptoms may be exacerbated by systemic medications such as diuretics, antihistamines, anticholinergics, antidepressants, HMG co-A reductase inhibitors such as Zocor or Lipitor, chemotherapy, systemic retinoids, and isotretinoin (Moss 2000). Dry eye also may be made worse by environmental factors that include exogenous irritants and allergens, as well as wind, drafts, air conditioning, heating, and reduced humidity.

Systemic diseases associated with dry eye include Sjögren's syndrome, rosacea, viral infections such as acquired immune deficiency syndrome (Lucca 1990), hepatitis C (Abe 1999, Siagris 2002), primary and persistent Epstein-Barr virus infections (Pflugfelder 1987, Merayo-Lloves 2001, Pflugfelder 1993), cystic fibrosis (Sheppard 1989, Mrugacz 2004) and graft versus host disease in recipients of allogenic bone marrow or stem cell transplants (Ogawa 1999).

Sjögren's syndrome is a common autoimmune condition and may in childhood. It is described both as primary and secondary to other autoimmune diseases such as rheumatoid arthritis or lupus. In Sjögren's syndrome an inflammatory cellular infiltration of the lacrimal gland leads to deficient tear production. Rosacea is associated with posterior blepharitis, poor tear quality, accelerated tear film break up time (TBUT), and increased tear evaporation. Aqueous tear deficiency may develop in conditions such as lymphoma, sarcoidosis (Drosos 1989), hemochromatosis, and amyloidosis (Fox 1994) that result in infiltration of the lacrimal gland and replacement of the secretory acini. Sjögren's may also be secondary to sarcoidosis, cancer, or severe atopic disease.

Ocular cicatricial pemphigoid (OCP) and Stevens-Johnson syndrome (SJS) produce tear deficiency due to inflammation, scarring, and destruction of the conjunctival goblet cells. Children with hereditary basement membrane or bullous cutaneous diseases mimic the changes seen in OCP. Atopy may produce dry eye due to blepharitis and eczema, or systemic antihistamine use. Children may develop vernal keratoconjunctivitis and later become severely atopic.

Important ocular surface conditions associated with dry eye include eyelid malposition, lagophthalmos, trichiasis, entropion, ectropion, seborrhea, and blepharitis, as well as neuromuscular disorders that affect blinking, such as Bell's palsy (Deuschl 1998). Local trauma, including orbital surgery, radiation, periorbital hematoma, and blunt injury, also may cause dry eye.

Advanced conjunctival squamous metaplasia and punctate epithelial erosions of the conjunctiva and cornea develop in many patients who have moderate to severe dry eye. These changes are reversible if treated relatively early in the course of CDED. Rarely, patients with severe dry eye will develop complications such as ocular surface keratinization; corneal ulceration, scarring, thinning (ectasia), or neovascularization; microbial keratitis; and sterile corneal keratolysis, with possible perforation and severe visual loss.

RILEY-DAY SYNDROME (FAMILIAL DYSAUTONOMIA)

The Riley-Day syndrome is an inherited disorder that affects nerve function throughout the body. Symptoms are present at birth and grow worse over time. It is also known as familial dysautonomia, hereditary sensory and autonomic neuropathy - type III. Yatzu and Zussman introduced the eponymic term "Riley-Day syndrome".

Riley-Day syndrome is inherited as an autosomal recessive trait, thus inheriting a defective copy of the target gene from each parent. It is seen most often in people of Eastern European Jewish ancestry (Ashkenazi Jews), where the incidence is 1 in 3,700. The disease is caused by mutation of the *IKBKAP* gene on chromosome 9. It is rare in the general population.

Symptoms include poor growth, feeding difficulties, breath holding, sweating while eating, protracted emesis, low muscle tone, hypotonia, seizures, lack of responsiveness to painful stimuli, absent corneal sensation, recurring bouts of fever, recurring bouts of high blood pressure, poor coordination - unsteady gait, an unusually smooth tongue surface, decreased taste, diarrhea/ constipation, severe scoliosis, and skin blotching.

Newborns and infants with this condition have feeding problems and develop pneumonia caused by breathing food into their airways. Vomiting and sweating spells begin as the infant matures. Young children may also have breath-holding spells that produce unconsciousness, since they can hold their breath for long enough to pass out without feeling the discomfort that normal children would.

The sine quo non of Riley-Day syndrome is insensitivity to pain. This leads to unnoticed injuries or injuries that might not have occurred had the child sensed discomfort. Children do not feel the normal sensations that generally warn of impending injury, such as drying of the eyes, pressure over pressure points, and chronic rubbing and chaffing. Bone and skin pain, including burns, are also poorly perceived. However, they can feel visceral (internal) pain, like menstrual cramps. Intelligence is in the normal range.

Diagnosis of Riley-Day syndrome is made through identification of the classic signs and symptoms, and by molecular genetic testing of the *IKBKAP* gene located on chromosome 9. The detection rate in the Ashkenazi Jewish population is >99%. Such testing is used for diagnosis, carrier detection, and prenatal diagnosis. Diagnostic signs include:

- Absence of axon flare response after intradermal histamine injection.
- Absence of overflow tears with emotional crying
- Tiny pupils after administering methacholine or pilocarpine into the eye
- Parents of Ashkenazi Jewish ancestry
- Dry eye and dry mouth
- Neurotrophic keratitis
- Decreased deep tendon reflexes: In 95% of patients, knee jerk is absent

Treatment may include protection from injury treatment of aspiration pneumonia, anticonvulsant therapy if seizures are present, liquid tears and bethanechol to prevent drying of eyes and the oral mucous membranes, and anti-emetics may be used to control emesis. Postural hypotension can be managed with increased fluid and salt intake, caffeine, and waist-high elastic stockings. With advances in diagnosis and treatment, survival continues to improve. Currently, a newborn with Riley-Day has a 50% chance of reaching age 30.

Complications of Riley-Day syndrome include crises, which may be accompanied or heralded by a number of symptoms. These symptoms of "autonomic crises" occur in about 40% of patients and include excessive sweating of the head and torso, blotching of the face and torso, mottling of the hands and feet, hypertension and tachycardia, nausea/vomiting, severe dysphagia/drooling, irritability, insomnia, and worsening of muscle tone.

Detection may be indicated in individuals of Eastern European Jewish background and families with a history of Riley-Day syndrome when considering having children. These families can seek genetic counseling to discuss risk and undergo testing where appropriate.

Genetic testing is now very accurate for Riley-Day syndrome and may be used for diagnosis of affected individuals and also for carrier detection and prenatal diagnosis.

Management of Severe Dry Eye

The centerpiece of dry eye therapy has always been aqueous tear replacement with artificial tears. Recent thinking extends therapeutic options well beyond this palliative course. Currently available tear substitutes replicate and replace tears, but their use is only briefly temporary, helping manage dry eye through short-term symptomatic relief. Anti-inflammatories reduce ocular surface effects of the underlying cause of dry eye, thereby for the first time treating the disease and not the symptoms. Secretagogues address specific deficiencies in the tear film. In addition, other classes of treatments include nutritionals, hormonal agents, anti-evaporatives, mucomimetics and improved polymers. Thus, numerous strategies are involved with the treatment of chronic dry eye disease and, while treatment algorithms and priorities differ between patients and practitioners, the approximate order of intervention presents as follows:

1. Preserved artificial tear substitutes
2. Vanishing preservative tear substitutes
3. Preservative free tear substitutes (in Single Dose Units, or SDUs)
4. Environmental control (wind, humidity, allergens, fumes, smoke, vapors)
5. Ocular surface antiinflammatory (Restasis, Loteprednol etabonate)
6. Systemic medication control (less diuretics, anti-histamines, anti-depressants, HMG co-A reductase inhibitors)
7. Punctal occlusion (collagen, plastic or silicone, cautery)
8. Oral secretagogues (Pilocarpine, Salagen, Evoxac)
9. New medication categories (Androgens, Diquafosol, 5-HETE)

Pediatricians should also keep in mind that sometimes the physical findings do not correspond to the patient's state of mind or complaints. Some patients' eyes may look awful but not feel very irritated, while others' feel terrible but look relatively healthy. Of greatest concern are these more paradoxical patients, since those without symptoms may also be neurotrophic, with clearly inadequate corneal sensation. Recent revelations regarding the interactive processes occurring between the ocular surface tissues and the corneal nerves indicate that neurotrophic corneas perpetrate the cycle of aqueous deficiency, inflammation, and further decreases in beneficial neurosensory output and epithelial neuropeptide production. In addition, if a patient has significant punctate keratopathy, or severe conjunctival disease as evidenced by lissamine green staining, intervention is indicated regardless of how he or she feels. Those patients with significant epithelial damage are very alarming, since irregular astigmatism, epithelial healing defects, and bacterial keratitis are more likely.

Poor tear quality results from ocular surface inflammation, meibomian dysfunction, evaporative tear loss, neurotrophic down-regulation, and mucin deficiency in addition to aqueous hyposecretion. Thus, a multitude of strategies to improve the condition of the ocular surface in dry eye have arisen. The litany of therapeutic pharmaceutical options can be divided into 6 categories:

1. Antiinflammatory topical agents:
   a. Cyclosporin (Restasis, Allergan)
   b. Tacrolimus (FK506, Protopic, Fujisawa)
   c. Pimecrolimus (Elidel, Novartis) research halted due to potential carcinogenesis of the topical compound
   d. Rebamipide (Novartis, Otsuka)
   e. NSAIDs (nonsteroidal antiinflammatory drugs) including Ketoprofen (Acular), Nepafenac (Nevanac), and Bromfenac (Xibrom)
2. Topical steroid agents:
   a. Loteprednol Etabonate (Bausch & Lomb)
   b. Rimexolone (Alcon)
   c. Fluorometholone (Allergan)
   d. Prednisolone Acetate (Allergan)
3. Secretagogues:
   a. INS-365 (Diquafosol 2%, Inspire)
   b. 15(S)-HETE (Alcon)
   c. Pilocarpine (Salagen, MGI)
   d. Cevimeline (Evoxac, Daiichi)
4. Oral nutritional agents:
   a. HydroEyes (Science based health)
   b. Theratears Nutritional (Advanced therapeutics)
   c. Fish oil, Cod liver oil, Flaxseed oil (Generic)
5. Topical androgens (1% Testosterone, Allergan)
6. Improved polymers:
   a. Refresh Endura (Allergan)
   b. Systane (Systane)
   c. Sooth (Alimera sciences, distributed by vistakon)
   d. Sodium Hyaluronate ("Healon" tears, santen and others)

It is essential to aggresively treat dry eye in cases of drug-induced dry eye or vitamin A deficiency. Management of blepharitis and meibomitis by teaching the child's parents to massage the child's lids and to clean the lid margins using diluted baby shampoo or a commerical lid scrub preparation (Eye Scrub, Ocusoft). Application of an antibiotic/corticosteroid combination ointment to the lid margin or topical combination antibioticsteroid drops (Zylet, Tobradex, Blephamide) may arrest further complications if given during the early stages of treating blepharitis.

Environmental control is important to dry eye management. Prevent tear loss by avoiding dry climates, humidifying living and sleeping areas, vacationing in humid locations and considering punctual occlusion, if necessary. Permanent occlusion is not recommended in most pediatric cases, so collagen or silicone plastic plugs are often employed

Vanishing preservative (refresh plus, refresh liquigel, celluvisc, genteal, Systane Free) or preservative-free artificial tears/rewetting agents are the most frequently used treatment for CDED. Rewetting agents are important components of the base compound.

In more severe cases, consider tarsorrhaphy especially when associated with corneal hypesthesia. Lid padding, taping, or cyano-acrylate glue temporary tarsorrhaphy may be urgently needed when the cornea is exposed, though these require careful execution and postoperative control. Sometimes it is beneficial to treat excess mucus production with 10% acetylcysteine drops q.i.d. Topical restasis (Cyclosporine 0.05% emulsion) is now successfully prescribed to children who have Sjögren's syndrome.

Multiple Concomitant Therapies

Any patient with dry eye, whether he or she has Sjögren's syndrome or a non-Sjögren's associated systemic inflammatory disease, will respond to anti-inflammatory therapy. Therefore, the first action is to place the patient on some type of antiinflammatory therapy, be it a safe steroid such as loteprednol (Lotemax; Bausch and Lomb, Rochester, NY) or cyclosporine emulsion (Restasis). Both are safe for children when conscientiously supervised by an experienced clinician. The antiinflammatory approach has drastically altered the original paradigm: aggressive tear conservation strategy first with punctal occlusion is now secondary, while antiinflammatory treatment comes first so as not to trap poor-quality or artificial tears.

At virginia eye consultants, we are in the midst of a Restasis cessation study to evaluate the necessity for continued use of Restasis and examine the effects of discontinuation of Restasis after at least one year of usage. Early results indicate minor regressions in signs but significant deterioration in symptoms after Restasis cessation. These symptoms seem to improve after reinstitution of Restasis therapy. There has been considerable difficulty in patient recruitment for this study because most of the women we recruit do not want to stop their Restasis therapy.

Filamentary keratopathy can be treated with debridement of the filaments or application of topical mucolytic agents, including specially prepared sterile n-acetyl cysteine (10% Mucomist) drops. Soft contact lenses are also effective in preventing recurrence of filamentary keratopathy, but may be poorly tolerated if the patient has severely dry eyes. If the patient has associated neurotrophic keratopathy, contact lenses should be avoided (AAO 2003).

Patients with systemic disease such as primary Sjögren's syndrome or connective tissue disease such as rheumatoid arthritis should be managed in conjunction with the appropriate medical specialist. Antiinflammatory or immunosuppressive therapy may be appropriate for patients with a systemic disease such as rheumatoid arthritis (AAO 2003). Surgical treatment is generally reserved for patients with symptomatic, moderate, or severe disease, and for whom medical treatment has been inadequate or impractical (AAO 2003).

Aqueous enhancement by means of punctal occlusion can be accomplished surgically with semipermanent plugs (silicone or thermal labile polymer) that are lodged at the punctal orifice (AAO 1997, AAO 1998, AAO 2003), or by permanent occlusion with thermal or laser cautery. Prior to permanent or semi-permanent punctual occlusion, temporary slowly dissolving collagen punctual plugs can be readily placed in most patients lower punctums. Because an occluded punctum can trap inflammatory mediators, inflammation should logically be controlled prior to punctal occlusion. Nevertheless, many patients with successful or partially helpful punctual occlusion procedures obtain additional benefit from subsequent or primary initiation of topical anti-inflammatory therapy.

Eyelid abnormality as a result of blepharitis, trichiasis, or lid malposition (e.g., lagophthalmos, entropion/ectropion) should be corrected prior to permanent punctal occlusion (AAO 2003).

Semipermanent plugs are reversible if the patient develops symptoms of epiphora, while cautery is not readily reversible. Therefore, a trial occlusion with collagen plugs should be performed first. To minimize the possibility of epiphora, no more than one punctum should be cauterized in each eye. The lower punctum is preferable for occlusion, as it is usually larger and more accessible. It is important to inspect the upper punctum first for both patency and integrity, before occluding the lower punctum. In general, laser cautery is not as effective as thermal cautery in achieving permanent, complete occlusion and is more expensive.

Pediatric Refractive Surgery

Refractive surgery has been more readily adapted to the pediatric population, particularly where amblyopia is threatened. The preoperative approach dictates that one always treat a patient's dry eye problem before performing surgery. This strategy disappoints those patients who impulsively seek urgent refractive surgery before a particular date or event, but it is necessary for an optimal surgical outcome. Healing an ocular surface can take 3 months or longer in an adult, but fortunately less time in children, depending on how severe the damage has been, which includes reinnervation of the ablated surface in the case or PRK. Restasis and/or a steroid remain important. If the patient's inflammatory response is severe, induce topical therapy with initial steroid treatment and then switch to Restasis for long-term maintenance. Although Restasis reaches its maximal effect at 6 months, by 1 to 3 months of use, most patients are ready for most types of refractive surgery. Epi-Lasek may present the biggest challenge to the ocular surface epithelium.

There is no absolute standard postoperative regimen, because every patient is different. Titrate my postoperative therapy to the patient's needs. Depending on the patient's response, underlying risk, and the results of initial Schirmer's testing and corneal staining, tailor an antiinflammatory therapy for each individual. Ofcourse, the surgeon must also consider such issues as the amount of expense and interference with the patient's daily lifestyle from frequent medication administration. Because corneal nerve regrowth takes approximately 6 weeks in the PRK patient and as long as 6 months in the LASIK patient, the surgeon can maximize refractive patients' therapy for at least that long under reasonably close observation.

Treatment Persistence

The clinician always administer long-term regimens according to the confines of patient compliance and tolerability. Also, remain committed to maintaining individuals on antiinflammatories for their entire lifetimes if needed, acknowledging the chronic nature of keratitis sicca. It is quite reassuring to be able to use a therapy such as cyclosporine that has no known long-term deleterious effects, even in children, without any detectable systemic absorption. Although there is always minor concern as to the long-term safety of the loteprednol steroid in low doses, the initial FDA trials and anecdotal reports have all shown minimal toxicity in long-term patients. In addition, the lower strength Alrex (0.2%) can be utilized successfully in many cases for added protection.

Children with dry eye require careful observation, diligent care, and dedicated parents. Most conditions in childhood will not resolve with time, so the establishment of outstanding therapeutic habits is central to vision preservation.

Chapter EIGHT

Hyphema

Earl R Crouch
Eric Crouch (USA)

Introduction

Blunt trauma to the eye may result in injury to the iris, angle structures, and other intraocular structures. Hemorrhage into the anterior chamber, or hyphema, is common in children. Generally, a projectile that strikes the eyeball produces the hyphema. A great variety of projectile missiles and objects have been commonly found to cause hyphema including balls, rocks, projectile toys, air gun, paint balls, bungee cords, and the human fist. With the increase of child abuse, fists and belts have started to play a prominent role. Boys are involved in three-fourths of cases.

Rarely, spontaneous hyphemas occur and may be confused with traumatic hyphemas. Spontaneous hyphemas are secondary to neovascularization, ocular neoplasms (retinoblastoma), and vascular anomalies (juvenile xanthogranuloma). Vascular tufts that exist at the pupillary border have been implicated in spontaneous hyphema. A traumatic hyphema may be graded by measuring the height of the layered hyphema in the anterior chamber in millimeters. A hyphema is an ocular emergency and should be referred immediately.

History

An exact history of the trauma should be obtained to assess the velocity involved, which in turn may indicate the extent of ocular damage that may have occurred. Inquiry must be made to determine if visual acuity changes occurred immediately after the injury. Flashing lights are often seen at the instant of injury and indicate irritation of the retina, as any message to the brain from the retina is perceived as light. Persistent blurred vision is indicative of a more serious injury. It may indicate blood in the anterior chamber that is suspended in the aqueous humor. Free-floating blood in the anterior chamber can generally not be appreciated by direct ophthalmoscopy. A slitlamp is necessary to observe the suspended red blood cells in the anterior chamber.

Examination

A hyphema may be graded by the following system: grade 1—layered blood occupying less than 1/3 the anterior chamber, grade 2—blood filling 1/3 to 1/2 of the anterior chamber, grade 3—blood filling more than 1/2 but less than the total anterior chamber, and grade 4—total clotted hyphema filling the anterior chamber, often referred to as an blackball or "eight ball" hyphema. Alternatively, hyphemas may be graded by measuring the height of the hyphema in millimeters from the inferior limbus. These grading systems enable the ophthalmologist to monitor the progress of the hyphema resolution.

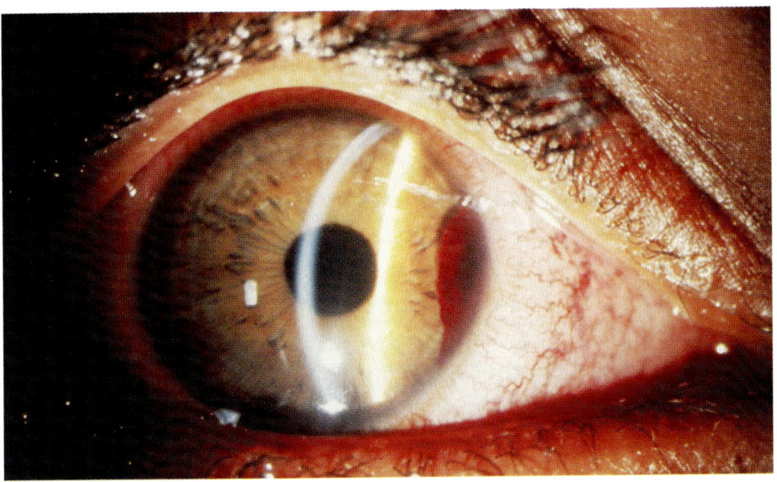

Fig. 1: Traumatic hyphema

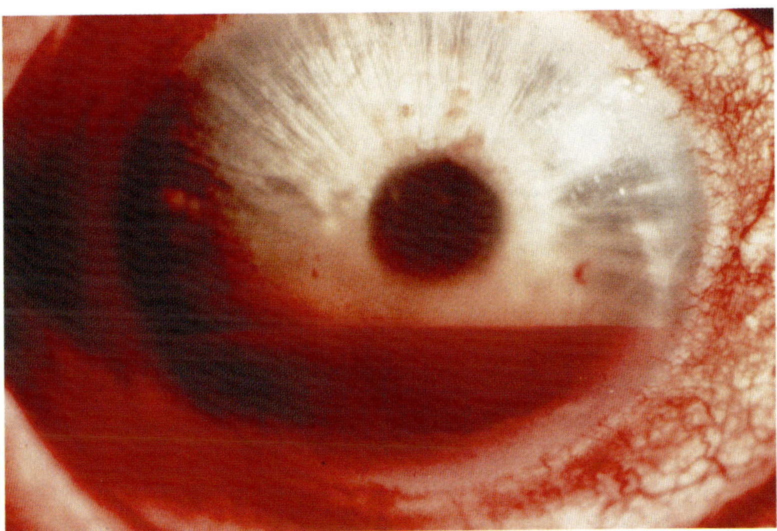

Fig. 2: Traumatic hyphema—grade 2

Secondary hemorrhage associated with traumatic hyphema results in a markedly worse prognosis. Eventual visual recovery to an acuity of 20/50 (6/15) or better occurs in approximately 64% of patients with secondary hemorrhage compared with 79.5% of those in whom no rebleeding occurred. True secondary bleeding into the anterior chamber is indicated by an obvious increase in the amount of blood in the anterior chamber. Secondary hemorrhage occurs in approximately 22% of all hyphema patients (range 7 to 38%). The rate of secondary hemorrhage is Caucasians is between 8-10%. The incidence of secondary hemorrhage is higher in hyphemas that occupy 50% or more of the anterior chamber.

There are specific complications of traumatic hyphema. They are directly attributed to the retention of blood in the anterior chamber and include posterior synechiae, peripheral anterior synechiae, corneal blood staining, and optic atrophy. Optic atrophy may result from either acute, transiently elevated intraocular pressure or chronically elevated intraocular pressure.

Posterior synechiae may form in patients with traumatic hyphema. They are secondary to iritis or iridocyclitis. Posterior synechiae are uncommon in patients treated medically but occur more frequently in patients who have had surgical evacuation of the hyphema. Peripheral anterior synechiae occur frequently in medically treated patients in whom the hyphema has remained in the anterior chamber for a prolonged period (9 days or more).

Corneal blood staining occurs primarily in patients who have a total hyphema and associated elevation of intraocular pressure. Factors that may increase the likelihood of corneal blood staining are: (i) initial state of the corneal endothelium (decreased viability resulting from trauma or advanced age, e.g. cornea guttata); (ii) surgical trauma to the endothelium; (iii) a large amount of formed clot in contact with the endothelium; and (iv) prolonged elevation of intraocular pressure. Each of these factors affects endothelial integrity. Corneal blood staining may occur with low or normal intraocular pressures; it may also occur in hyphemas that are less than total. Corneal blood staining has a larger potential for occurrence in patients who have a total hyphema that remains for at least 6 days with concomitant, continuous intraocular pressures above 25 mm Hg. Corneal blood staining may require several months or more to clear.

Nonglaucomatous optic atrophy in hyphema patients may be due either to the initial trauma or to transient periods of markedly elevated intraocular pressure. Diffuse optic nerve pallor is the result of transient periods of markedly elevated intraocular pressure; it occurs with constant pressure of 50 mm Hg or higher for 5 days or 35 mm Hg or higher for 7 days. We have observed a number of patients with sickle cell trait who developed a nonglaucomatous optic atrophy with relatively small elevations of intraocular pressure (35 to 39 mm Hg) that lasted 2 to 4 days. Despite maximum medical therapy, final visual acuity was less than 20/400 in all patients. We continue to observe optic atrophy in sickle cell trait patients referred to our institution

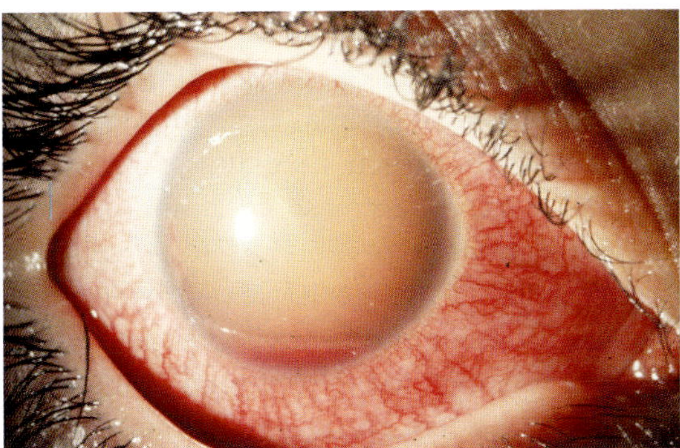

Fig. 3: Traumatic hyphema—grade 4

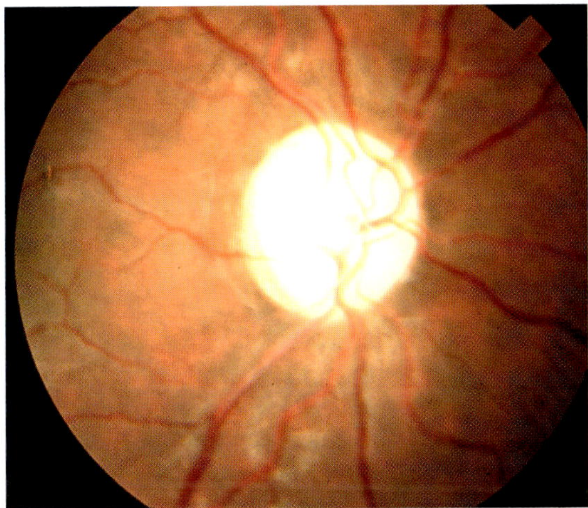

Fig. 4: Optic atrophy secondary hyphema-induced glaucoma

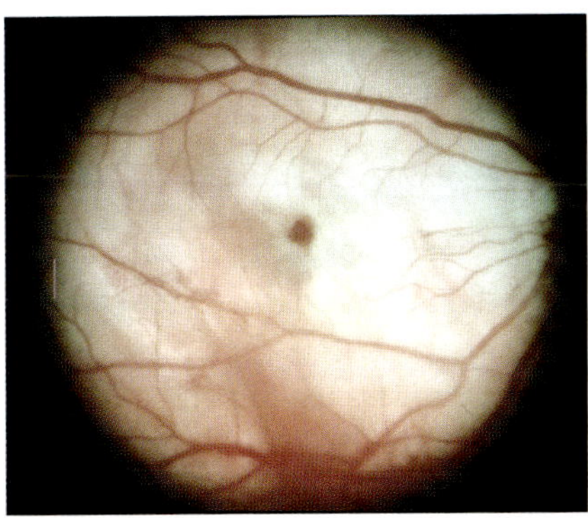

Fig. 5: Commotio retinae associated with hyphema

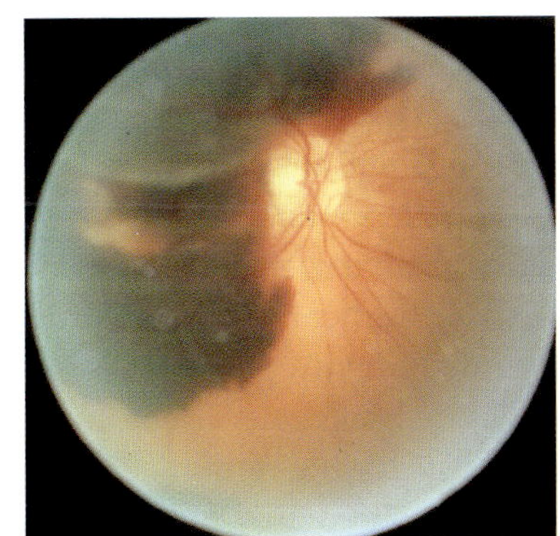

Fig. 6: Retinal detachment with subretinal hemorrhage

that have not had vigorous control of intraocular pressure and/or delay in paracentesis. Other studies indicate that patients with sickle cell hemoglobinopathies and anterior chamber hyphemas have more sickled erythrocytes in their anterior chambers than in their circulating venous blood. The sickled erythrocytes obstruct the trabecular meshwork more effectively than normal cells, and there is a concomitant elevation of intraocular pressure to higher levels with lesser amounts of hyphema. Moderate elevation of intraocular pressure in patients with sickle cell hemoglobinopathy may produce rapid deterioration of visual function due to profound reduction of central retinal artery and posterior ciliary artery perfusion.

Associated Exam Findings

There are a variety of complications associated with hyphema and blunt globe trauma. External examination may reveal a contusion of the lids and periorbital tissues. A black eye may be serious or relatively minor. If accompanied by severe pain, bleeding, or constant blurred vision, more serious eye trauma must be considered. An orbital CT scan and ophthalmologic consultation should be considered to rule out a ruptured globe. Depending on the mechanism of injury, corneal and scleral lacerations may also occur. Frequently, signs of corneal and scleral lacerations include unequal pupils, decreased intraocular pressure, iris prolapse, or hyphema. Frequently, a corneal laceration also involves the lens. Almost all ocular trauma cases include bleeding or dilation of blood vessels on the surface of the eye resulting in the formation of subconjunctival hemorrhages. This sign may be observed with any degree of eye injury. For instance, a subconjunctival hemorrhage may be spontaneous and often indicates minor injury. In the presence of a hyphema, a subconjunctival hemorrhage suggests more serious injury and necessitates the evaluation for a possible occult ruptured globe.

Hyphema may result in lacerations of the sphincter muscle of the pupil. They are manifested by traumatic mydriasis. Unlike the unequal pupils seen with congenital anisocoria, traumatic mydriasis is characterized by recent onset of unequal pupils and by the irregularity of the dilated pupil. Although traumatic mydriasis by itself is not harmful, it suggests severe blunt trauma and is an indication for a careful assessment of other ocular structures, including the vitreous and retinal periphery.

Ophthalmologists should consider posterior injuries to the globe may be present, including retinal detachment, retinal tear, and vitreous hemorrhage. An increase in previous floaters or the onset of new floaters may occur with hyphema. In such cases, a complete eye exam including either dilation should be performed to evaluate for a retinal detachment. In cases of hyphemas that obscure direct visualization of the posterior segment B-scan ultrasonography should be completed. Additional evaluations may include orbital CT imaging

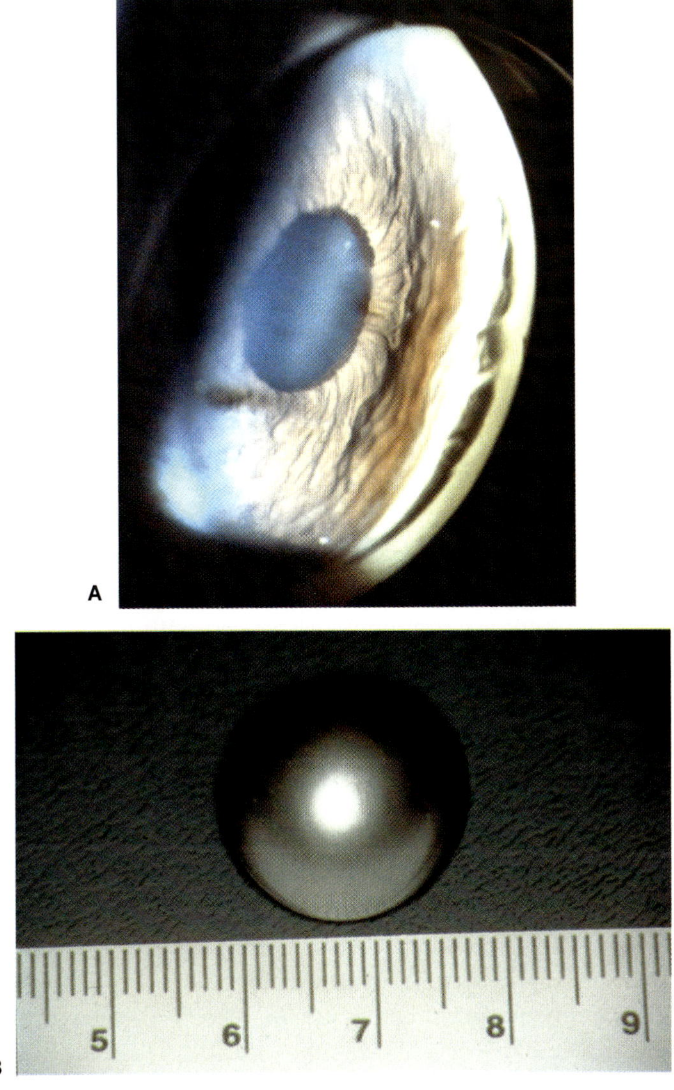

Figs 7A and B: (A) Angle recession, (B) Ball relative size

to evaluate for associated orbital fracture. Traumatic detachment of the retina can be observed after blunt eye injury, especially in older individuals. The patient may complain of reduced overall brightness in the involved eye or may have continuous light flashes, indicating retinal traction. After eye trauma it is imperative to inspect not just the central portions of the retina but the peripheral portions as well. Other serious post-traumatic injuries are traumatic tears of the iris, subluxation or dislocation of the lens that occasionally displaces into the anterior chamber, and blowout fracture of the orbit that present with impaired eye movement in the upward direction because of entrapment of the inferior rectus muscle. These serious injuries are generally readily identified.

Patients presenting with hyphema should also have evaluations to rule out penetrating injuries of the globe, acute angle closure glaucoma, pupillary block, corneal foreign body, and acute iritis. Blunt trauma may also result in vitreous hemorrhage, posterior vitreous detachments, and commotio retinae.

Prognosis and Treatment of Hyphema

Cataract, choroidal rupture, vitreous hemorrhage, angle recession glaucoma, and retinal detachment are commonly associated with traumatic hyphema, compromising the final visual acuity. It is important to recognize that the prognosis for visual recovery from traumatic hyphema is directly related to three factors:

1. Amount of associated damage to other ocular structures (i.e. choroidal rupture or macular scarring)
2. Whether secondary hemorrhage occurs
3. Whether complications of glaucoma, corneal blood staining, or optic atrophy occur.

Treatment modalities should be directed at reducing the incidence of secondary hemorrhage and the risk of corneal blood staining and optic atrophy. The success of hyphema treatment, as judged by recovery of visual acuity, is good in approximately 75% of patients. Approximately 80% of hyphema patients with less than one-third filling of the anterior chamber regain visual acuity of 20/40 (6/12) or better. Approximately 60% of those with more than half but less than total hyphema regain 20/40 or better, whereas only approximately 35% of those with initially total hyphema have good visual results. Approximately 60% of hyphema patients below age 6 years have good visual results; older age groups have progressively higher percentages of good visual recovery.

Hyphema should be carefully managed with bed rest, shielding the injured eye, and appropriate treatment either pharmacologically or surgically in order to minimize potential complications. Patients with sickle cell disease or sickle cell trait should be closely monitored for possible elevated intraocular pressure and rebleeding events. Some ophthalmologists use aminocaproic acid or oral steroids in addition to topical treatment with steroids and mydriatics. Some

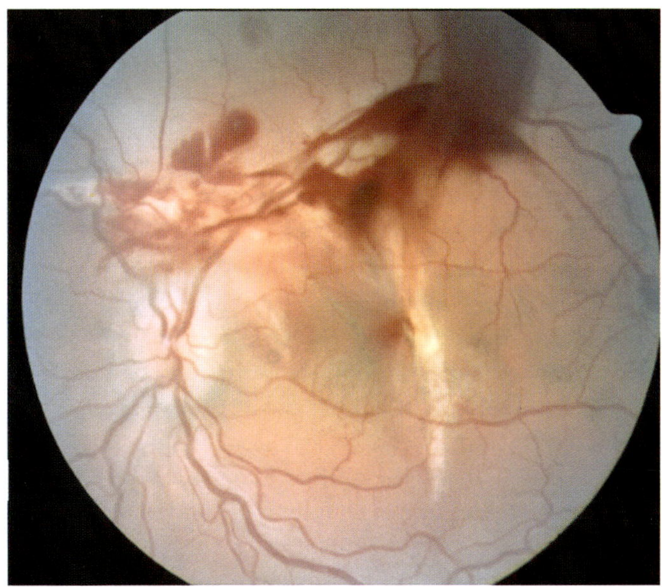

Fig. 8: Choroidal rupture with macular scar and retinal hemorrhage

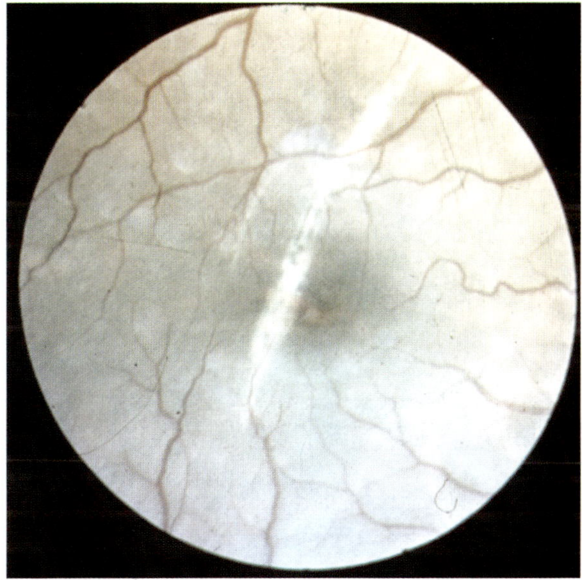

Fig. 9: Choroidal rupture involving macula

studies have demonstrated a lower incidence of secondary hemorrhage with aminocaproic acid treatment. Patients with hyphema and angle recession require life-long evaluation for possible glaucoma. Common treatment plans include atropine sulfate 1% 3 times a day for 7 days and topical dexamethasone 0.1% 4 times a day. Additionally, treatment includes a protective shield for the involved eye.

In general, hyphemas are best managed with medical treatment followed by surgical treatment as indicated. Surgical management can be difficult and is associated with a series of potential complications. Surgery is best reserved for severe hyphemas or thus unresponsive to medical management. Surgery is often unnecessary when less than 50% of the anterior chamber is involved. In general, corneal staining with blood resolves, but may take several weeks. Even total hyphemas should be conservatively managed for 4 days before considering surgery. Spontaneous resolution often occurs rapidly during this period. After surgical intervention is usually indicated on or after the fourth day for total hyphemas. Surgical indications also include: intraocular pressure of 50 mmHg or greater for 4 days, Grade III hyphemas lasting 6 days or with pressures of 25 mmHg, or Grade II hyphemas lasting longer than 8 days. Also, special attention should be given to sick cell trait and sickle cell disease patients. In these patients, an intraocular pressure greater than 35 mmHg for more than 24 hours increases the need for surgical evacuation.

Complications of hyphema surgery include damage to the corneal endothelium, lens, or iris; prolapse of the intraocular contents; rebleeding; and increased synechiae formation. The preferred technique is evacuation of the hyphema with vitrectomy instrumentation. The initial clear corneal incision is fashioned and a vitrectomy hand piece is gently placed into the anterior chamber. Extreme care is required to avoid any contact with the iris, the lens, or the corneal endothelium. Intraoperative secondary hemorrhage may occur. Raising the infusion bottle to approximately 70 cm above the eye for several minutes provides tamponade in most cases. At the end of the surgical procedure, filling the anterior chamber with an air bubble is helpful. Standard closure is created with 10-0 nylon corneal sutures.

In patients with total hyphema, some surgeons advocate trabeculectomy with peripheral iridectomy. The trabeculectomy is performed through a partial thickness sclera incision. Peripheral iridectomy is performed with the trabeculectomy. Two 10-0 nylon scleral flap sutures are used to close the trabeculectomy site. Because these surgical procedures have a variety of associated complications, the surgeon should approach each case with a patient-specific treatment plan.

Chapter NINE

Pediatric Iris Abnormalities

Arif Adenwala (UAE)
Mahesh Dalvi (India)

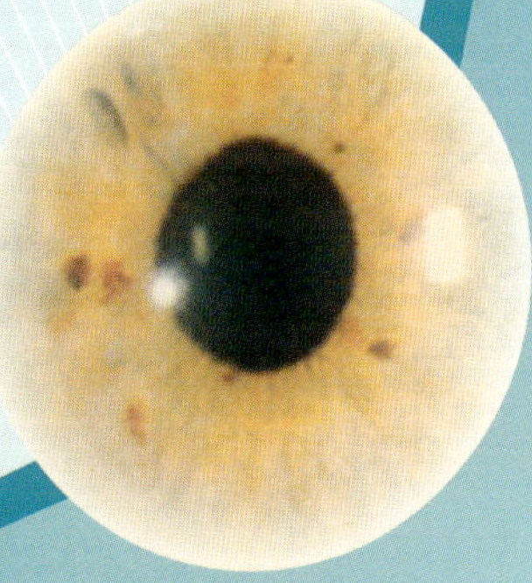

Aniridia

It represents a spectrum of disorder with iris hypoplasia. It may occur due to anomalous development of neuron ectoderm or neural crest cells.

Histology

Iris is reduced to small stub and smooth muscle is usually absent. Angle may also be poorly developed.

It is defines as absence of iris tissue. But it is misnomer as at least a rudimentary tissue is present.

It is bilateral disorder.

Additional Abnormalities

- Foveal and optic nerve hypoplasia are present leading to congenital sensory nystagmus
- Decreased visual acuity is seen due to multiple risk factors like light scatter, corneal or lenticular opacities, severe glaucoma optic nerve and macular hypoplasia
- Cataract
- Glaucoma and
- Corneal opacity.

Typical Clinical Presentation

- Nystagmus
- Dilated fixed pupil
- Photophobia
- Anterior polar cataract—persistent pupillary membrane.

Cause

Sporadic or Familial

- Defect in PAX6 gene on chromosome 11. PAX6 gene is localized to band 11p13.
- Chromosomes 1 and 2 play an important role in dominant of congenital aniridia.

Familial

It is autosomal dominant with complete penetrance and variable expressively.

Sporadic

Common association with Wilm's tumor. All cases of anirdia should get chromosomal analysis for Wilm's tumor gene defect.

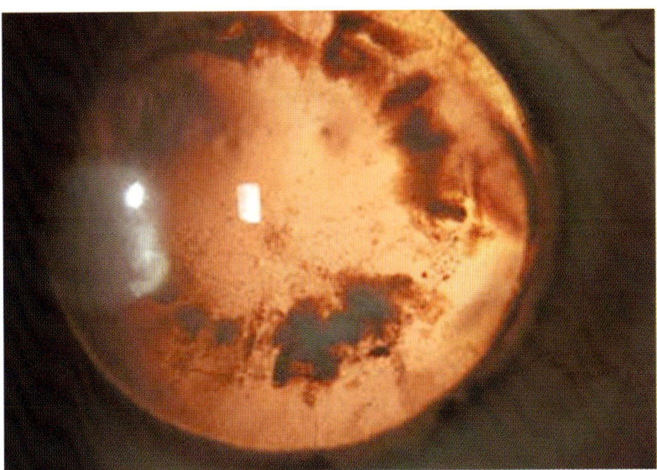

Fig. 1: Aniridia (*Courtesy:* Online Journal of Ophthalmology)

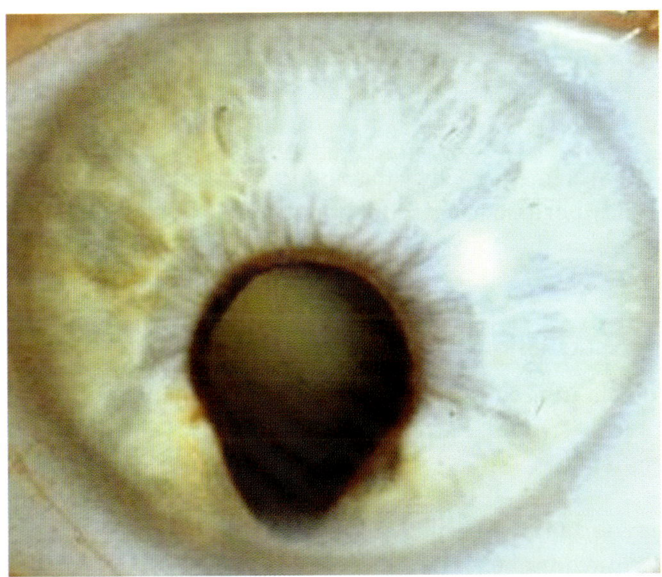

Fig. 2: Coloboma of iris (*Courtesy:* Online Journal of Ophthalmology)

There is also association with genitourinary abnormalities and mental retardation (ARG).

Cataract surgery in aniridia is slightly complicated. But nowadays with recent advances the success rate is good. Special aniridia intraocular lenses are used in these patients.

Occluder contact lenses with pupillary aperture is indicated for optical correction of refractive errors

Coloboma Iris

It is defined as partial absence of iris tissue. It is classified depending on the site of absence.

Typical

Coloboma is seen in inferonasal quadrant. It is caused by failure of closure of the embryonic fissure in 5th week.

The shape of the pupil is light bulb, keyhole or inverted tear drop.

It involves the ciliary body, choroid, retina and optic nerve.

Atypical

Coloboma is seen in areas other than inferonasal quadrant.

It is usually not associated with more posterior uveal coloboma.

It results from the fibrovascular remnants of the anterior hyaloids system and pupillary membrane.

Common Association

Iris colobomata are seen with almost any chromosomal abnormalities. The most common being. Trisomy 13, Trisomy 18, Triploidy, Klinefelter syndrome, cat eye syndrome, etc.

Common syndromes associated are:

- CHARGE syndrome:
  C: Ocular coloboma.
  H: Heart defects.
  A: Choanal atresia.
  R: Mental retardation.
  G: Genitourinary abnormalities and
  E: Ear abnormalities.
- Aicardi syndrome
- Goldenhar syndrome
- Rubinstein-Taybi syndrome.

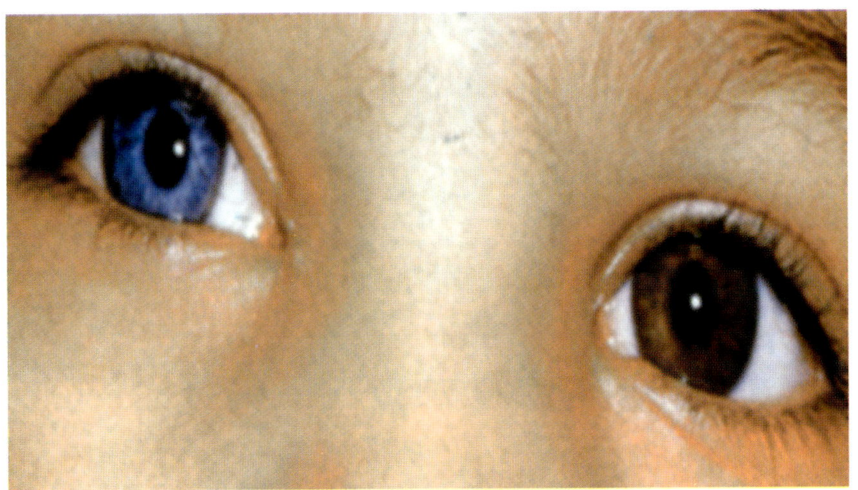

Fig. 3: Heterochromia iridium

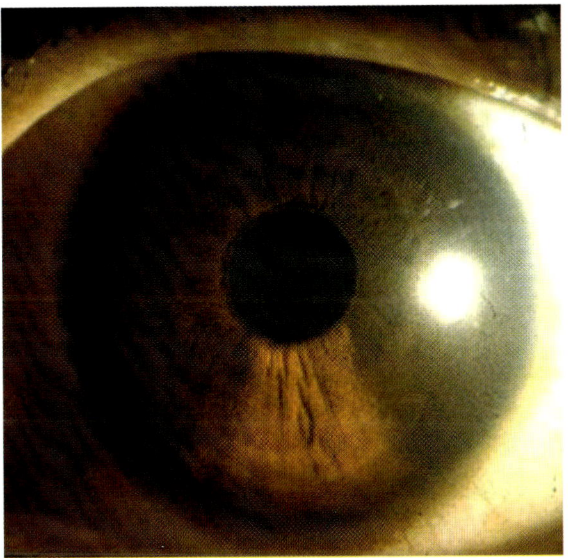

Fig. 4: Ocular melanosis
(*Courtesy*:Ritch, Robert, MD, Online Journal of Ophthalmology)

Heterochromia Iridis

A difference in iris color between both the eyes is known as heterochromia iridis. It can be congenital or acquired.

An abnormal eye may be either darker/lighter than the other eye.

Congenital

Involved iris can be either dark or light in color.

Involved Iris Dark

It is seen in ocular melanocytosis or ocular dermal melanocytosis or secondary to iris hamartomas.

Involved Iris Light in Color

It is seen in Horner's syndrome and Waardenburg syndrome. Congenital Horner's syndrome includes ipsilateral hypopigmentation, miosis and ptosis.

Waardenburg Syndrome

It is autosomal syndrome inheritance. Features include lateral displacement of inner canthus, prominent root of the nose, deafness, white forelock, and heterochromia iridis.

Acquired

Involved Iris Dark

Usually results from infiltration process like nevus or melanomatous tumor or secondary to sideroses.

Involved Iris Light

It is commonly seen in Fuch's heterochromic iridocyclitis, Juvenile Xantho Granuloma, or metastatic malignancies.

William Syndrome

There is stellate pattern of iris. Associated features includes prominent lips, mental retardation, growth retardation, cardiac defect.

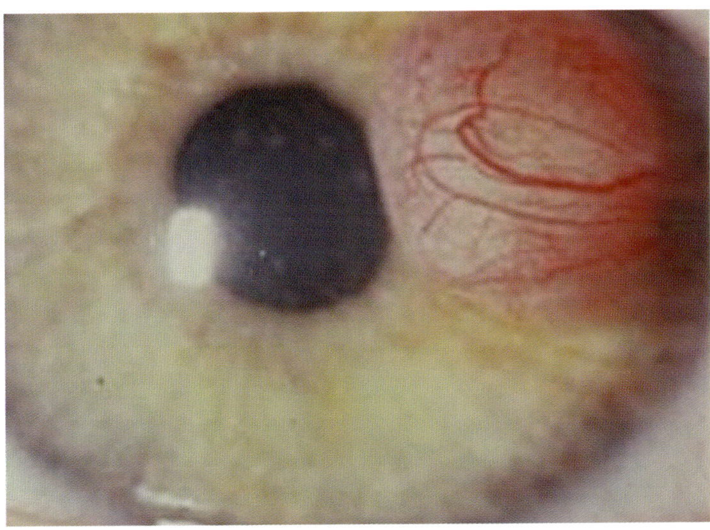

Fig. 5: Juvenile xanthogranuloma
(*Courtesy:* Online Journal of Ophthalmology)

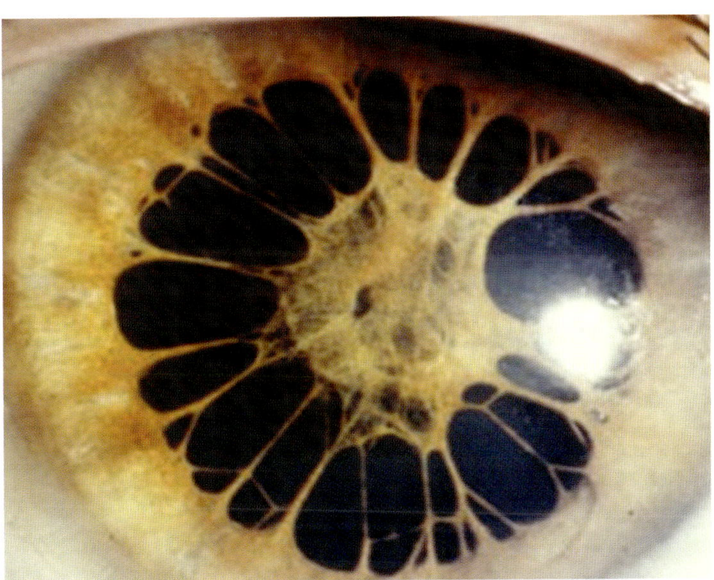

Fig. 6: Persistent pupillary membrane (PPM)
(*Courtesy:* Online Journal of Ophthalmology)

Iris Nodules

Lisch Nodule

These are neural crest hamartomas. It is seen in association with NF-1.

It is raised swelling and usually tan in color. The prevalence in NF-1 increases with age.

Juvenile Xanthogranuloma (JXG)

It is mainly cutaneous disorder. It had increase predilection for head and face.

It presents as discrete yellowish nodules/dense infiltration causing heterochromia.

Vascular iris lesion can lead to spontaneous hyphema.

Primary Iris Cysts

Primary iris cysts are rare swelling arising from pigmentary epithelium or stroma.

Iris Pigment Epithelium Cysts

These are unilateral, solitary dark brown swelling.

It occurs due to separation of two layers of epithelium anywhere between pupil and ciliary body.

It is stable condition and rarely causes any complication. It has feature of trans illumination and it may dislodge and float freely in anterior chamber or vitreous.

Central Cysts (Pupillary)

- Usually hereditary
- It can be seen at any age group
- It is caused by the use of miotic eye drops mainly phenylepherine
- Rupture of the cyst can cause formation of iris flocculi.

Cyst Iris Stroma

It is caused by sequestration of the epithelium during embryologic development. It is seen commonly in infants and young children and usually presents in first year of life.

They are solitary swelling having smooth, translucent anterior wall filled with fluid.

These cyst may contain goblets cells and when enlarges it causes obstruction of the visual axis, glaucoma, corneal decompensation.

Preferred treatment of choice is surgical excision of the lesion although spontaneous regression may occur.

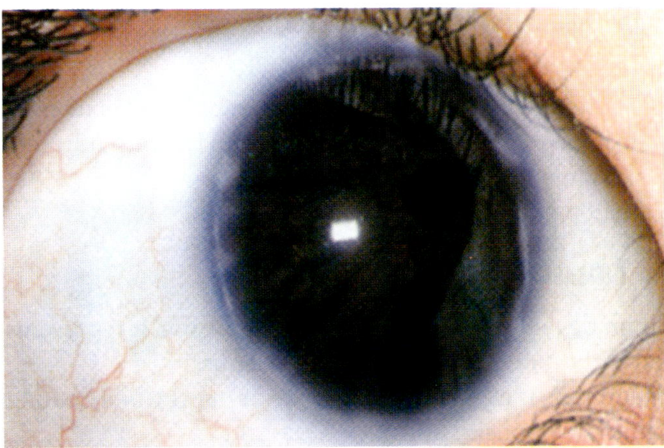

Fig. 7: Rieger's anomaly with posterior embryotoxon and polycoria
(*Courtesy:* John Elston: Textbook of Paediatric Ophthalmology: David Taylor)

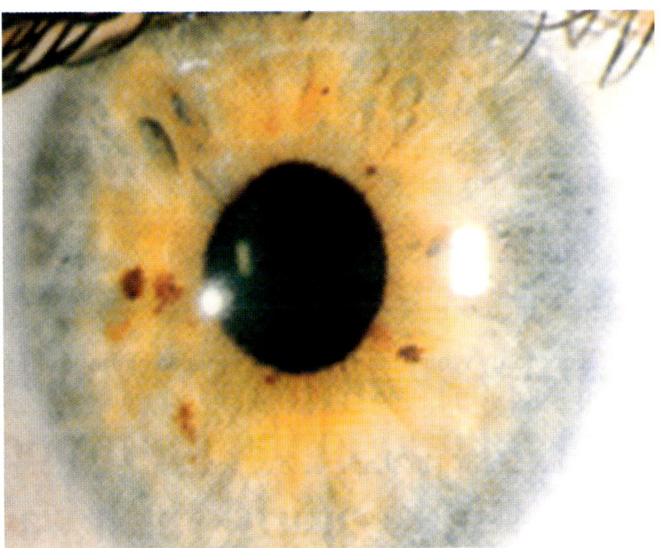

Fig. 8: Rieger's anomaly with focal iris hypoplasia
(*Courtesy:* John Elston: Textbook of Paediatric Ophthalmology: David Taylor)

Rieger's Syndrome

This includes combination of Rieger's anomaly with somatic features. These include:

- Facial abnormalities like maxillary hypoplasia and short philtrum
- Dental abnormalities which affect primary and secondary dentition with widely spaced cone shaped teeth
- Other features include umbilical hernia and hypospadias
- Rieger's syndrome is an autosomal dominant condition. Glaucoma is seen in 20 to 25% of affected individuals
- It is associated with abnormalities in chromosome 6 and with isolated growth hormone deficiency.

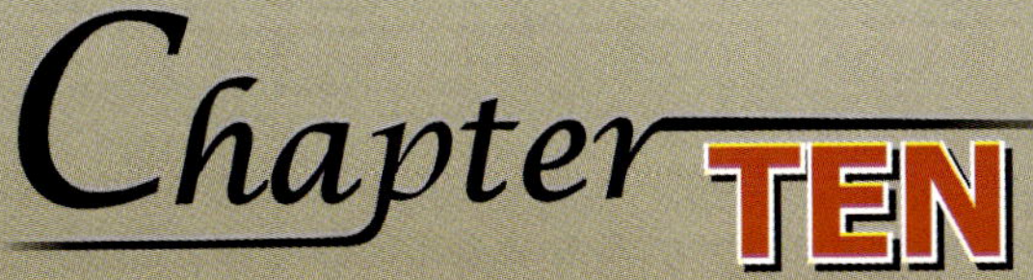

Chapter TEN

Anterior Segment Tumors

Flavio A Marigo
Paul T Finger (USA)

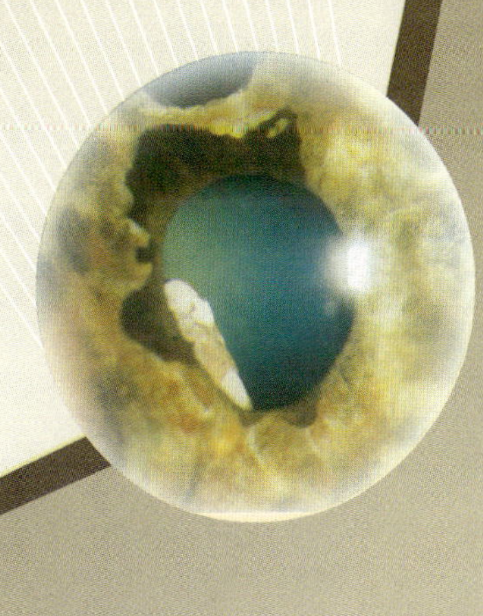

Introduction

Anterior segment tumors primarily originate from the iris and/or ciliary body. The majority of the anterior segment neoplasms are iridociliary cysts, which are benign and frequently undetected in routine examination. However, anterior segment cysts may enlarge enough to cause compression and dislocate surrounding structures.

Malignant melanoma is the most frequent primary malignancy in the anterior segment. Compared to posterior uveal melanomas, iris melanomas tend to be smaller and visible, so they are detected early and rarely metastasize. In contrast, ciliary body melanomas are considered more malignant. Hidden behind the iris, ciliary body melanomas are usually detected after they have become relatively large. Size (primarily largest tumor dimension) continues to be the best predictor for metastases.

The basic work-up for anterior segment tumors involves slit lamp biomicroscopy, gonioscopy, transillumination and ophthalmoscopy. There have been several recent advances in diagnosis and treatment of ocular tumors. Anterior segment tumor diagnosis has been greatly enhanced by fine-needle aspiration biopsy (FNAB), and high-frequency ultrasonography (UBM) as well as computerized tomography (CT), and MRI.

Tumor diagnosis and treatment are influenced by its location, size, local extension, patterns of growth and secondary complications (e.g. glaucoma). High-frequency ultrasound (UBM) has provided unique and important high-resolution images of tumors previously hidden within and behind the iris. Unique cross-sectional images in which tumor surface, internal reflectivity and borders have been revealed. These features have made UBM an indispensable tool for evaluating anterior segment tumors.

Treatment of anterior segment tumors include local resection (e.g. sector iridectomy), by lamellar sclerouvectomy, and ophthalmic plaque radiation therapy. If all else fails or for uncontrollable secondary glaucoma, enucleation is also employed. Fine-needle aspiration biopsy (FNAB) and high-frequency ultrasonography continue to play important roles in evaluation and for planning surgery and radiation therapy.

This chapter highlights the unique role of UBM for the diagnosis and treatment of anterior segment tumors as well as an overview of basic knowledge used in the management and treatment of the anterior segment tumors.

Iris Nevus

Introduction

Iris nevi are benign, pigmented lesions that are commonly visible at the iris surface. These lesions are composed by a cluster of atypical, but benign-appearing, small spindle and dendritic nevus cells within the iris stroma.

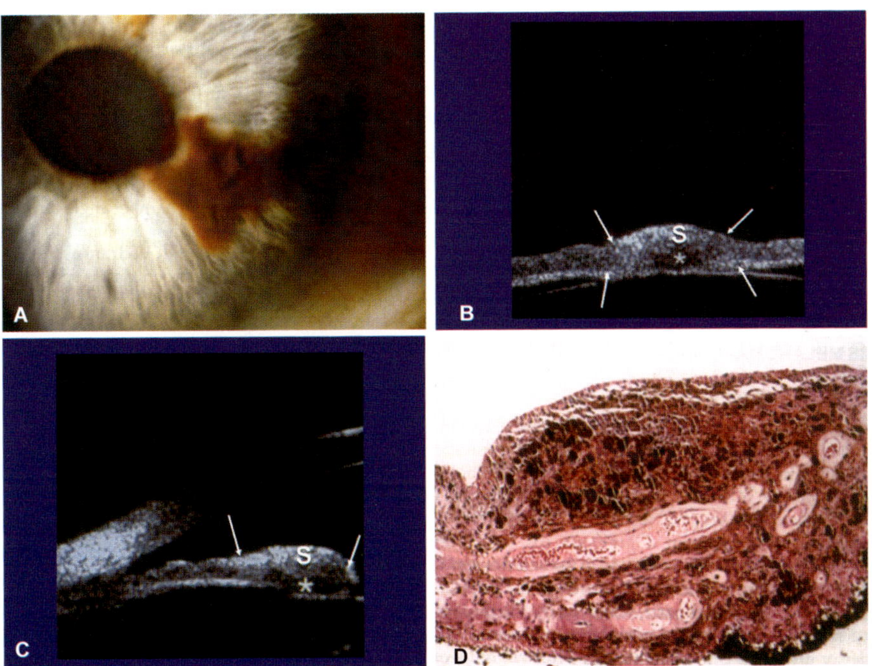

Figs 1A to D: Iris melanoma: (A) There is a pigmented lesion in the superonasal quadrant near the pupillary border, correlation between UBM, (B) radial section, and (C) transverse section and histopathology, (D) light microscopy, hematoxylin-eosin, original magnification 33 × shows that diffuse thickening of the iris stroma (S) is determined by neoplastic melanocytic cells. Bowing of iris anterior surface (outlined by arrows) is related to involvement of the anterior iris border by tumor cells. The large hypoechoic, 'cystic' space (*) in posterior stroma correlates with exaggerated enlarged vessels

Diagnosis

Iris nevi present as a focal areas of iris pigmentation are flat or slightly elevated. Typically these tumors do not distort the iris stroma and do not grow. However, some iris nevi can grow and infiltrate the iris and other anterior segment structures. When iris nevi present with iris infiltration and distortion, ectropion uvea and sector cataract they must be differentiated from iris melanomas.

High-frequency ultrasonography (UBM) has been employed to help delineate and follow suspicious iris nevi for evidence of growth. More typically, iris nevi appear as a low reflective surface plaque overlying the iris stroma, or an area of iris thickening with a bowed appearance.

Other ultrasonically-defined morphologic features include: a fusiform thickening of the iris, a diffuse elongated thickening of the iris, a focal thickening of the iris surface with a distinct, sharp border between the lesion and the iris, the so-called "stuck-on appearance", and a collar-button shape similar to that of choroidal melanomas. UBM can be used to define the boundaries of a lesion as well as its shape and internal reflectivity.

Iris tumors should be scanned in a cross-sectional pattern. This will allow for both a horizontal and longitudinal assessment of tumor thickness and extent.

Special forms of Iris Nevus

Iris Freckles

Iris freckles are caused by increased pigmentation of the anterior border layer melanocytes (without an increase in the number of cells). Therefore, they present as flat plaques of increased pigmentation of the iris surface without alteration of the iris architecture. In contrast to the iris nevus, iris freckles have no associated thickening or nodule formation.

Lisch Nodules

In neurofibromatosis type I, the iris may contain several lightly pigmented, nodular nevi in a diffuse distribution (Lisch nodules). These lesions are characteristically bilateral and appear after age 16. Other ophthalmic manifestations of neurofibromatosis type I include eyelid neurofibromas which if in the upper lid may cause a typical "S-shaped ptosis", prominent corneal nerves, congenital ectropion uveae, glaucoma and choroidal hamartomas. Orbital features include optic nerve glioma, neural tumors and spheno-orbital encephalocele.

Cogan-Reese Syndrome

The Cogan-Reese syndrome (CGS) is characterized by small, darkly pigmented, pedunculated nodules which can take either a diffuse or focal distribution on

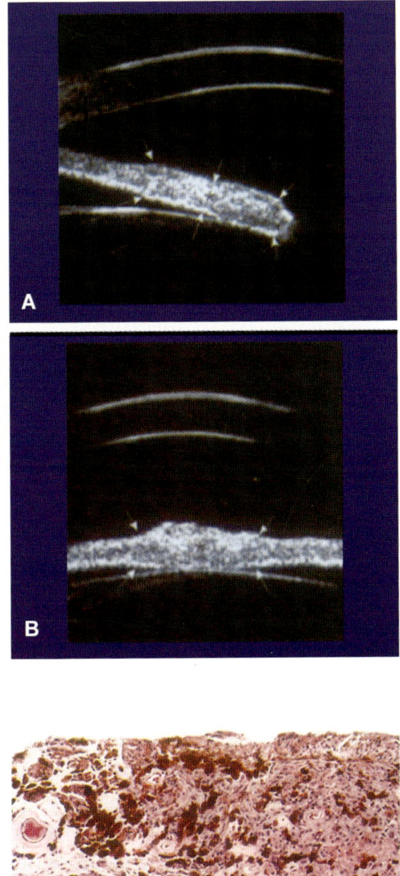

Figs 2A to C: Iris melanoma: (A) UBM, radial section, (B) transverse section, (C) light microscopy, hematoxylin-eosin, original magnification 33 ×. Iris thickening (*) is determined by spindle shaped and atypical cells extending in the iris stroma. UBM images bowing of the iris surfaces which are involved by tumor (arrows)

the iris surface. CGS is unilateral. Other anterior segment findings include essential iris atrophy, endothelial corneal abnormalities which may lead to corneal edema (Chandler's syndrome), peripheral anterior synechiae, and secretion of a new Descemet's membrane. Proliferation of an endothelial membrane over the iris and the anterior segment angle structures will include glaucoma.

Nevus of Ota (Oculodermal Syndrome)

The nevus of Ota (NO) affects woman in 80% of cases and generally becomes evident during adolescence or early adulthood. It is typically unilateral and associated with pigmentation of skin within the distribution of the first and second branches of trigeminal nerve (including the skin of the lids and periorbital skin). Nevus of Ota is also associated with increased pigmentation of the episclera, sclera and rarely the conjunctiva. The iris presents a sector or diffuse hyperpigmentation resulting in heterochromia. The angle is heavily pigmented with persistence of pectinate ligaments. Secondary glaucoma and uveal melanoma can be associated with NO. Orbital and intracranial melanomas have also been reported.

Treatment

Iris freckles and nevi do not need to be treated. Suspicious lesions are typically monitored for growth (with photography and high-frequency ultrasonography) prior to considering treatment. If growth is definitively documented, excisional biopsy (sector iridectomy or iridocyclectomy) can be performed as needed.

Prognosis

Iris freckles and nevi are benign lesions and are not considered to be a risk factor for melanoma metastasis. However, nevus of Ota is associated with an increased risk of uveal melanoma. Those patients must have a careful follow-up with indirect ophthalmoscopy.

Ciliary Body Nevus

Introduction

Ciliary body nevi are very infrequent comparing to choroidal nevus. Due to their location behind the iris, they are usually missed during routine examination.

Diagnosis

Ciliary body nevi typically present as small, discoid, relatively avascular, and pigmented lesions. High-frequency ultrasonography has revealed many more ciliary body nevi. Rare histopathologic evaluations have revealed benign melanocytic nevus cells.

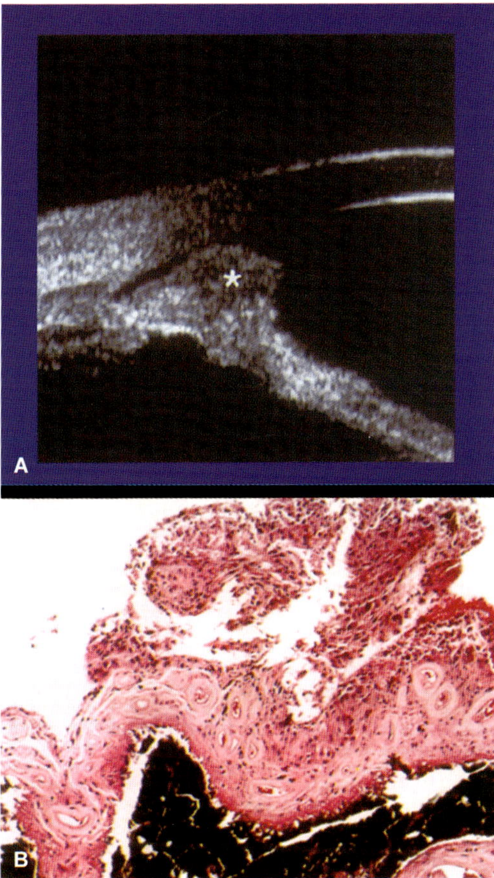

Figs 3A and B: Iris melanoma: (A) UBM, radial section, (B) light microscopy, hematoxylin-eosin, original magnification 33 ×. UBM images a nodular lesion (*) on the iris surface corresponding to an epithelioid malignant melanoma

including heterochromia, spontaneous hyphema, and chronic uveitis have been associated with iris melanoma.

High-frequency ultrasonography provides high-resolution cross-sectional images in which tumor surface, internal reflectivity and tumor borders can be visualized. Additionally, UBM allows quantitative follow-up evaluations of tumor size and thickness. This ability is often crucial to tumor diagnosis.

Iris melanomas (as imaged by UBM) are typically low to medium echoic and nodular arising from the peripheral iris surface with a medium to hyperechoic thickening of the iris stroma. Displacement of iris surfaces results in a bowed profile, which indicates infiltration of the iris stroma. Additionally, the presence of hypoechoic, "cystic" spaces in the iris stroma correlates to blood vessels. Small projections attached to the main tumor may extend to the angle and ciliary body, and change the prognosis for metastasis.

Fluorescein angiography can demonstrate the vascular pattern of the lesion but it is of little help. Conventional water-bath ultrasound examination also provides additional information but with limited resolution.

Diagnosis of an iris melanoma depends on features that are suggestive of tumor malignancy: tumor size, distortion of iris, ectropion uveae, and sector cataract. However, documented growth is the most important feature for diagnosis. Suspicious lesions should be photographed and measured with ultrasound, then carefully followed up at 3 to 6 months intervals monitoring for growth. We suggest high-quality slit lamp and goniophotographs together with either a video of the UBM and/or representational cross-sectional images with measured tumor height and thickness. The ciliary body in the quadrant of the tumor should be visualized as well as the other quadrants (looking for evidence of a ring melanoma). Clearly, changes in tumor size and internal reflectivity suggest malignancy.

The main differential diagnosis of the iris melanomas include: iris nevi, iris cysts, leiomyoma, metastases and juvenile xanthogranuloma. However, differentiation between benign and malignant lesions, mainly those located in the iris, is still a challenge. Histopathologically "benign" lesions such as nevi can grow and invade adjacent tissues and even recur after excision. Therefore, the definitive diagnosis is both clinical and histopathologic.

Treatment

Sector iridectomy is the procedure of choice for suspicious lesions and may be combined with cataract surgery when necessary. Lesions which extend to or invade the ciliary body are treated with iridocyclectomy or ophthalmic plaque radiation therapy. For diffuse tumors with intractable glaucoma, enucleation is commonly employed.

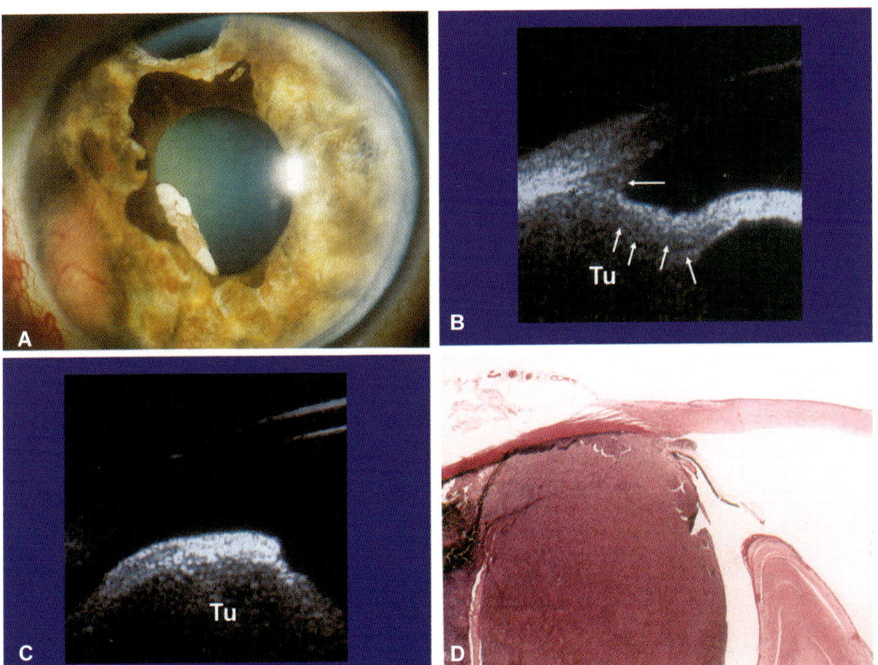

Figs 5A to D: Ciliary body melanoma: (A) slit lamp photo, (B and C) UBM, radial section, (D) light microscopy, hematoxylin-eosin, original magnification 6.6×—Slit lamp examination revealed engorged episcleral vessels nasally, ectropion uveae inferonasally and a mass located behind the iris. UBM images a large ciliary body tumor (Tu) invading the iris root near its posterior surface (hollow arrows). Note interruption of the iris pigment epithelium (arrow) and infiltration of iris stroma. The anterior chamber angle is also compromised (arrowhead). Observe scleral spur (*). More than half of the posterior chamber is occupied by tumor

Prognosis

Iris melanomas are usually diagnosed early or when they are small. This is probably because the iris is visible and the tumors are easily noticed. Since most are spindle cell melanomas and are typically located far from points of egress from the eye, iris melanomas rarely metastasize. The reported mortality rate for iris melanomas is low, calculated to be 4 to 8%.

Ciliary Body Melanoma

Introduction

Ciliary body melanoma is less frequent than either choroidal melanoma or iris melanomas. The age of presentation is usually during the sixth decade of life, being rare after the age of 80 years and before the age of 30 years. The tumor is rare in black patients. It may be primary located in any quadrant of the ciliary body. Bilateral tumors are rare, and association with other tumors is even rarer.

Diagnosis

Ciliary body melanomas usually present as a ciliary body mass causing either sector cataract, irregular astigmatism, extrascleral extension or a visual field defect. They can be darkly pigmented or amelanotic with evidence of vascularization.

Ciliary body melanoma can present with anterior, posterior and extrascleral extension. The tumor is frequently hidden behind the iris, with growth that can cause anterior displacement and/or infiltration of the iris. Clinical signs suggestive of the malignancy include: engorged episcleral "sentinel" vessels, anterior bulging of the iris, iris infiltration, pupillary distortion, ectropion uveae, sector cataracts, displacement of the lens, and pigment dispersion.

Posteriorly, ciliary body melanomas grow to affect the lens and into the choroid (ciliochoroidal melanoma). In certain cases, the primary origin of the melanoma cannot be determined.

Diffuse melanoma is a rare but distinct clinical presentation of ciliary body melanoma. It usually originates from a ring melanoma. It differs from more typical, localized or diffuse melanoma. As tumor growth is slow, the neoplastic cells adhere and proliferate into the vitreous, hyaloid interface, and local retinal surface infiltrating the nearby neurosensorial retina and optic nerve but not the choroid and the non-adjacent retina.

Extrascleral extension has been associated with a greater incidence of metastatic disease. The tumor typically exits through scleral emissary channel or by direct infiltration of the sclera. Other lesions that may simulate ciliary body melanoma with extrascleral extension include staphyloma, occult foreign body and melanocytoma.

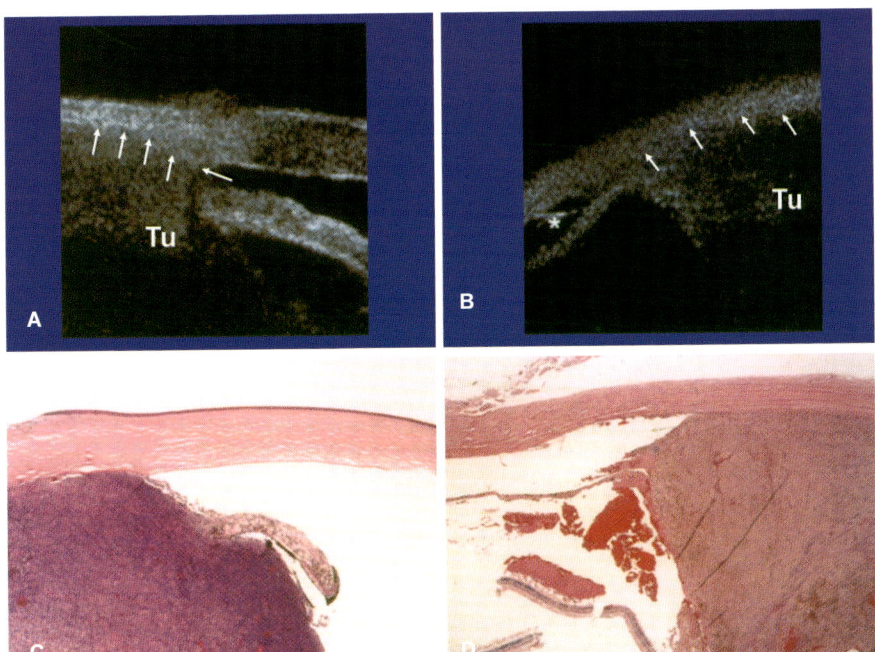

Figs 6A to D: Ciliary body melanoma: (A) UBM, anterior radial section, (B) posterior radial section, (C and D) light microscopy, hematoxylin-eosin, original magnification 6.6 ×. Tumor is seen invading the iris root and the anterior chamber angle (arrowhead, Figure A). Minimal scleral infiltration is observed in tissue sections, correlating with an irregular scleral-choroidal interface in UBM (arrows). There is a serous retinal detachment (*)

Conventional "low frequency" ultrasound examination continues to be the standard method to define the tumor's posterior extent. B-scan evaluations of ciliary body melanomas typically reveal a homogeneous color-button or dome-shaped mass with low internal reflectivity. Internal echolucent areas are not atypical.

UBM offers unique views of ciliary body melanomas. High-frequency examination images the base of the tumor, extension into the iris root and lenticular displacement. Though basal dimensions of most ciliary body melanomas can be defined by transscleral or transpupillary transillumination, tumor shadows can merge with the ciliary body band. Therefore, sequential clock-hour imaging of ciliary body melanomas offers an additional method to evaluate lateral tumor spread within the ciliary body. This technique may be of particular value in assessment of ring melanomas.

Characteristically, ciliary body melanomas are imaged by UBM as a moderately echogenic ciliary body mass. Infiltration of the iris is characterized on UBM by disruption of the hyperechoic line representing the iris pigment epithelium. Subsequent stromal invasion is represented by a change in the echogenicity of the affected area compared to the normal appearing iris. Disruption of the iris pigment epithelium is a characteristic which suggests malignancy.

Invasion of the anterior chamber angle is observed by UBM in the initial cases, as a loss in the normal acute shape of the angle, which assumes a convex or linear shape. In more advanced cases, a moderately echolucent tissue can be seen in the anterior chamber. The scleral spur and the Descemet's membrane are important landmarks when evaluating the trabecular meshwork and cornea for infiltration by tumor cells. This information is significant when radioactive plaque therapy is being considered. Plaque size and position relative to the tumor and other landmarks can be determined by UBM to provide optimum irradiation to the neoplasm avoiding unnecessary irradiation of unaffected structures.

UBM allows for an assessment of posterior chamber extension of anterior uveal tumors. These tumors can extend to the lens equator or lenticular surface. The tumor can eventually encroach and dislocate the lens, disrupting the lenticulopupillary axis. In these cases, UBM can help in planning treatment, by demonstrating that complete local resection may not be technically possible to perform.

Serous retinal detachment can be associated with uveal melanomas. The detachment can be imaged as a highly echogenic line delimiting a small fluid-containing sonolucent space. Relatively small and previously obscure secondary serous detachments can be imaged with UBM. Scleral invasion appears either as a localized loss of integrity in the chorioscleral interface, a decreased scleral reflecticity, or as a sonolucent line that is thought to represent tumor within an emissary canal.

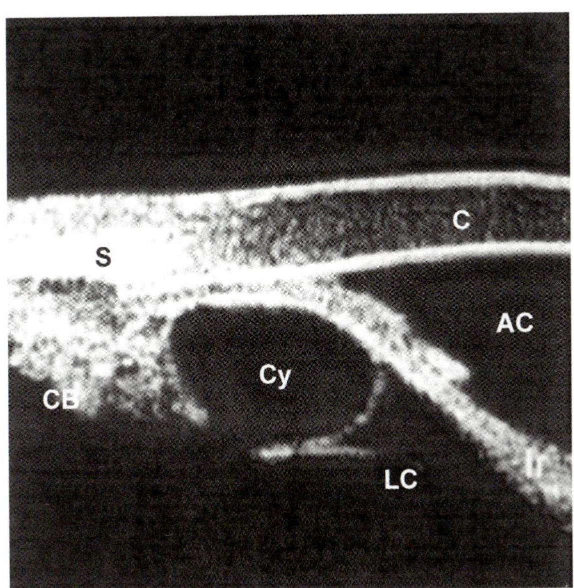

Fig. 7: Iris and iridociliary cyst—UBM radial section. The cysts (*) located in the iris and iridociliary junction pushes the iris root anteriorly, which causes angle closure (AC—anterior chamber, C—cornea, CB—ciliary body Ir: iris, LC—lens capsule)

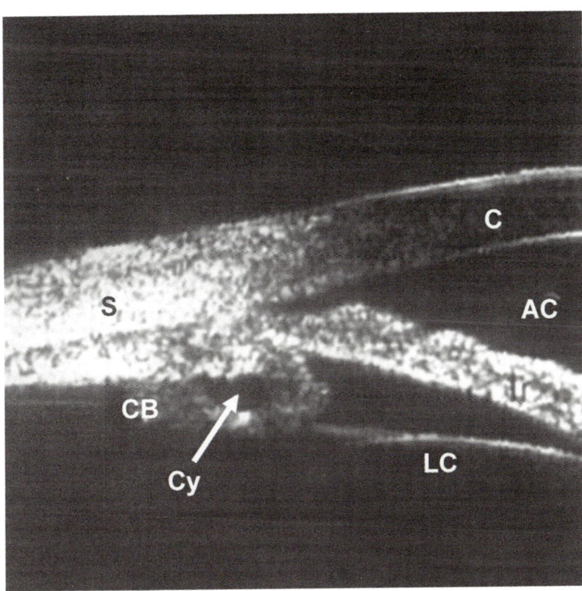

Fig. 8: Pars plicata cyst—UBM radial section. Ciliary body cyst (Cy) can be recognized among the ciliary processes (CB) (AC—anterior chamber, C—cornea, Ir—iris, LC: lens capsule, S—sclera)

Differential diagnosis of ciliary body melanoma includes: ciliary body cysts, neuroepithelial and implantation cysts, metastasis, leiomyoma, Schwannoma, neurofibroma, melanocytoma, adenoma of the ciliary body epithelium, adenocarcinoma, pseudoepitheliomatous hyperplasia (Fuch's adenoma) medulloepithelioma and lesions that simulate extrascleral extension such as staphyloma and occult foreign body.

Treatment

Ciliary body melanomas were typically treated by enucleation due to tumor size and local infiltration. However, in more recent years, treatment has changed to emphasize the preservation of the eye and sparing of vision.

Enucleation is the treatment of choice for large melanomas in eyes without useful vision or extra-large melanomas. These tumors are not typically irradiated because the volume of tumor and therefore the area of irradiation is so large, the eye will not tolerate standard doses. Pre-enucleation external beam radiation therapy has not proved to decrease the incidence of metastatic melanoma.

Radiation plaque therapy (RPT) involves attaching a radioactive device onto the episclera beneath the intraocular tumor and leaving it in place (typically for 5 to 7 days) prior to removal. The main radionuclides (isotopes) within the plaque are iodine-125 and ruthenium-106. Radiation plaque therapy has been shown to stop tumor growth or induce tumor shrinkage in more than 90% of cases. In a multinational multicenter prospective randomized clinical trial, the collaborative ocular melanoma study is investigating if enucleation or plaque radiation therapy is better for patient survival due to metastatic choroidal melanoma. The main complications reported are cataracts, radiation retinopathy, vitreous hemorrhage, glaucoma, corneal lesion and scleral necrosis.

Charged-particle external beam "proton" radiotherapy is also used for ciliary body melanomas. Since the treatment zone is moved into the anterior segment for this technique, the incidence of eyelash loss, dry eye, keratopathy, neovascular glaucoma, and cataract are greatly increased.

Partial lamellar sclerouvectomy has been employed for small tumors, with less than 15 mm in diameter. It involves the resection of the neoplasm with a rim of healthy uvea under a scleral flap. However, it is a difficult technique and possible complications include cataracts, vitreous hemorrhage, retinal detachment and tumor recurrence. Secondary enucleations are not uncommon. Though (with this technique) tumor seeding of the orbit is inevitable, local orbital recurrences have not been reported.

Exenteration (removal of the eye and all orbital tissues) has been employed for cases with massive extraocular extension. Smaller extraocular extensions can be managed by post-enucleation external beam radiotherapy.

A palliative treatment consists of chemotherapy and immunotherapy for patients with metastasis.

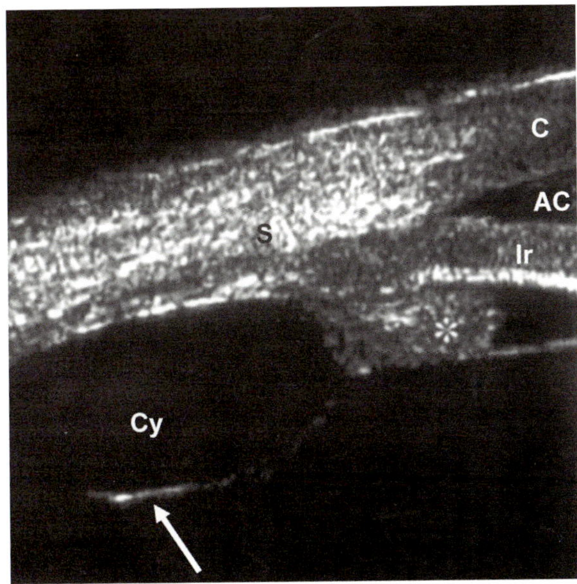

Fig. 9: Pars plana cyst—UBM radial section. Pars plana cysts (Cy) are usually large and dome-shaped (AC—anterior chamber, C—cornea, Ir—iris, S—sclera, arrow: cyst wall, asterisk: ciliary process)

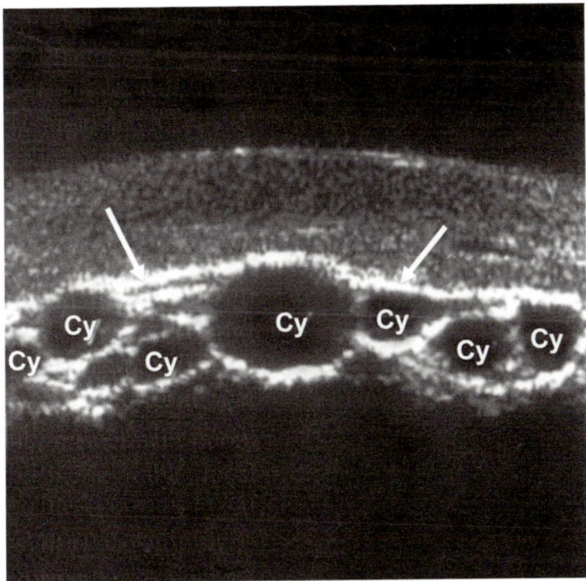

Fig. 10: Multiple iridociliary cysts—UBM transverse section. Multiple cysts (Cy) can be found at the iridociliary junction and may cause angle-closure glaucoma. Note the iris pigmented epithelium (arrows)

Prognosis

Ciliary body melanomas are considered to be more malignant due a higher rate of distant metatasis or extrascleral extension. The 5-year survival rate is about 59%.

Factors that influence the metastatic potential are:

- Cell type—spindle cell melanomas are least likely to metastasize. Tumors which contain mixed cell-types, necrotic-areas, and epithelioid-cell carry a worse prognosis.
- Tumor size—large tumors have a worse prognosis than the smaller ones. The greatest diameter of the tumor is considered to be the most important predictor of metastasis and death.
- Tumor extension—extrascleral tumor extension increases metastases.
- Growth patterns—a diffuse growth pattern carries a worse prognosis.
- Age of the patient—patients over the age of 65 years have worse prognosis than the younger patients.

Anterior Segment Cysts

Introduction

Cystic lesions occurring within the anterior segment may be classified as primary or secondary. Primary cysts are of neuroepithelial origin, while secondary cysts may result from implantation, metastasis, parasites or miotic therapy. Neuroepithelial cysts involve the pigment epithelium of the iris and the ciliary body. When large, they may produce focal angle-closure glaucoma. Secondary cysts are more problematic and may lead to corneal edema, uveitis, glaucoma, and decreased visual acuity.

Diagnosis

Cysts can be found in a variety of locations within the anterior segment and can have different etiologies. Neuroepithelial cysts are the most common and are usually located at the iridociliary junction. They are round or oval with thin walls and sonolucent contents (as imaged by UBM). It is generally accepted that the high reflectivity of the cyst wall is caused by its epithelial cell lining and that its sonolucent core is consistent with a fluid content. Cysts restricted either to the iris or ciliary body are less common.

Iridociliary cysts can displace the iris root anteriorly. This can induce a pseudoplateau configuration with or without angle-closure. While single cysts are more common, multiple cysts are found in about one-third of cases. When multiple cysts involve more than 180 degrees of the iris, as it does in 10% of patients, angle-closure glaucoma may develop.

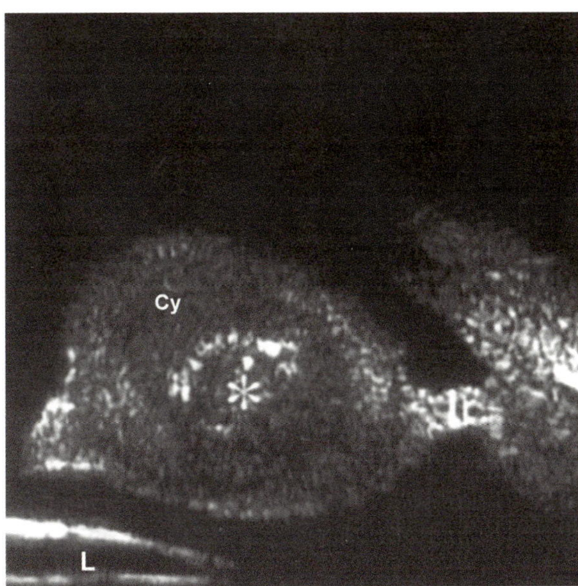

Fig. 11A: Pearl cyst, UBM, radial section. Pearl cysts have moderately echogenic content (Cy) and hyperechoic core (asterisk): Ir—iris, L—IOL

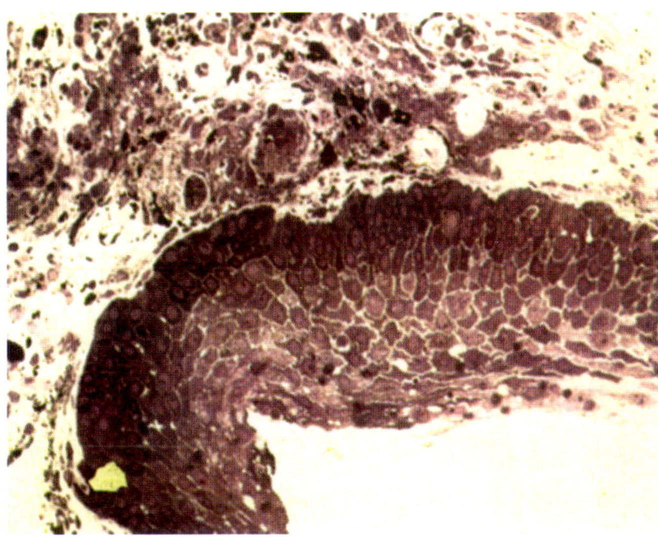

Fig. 11B: Pearl cyst, light microscopy, hematoxylin-eosin, original magnification: 66×. Pathology revealed stratified squamous cell lining cyst. Acute and chronic inflammatory cells infiltrated the iris stroma

Most of the uveitic cysts are commonly bilateral and located within the posterior iris and ciliary body epithelium (at the iridociliary junction or anterior ciliary body). Most of these iris cysts are associated with nongranulomatous uveitis and some patients have been found to be HLA-B27 positive. These figures can explain the younger age of the affected patients. Uveitis may be responsible for the lower IOP found in these eyes, when compared to those with spontaneous neuroepithelial cysts.

Implantation of epithelial surface cells from the cornea, conjunctiva or skin may occur by entrance of these cells into the eye during surgical or perforating trauma or through a poorly closed surgical wound. Prolonged postoperative hypotony or incarceration of iris or lens capsule are considered risk factors. Although normal aqueous is supposed to inhibit growth of these cells, the iris provides a more than adequate environment for cell proliferation.

Three types of proliferation are classically recognized: (i) pearl cyst, (ii) serous cyst, and (iii) epithelial downgrowth. Pearl cysts are rare. They are usually small, white and solid tumors with opaque walls located in the iris stroma. Pearl cysts are imaged by UBM as solid round to ovoid tumors containing three concentric layers. The external layer has moderate reflectivity and correlates with the cystic epithelial lining. The intermediate layer has lower reflectivity corresponding to degenerated epithelial cells, mucus and inflammatory debris. Finally, a central, highly reflective core has been correlated to keratinous debris in the center of the cyst contents and cholesterol crystals derived from degenerative keratinized cells.

Serous, translucent cysts are more common and can erode through the iris and invade the posterior chamber. Their growth rate is variable; they can grow for some period and suddenly become stationary. They tend to have large diameters which cause iris atrophy by compression. These cysts are typically imaged by UBM as round or elliptic lesions with thick walls and a sonolucent cavity, or they can be septate. Dense fluctuating particles have been observed within cystic cavity.

Epithelial downgrowth is detected as a thin translucent membrane usually on the posterior surface of the cornea. A fine gray line can be noticed at the borders of the membrane. The adjacent cornea is generally edematous and new vessels can be present in the deep layers of the stroma. The membrane can extend to the iris, where it is noticed as a thin translucent film covering the anterior surface of the iris, with a slight loss of normal iris topography. A mild iridocyclitis can be present. If the membrane grows to the trabecular meshwork, intractable glaucoma can develop. Epithelial downgrowth is detected by UBM as a moderately echogenic membrane arising on the posterior corneal surface.

Cavitation within ciliary body tumors must be distinguished from large blood vessels within the tumor and slit-like spaces of supraciliary effusion that can be found in ciliary body melanomas. These cavities may be empty or they may contain erythrocytes, serous fluid, pigment-laden macrophages, or necrotic debris.

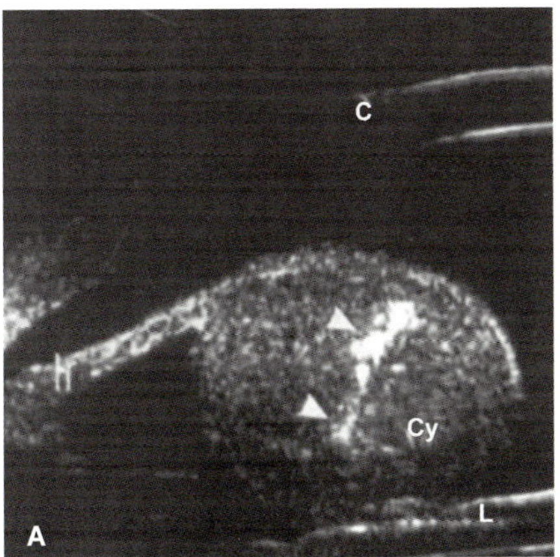

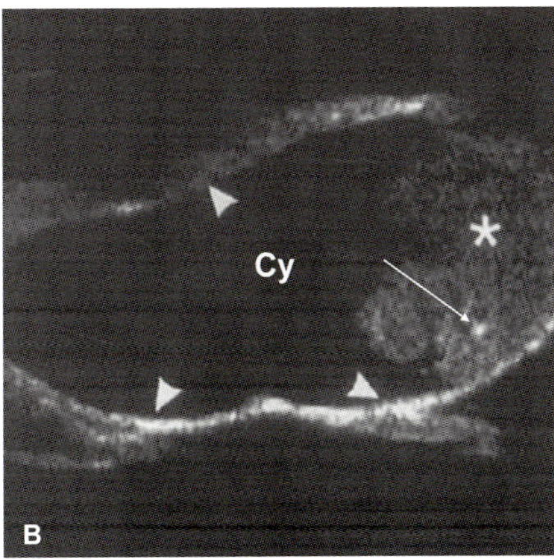

Figs 12A and B: (A) Mixed cyst, UBM, radial section,The cyst (Cy) was filled by moderately echogenic material with a hyperechoic core (arrowheads). It was located on the posterior iris (Ir) surface: C—cornea, L—IOL (B) Mixed cyst, UBM, transverse section. On transverse section, it was possible to observe that the moderately echogenic material (asterisk) was adherent to the cystic wall (arrowheads) and that part of the cyst (Cy) was also filled with sonolucent material. The hyperechogenic dot corresponds to the plan of the radial section shown in Figure A (arrow)

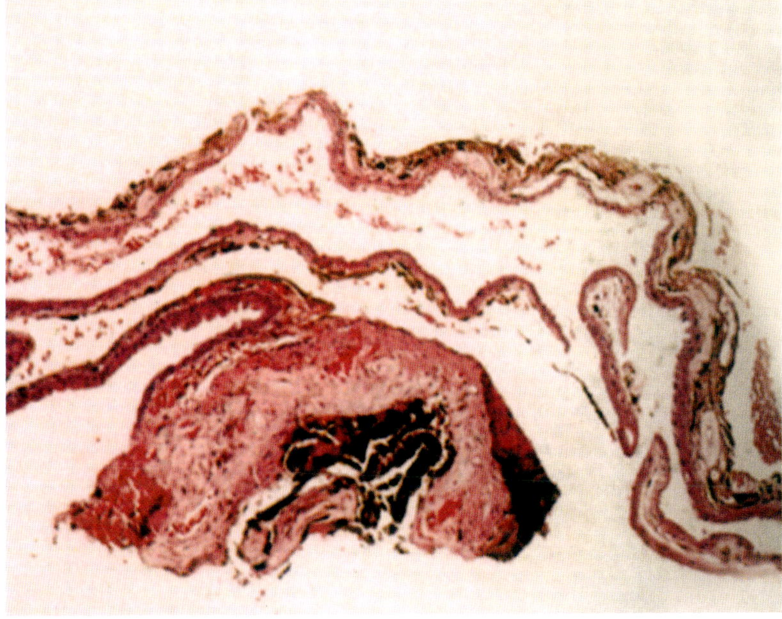

Fig. 12C: Mixed cyst, light microscopy, hematoxylin-eosin, original magnification: 25×. Light microscopy showed a non-keratinized squamous epithelial cell lining (arrowheads). Cyst's cavity (Cy) was filled with inflammatory debris. Cyst was adherent to the iris

Treatment

Implantation cysts are treated when they enlarge causing a decrease in the visual acuity, glaucoma, uveitis or cataracts. Treatment is controversial. Should one or more of these complications be noted, total excision is the best treatment. Treatment may also require a tectonic graft, aspiration of the cyst, and/or laser therapy.

METASTASIS

Introduction

Uveal metastases are more frequent than primary intraocular malignancies. Metastases to the eye most commonly originate from the breast in woman and the lung in men. Typically, there is a history of mastectomy or lung cancer at presentation. Eighteen to thirty percent of patients have no known or discoverable primary tumor. Other less frequent sites of origin include the gastrointestinal tract, the kidney, thyroid, and the testis. The prostate is an uncommon primary site.

Intraocular metastatases are typically discovered in the choroid, followed by the ciliary body and rarely in the iris. Ocular metastasis can be multifocal, bilateral, and they do not have a preference for affecting any specific quadrant.

Iris metastasis typically presents as pink or yellow solitary or multifocal tumors. Like ciliary body melanomas, ciliary body metastasis are generally large at the time of the diagnosis. They usually are diagnosed as a yellow, sessile, dome-shaped mass in the inferior quadrants. Metastasis to either iris or ciliary body can present as hyphema, anterior uveitis or as a pseudohypopyon.

Diagnosis

While fluorescein angiography will demonstrate early hyperfluorescence in the venous phase and late mottled hyperfluorescence, it is not typically helpful for differentiating metastatic lesions. Ultrasonography of metastasic tumor will demonstrate relatively high internal reflectivity and irregular shapes. If the clinical history and medical work-up are negative, transcorneal fine-needle aspiration or incisional biopsy can be helpful.

Treatment

Iris and ciliary body metastasis may be treated with systemic chemotherapy, but often prompt external beam radiation therapy offers the best hope for preventing secondary glaucoma. While radiation is a palliative treatment, the intraocular mass should not be irradiated if it is the only site which may help localize the source of the tumor. Enucleation is occasionally required for intractable glaucoma secondary to tumor invasion and/or occlusion of filtration.

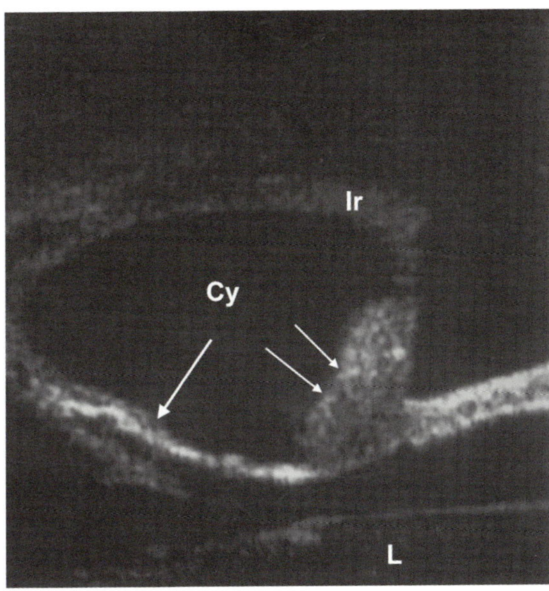

Fig. 13A: Serous cyst, UBM, radial section. Serous cysts (Cy) have sonolucent content and thick walls (arrowhead). Note the localized thickening of the cyst's wall (double arrowheads): L—lens, Ir—iris

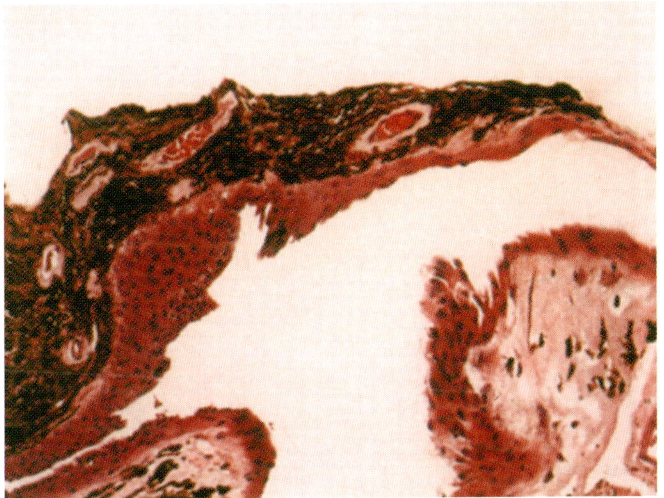

Fig. 13B: Serous cyst, light microscopy, hematoxylin-eosin, original magnification: 33×. Observe the stratified epithelial cell lining of the cyst. Note localized thickening of the cyst's wall determined by collagen. Iris stroma atrophied (Ir)

Prognosis

Prognosis for survival after uveal metastasis is poor, and computed tomography of the brain is recommended.

Tumors of the Non-pigmented Ciliary Body Epithelium

Medulloepithelioma

Introduction

Medulloepithelioma is a rare, congenital tumor of the non-pigmented epithelium of the ciliary body. Most patients present in the first decade of life.

Diagnosis

Medulloepithelioma usually presents as a mass lesion in the ciliary body. The lesion presents as internal cysts. Although benign, it is locally invasive and can erode to the anterior chamber or become externally visible. Glaucoma and cataracts may be associated. Most patients are diagnosed after enucleation.

Fuchs' Adenoma (Pseudoepitheliomatous Hyperplasia)

Introduction

Pseudoepitheliomatous hyperplasia is a benign, acquired lesion that arises in the non-pigmented epithelium of the pars plicata of the ciliary body. There is some discussion about the nature of the lesion. Probably, it is a proliferative disease rather than a tumor. Histopathologically, the lesion is composed by a nonvascular proliferation of the non-pigmented ciliary body epithelium which is rich in acid mucopolysaccharides. Some surveys have found pseudoepitheliomatous hyperplasia in as much as 25% of older people.

Diagnosis

The tumor is generally found incidentally during histopathological examination of an enucleated eye. It usually presents as a white glistening lesion arising in the pars plicata of the ciliary body. Depending on its size, it can cause a focal narrowing of the anterior chamber angle.

Other Tumors of the Nonpigmented Ciliary Body Epithelium

Adenoma and adenocarcinoma are very rare tumors that can only be differentiated of melanoma in a histopathological basis. Adenoma is suspected

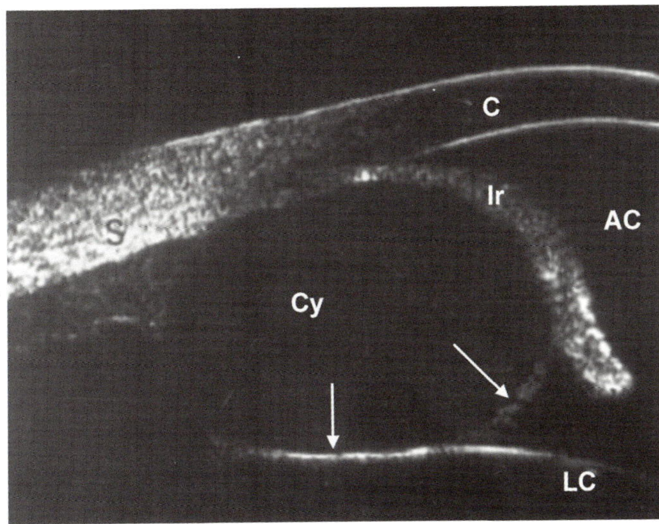

Fig. 14A: Congenital non-pigmented iris cyst, UBM, radial section. The cyst (Cy) was located on the posterior iris (Ir) surface, had a thick wall (thick arrow) and few moderately echoic dots within a sonolucent cavity. Note indentation on the anterior lens surface (arrow): S—sclera, C—cornea, LC—lens

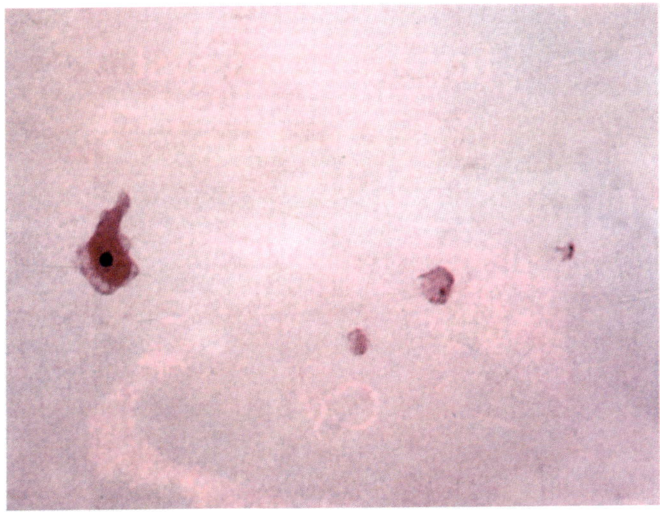

Fig. 14B: Congenital non-pigmented iris cyst, light microscopy, hematoxylin-eosin, original magnification: 132×. Pathologic examination of the fluid obtained by fine-needle biopsy revealed rare, exfoliated, non-keratinizing squamoid cells with occasional macrophages and melanin pigment

in cases of amelanotic ciliary body tumors with an irregular surface that transmits light well during transillumination. It is usually associated to uveitis. Ultrasonography shows high internal reflectivity. Adenocarcinoma should be suspected in women with persistent uveitis and a melanotic intraocular tumor that respond poorly to radiation plaque therapy. Both tumors are often managed by local excision.

Other Tumors

Leiomyoma

Leiomyoma of the uvea is an extremely rare iris or ciliary body tumor. Since the smooth muscle of the iris and the ciliary body is from neural crest origin, this tumor is considered to be from mesectodermal origin.

The leiomyoma occurs in younger patients and has a predilection for females. Leiomyomas are clinically indistinguishable of amelanotic melanomas. However, there are some features that help differentiate leiomyomas of melanomas: (i) as pointed before, leiomyomas tend to occur in young females, (ii) it tends to affect the ciliary body or the peripheral choroid and is rare in the posterior choroid, (iii) the tumor seems to grow in the supraciliary or supra-choroidal space between the uvea and the sclera and it does not seem to arise from the uveal stroma, and (iv) leiomyoma transmits light readily when transillu-minated, but melanoma produces a shadow.

The treatment consists in local resection by lamellar sclerouvectomy. Differently from melanoma, leiomyoma presents positive immunoreactivity for muscle markers and negative immunoreactivity for melanoma-specific antigen and neural markers.

Neurilemmoma (Schwannoma)

Neurilemmoma is a benign tumor that arises from a ciliary nerve. Likewise leiomyoma, neurilemmoma may simulate an amelanotic melanoma.

Neurofibroma

Neurofibroma is also a tumor derived from the neural crest. It arises from the ciliary nerves. Neurofibroma of the uvea is a very rare tumor. It is generally related to neurofibromatosis.

Hemangioma and Lymphoid Tumors

Hemangioma and benign or malignant lymphoid tumors are uncommon either in iris, ciliary body or choroid. When suspected, fine-needle aspiration biopsy (FNAB) may help in the diagnosis. External beam radiation therapy offers the best treatment (when necessary).

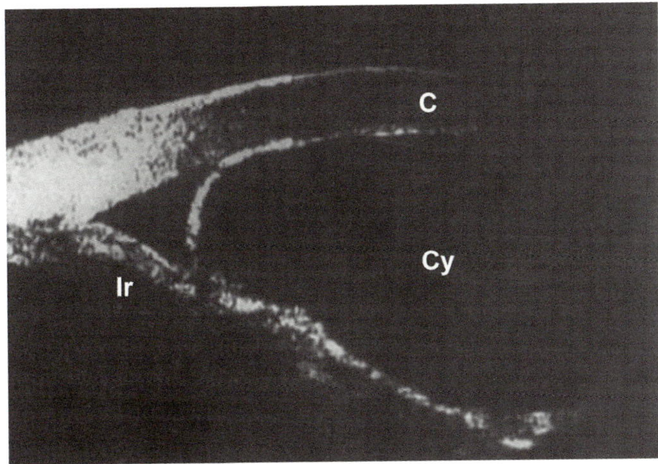

Fig. 15: Congenital non-pigmented iris cyst. UBM, radial section. Composite photo from two UBM images. A large cyst (Cy) was located on the anterior iris surface (Ir) and was adherent to the corneal endothelium (C)

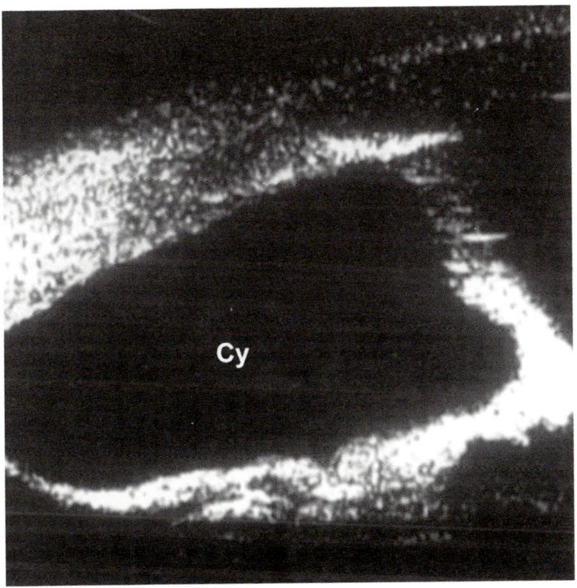

Fig. 16: Serous cyst. UBM, transverse section. A large epithelial cyst (Cy) was located in the anterior chamber secondary to cataract surgery

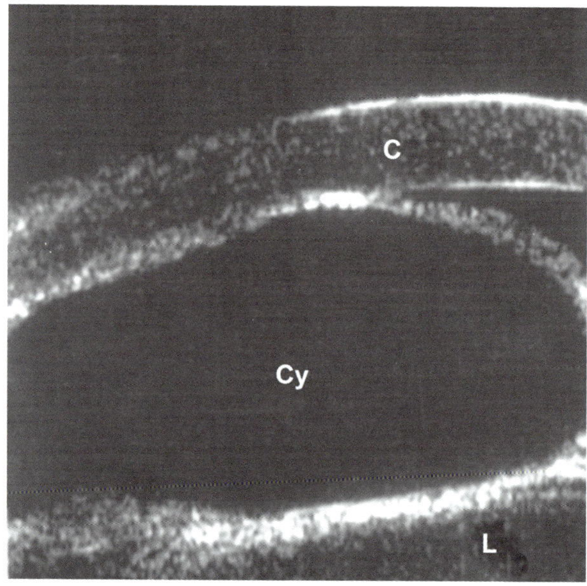

Fig. 17: Serous cyst. UBM, radial section. A large cyst (Cy) was adherent to corneal endothelium (C) and to anterior lens surface (L)

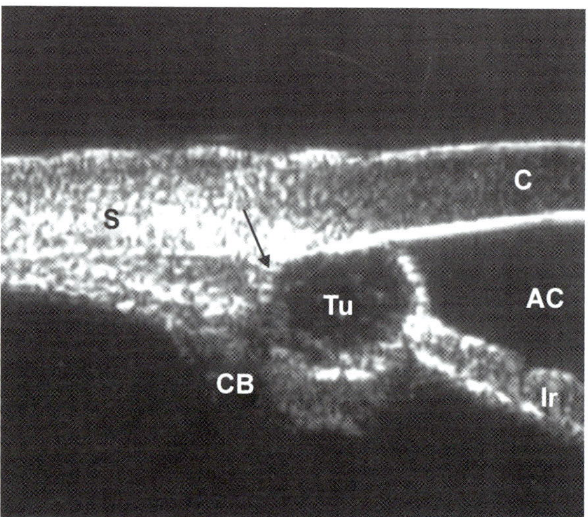

Fig. 18: Cavitated tumor—UBM radial section. A ciliary body (CB) mass with an echolucent cavity (Tu) infiltrating the iris root and extending to the angle was a cavitated melanoma (AC—anterior chamber, C—cornea, Ir—iris, S—sclera, arrow—scleral spur)

Chapter ELEVEN

Keratoplasty

- **Pediatric Keratoplasty**
  Anita Panda, Geeta Behera, Abhiyan Kumar (India)
- **Evolution of Keratoplasty through Centuries**
  Anita Panda, Sandeep Kumar, Shibal Bhartiya, Abhiyan Kumar (India)
- **Current Concepts in Pediatric Corneal Transplant Surgery**
  Ashok Sharma (India)

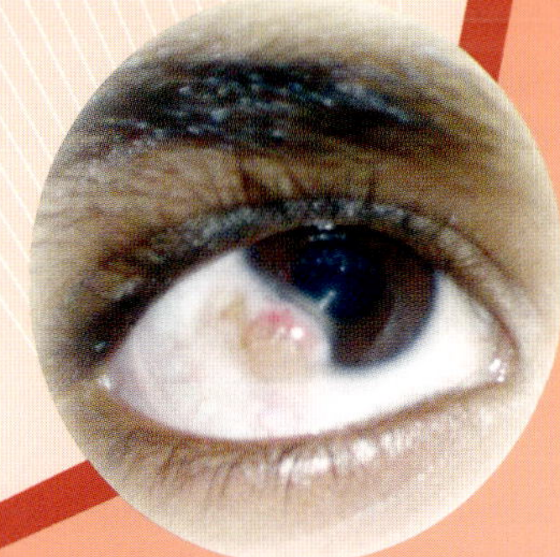

Pediatric Keratoplasty

Anita Panda, Geeta Behera, Abhiyan Kumar (India)

Introduction

Penetrating keratoplasty may be the necessary first step in preventing irreversible loss of visual function in a child, though the visual results of pediatric penetrating keratoplasty have been fairly disappointing. Many special difficulties encountered in the management of corneal transplantation in a child conspire to make these patients among the most challenging for the corneal surgeon.

Many aspects of an infant's or a child's preoperative, intraoperative and postoperative care differ from those of an adult undergoing a corneal transplantation. The child and the child's parents are usually very anxious when they present for preoperative evaluation. The difficulty in assessing the visual function of an infant, a child's inability to cooperate with the eye examination and the great variability in outcome all make the physicians decision regarding surgery more difficult.

Visual Assessment

Measuring vision in infants and children is a special skill. To start with, the examiner must create a rapport and gain attention of the child.

A normal child can fix and follow objects by 3 months of age, the blink response develops from 2 to 3 months, reaching out for objects begins by 6 months and binocular function develops by 3-7 months. The visual acuity of a normal child at birth is 6/120, at 6 months is 6/36, at 12 months at 6/18 and 6/6 at the age of 2 years.

WHO recommends that vision should be assessed at both distance and near with the same optotype. It should be recorded at 6, 4, 3 metres and 40 cm with a luminance of 80 and 160 candles/mm^2. Further, the distance and angle should be adjusted to fit the need of the child. Measuring the vision can be performed either directly or indirectly.

Direct

Up to 3 months of age by observing the baby recognize its mother's face, between 3-6 months by judging through colorful objects, between 6-12 months by its ability to differentiate details of small objects, between 12-36 months by Allen pictures, Lea symbols or Kay picture symbols and after 3 years and until 5 years by HOTV test, tumbling E test, Landolt broken ring test.

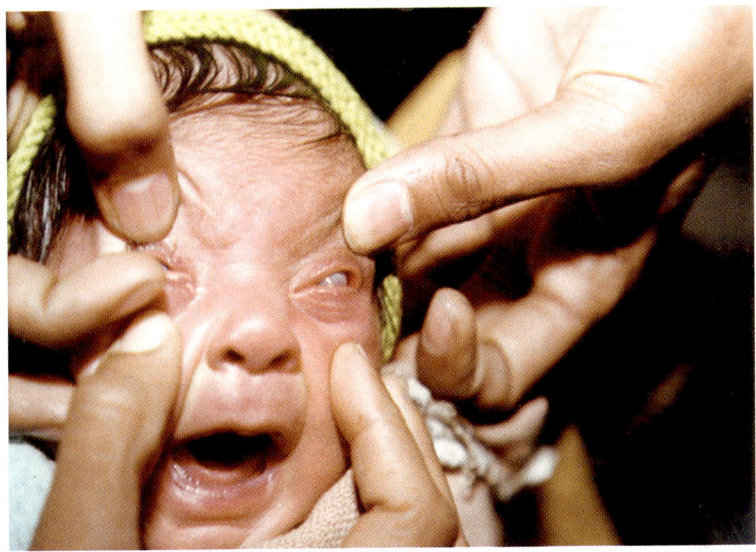

Fig. 1: Bilaterally blind infant

Indirect

Optokinetic (OKN) response, preferential looking techniques (PLT) and pattern evoked potentials.

Besides visual acuity, visual testing also includes assessing the pupillary reaction, fixation, ocular motility, fusion and color vision.

Ocular Examination

Like in adults, the ocular surface, anterior and posterior segment evaluation and adnexal examination are essential besides detailed corneal examination.

A full ocular evaluation under sedation or anesthesia is necessary involving refraction, tonometry, gonioscopy and fundoscopy. Because of the difficulty in determining any associated retinal or lens pathology in an infant with an opaque cornea, ultrasound for posterior examination and a single maximum intensity bright flash electroretinogram and visual evoked potential become essential.

Surgical Procedures

All surgery is carried out under general anesthesia. The surgery itself is technically more difficult because in infants the cornea and the anterior chamber are smaller, and the cornea is often thinner and more pliable, requiring more exacting surgical technique. Compared to an adult eye, the eye of a young keratoplasty patient is more likely to have scleral collapse and alarming posterior pressure. The iris of infants and children seems to have a greater tendency to adhere to the posterior corneal surface and the wound. Many young patients with congenital or traumatic corneal disease have significant anterior segment abnormalities, which may be difficult to anticipate but must be addressed during the surgery. In children requiring vitrectomy, the vitreous is more tenacious which makes its safe, rapid removal more difficult.

Infants and children in comparison to adults, appear to be more prone to a severe inflammatory response during the early postoperative period and more likely to have endothelial graft rejection or graft failure.

Again, the corneal wound heals more rapidly in infants and children, increasing the risks that sutures will loosen quickly, erode, vascularize and become infected. Therefore, all sutures must be removed early, making selective suture removal to minimize transplant astigmatism impossible.

The graft's success may eventually decrease if parents fail to understand the important role of postoperative management and difficulties thereof. Unless the surgeon is able to communicate to them the importance of constant supervision and the need for regular medication and follow-up, it is probably wiser not to attempt such surgery.

Postoperatively, infants and young children are unable to cooperate for examinations. Therefore, the examination must be either suboptimal or

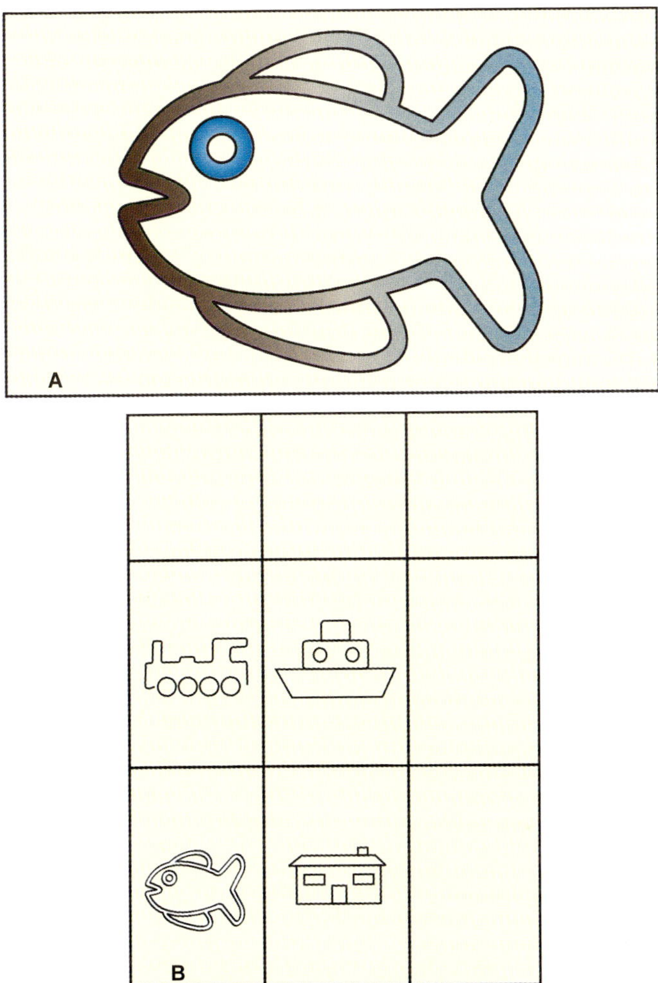

Figs 2A and B: Cardiff acuity cards

performed with the patients under restraint, under sedation or under anesthesia. Infants and children cannot effectively communicate that they have visual loss, pain or other symptoms that require evaluation. Therefore, compared to adults, they require more frequent examinations. Also, children are more likely to rub or traumatize their eye.

The greatest difference between the management of pediatric and adult corneal transplantation patients is that infants and young children with a visually significant corneal opacity develop visual deprivation amblyopia. The specter of amblyopia affects the decision to proceed with surgery. The timing of the surgery is very crucial. In fact, the fundamental goal of pediatric penetrating keratoplasty and all the postoperative care is to reverse or limit the effects of amblyopia. The duration of time the eye is capable of perceiving a clear, well-focused image and the effectiveness of amblyopia therapy during the initial years of life establish the eye's visual potential for the rest of the patient's life. Physician and parents should view the surgery itself, alike, as the first in a long series of interventions designed to treat amblyopia.

Indications

The indications for corneal grafting differ between the neonatal period and the age of 2 years. In the latter they may be somewhat similar to those for the adult. When there is a congenital corneal opacity and normal contralateral eye, the visual results following grafting are poor even in a technically successful surgery for a number of reasons. The grafting is usually done too late and there are difficulties with occlusion of the other eye. The more abnormal the cornea, the more abnormal the intraocular structure, and the use of vitreous cutters may be necessary. If there is abnormal recipient corneal tissue then a large graft may be necessary. The graft is likely to remain clear, the greater the normal tissue.

In such cases the parents are all important. If they cooperate, a vision of 3/60 may be achieved, which may provide the infant with a cosmetically acceptable spare eye. On the other hand, children with acquired corneal opacification should have surgery performed as soon as the condition has stabilized.

Congenital

- Sclerocornea
- Corneal dermoids
- Congenital hereditary endothelial dystrophy
- Peter's anomaly
- Glaucoma with corneal edema
- Posterior polymorphous dystrophy
- Mucopolysaccharidosis

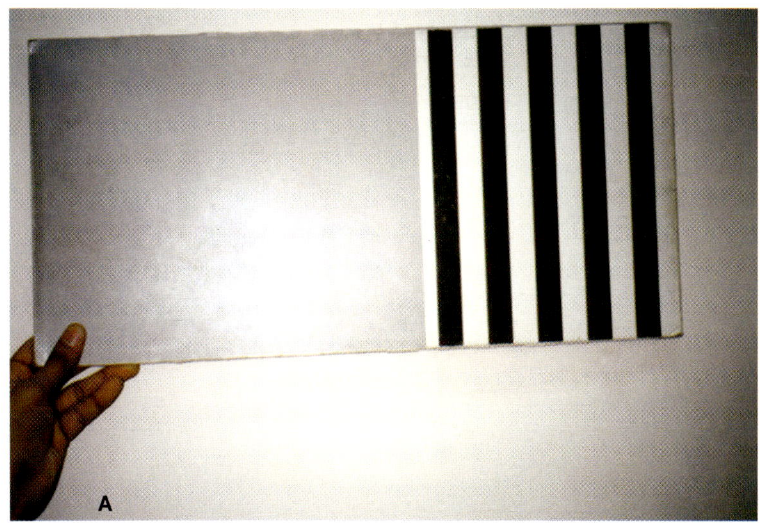

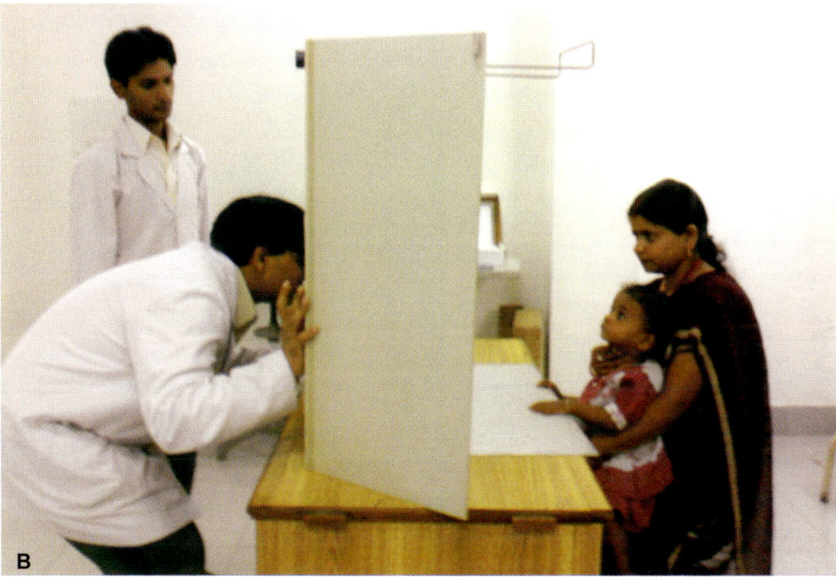

Figs 3A and B: Teller's acuity cards

Acquired, Non-traumatic

- Ophthalmia neonatorum
- Herpes simplex keratitis
- Bacterial keratitis
- Steven Johnson syndrome
- Keratoconus
- Neurotrophic keratitis
- Interstitial keratitis
- Fungal keratitis
- keratomalacia

Acquired, Traumatic

- Birth trauma
- Corneal or corneoscleral laceration
- Nonpenetrating injury with scar

Of the congenital anomalies, Peter's anomaly, sclerocornea and congenital glaucoma have a particularly poor chance of success, while patients with posterior polymorphous dystrophy and congenital hereditary endothelial dystrophy fare better. Traumatic causes of congenital opacities have a better prognosis than congenital. Of the acquired, non-traumatic causes, keratoconus and herpes simplex keratitis show a good graft survival while visual outcome is poorer in the infective and nutritional causes.

Though grafts in older children tend to do better than grafts in younger ones, amblyopia occurring thereof may severely compromise visual recovery. Also, first grafts survive longer than regrafts.

Surgical Management

Pediatic penetrating keratoplasty is performed using an operating microscope, with the patient under general anesthesia. The surgery in infants and children is marked, more than anything else, by scleral collapse and alarming posterior pressure. Particularly in infants, lens expulsion often seems common. Every available maneuver to reduce posterior pressure should be used. The anesthesiologist should be asked to hyperventilate the patient, which reduces intraocular pressure. Paralysis with a nondepolarising muscle relaxant monitored with a peripheral nerve stimulator eliminates the risk of movement and contraction of the extraocular muscles. Positioning the patient with the head slightly higher than the feet probably also decreases posterior pressure.

Digital massage reduces posterior pressure and endothelial cell loss during penetrating keratoplasty. Alternatively a Honan balloon should be applied at 30 mm Hg for 5 or more minutes. Care should be taken to ensure that the speculum, surgeon and assistant do not apply pressure to the globe.

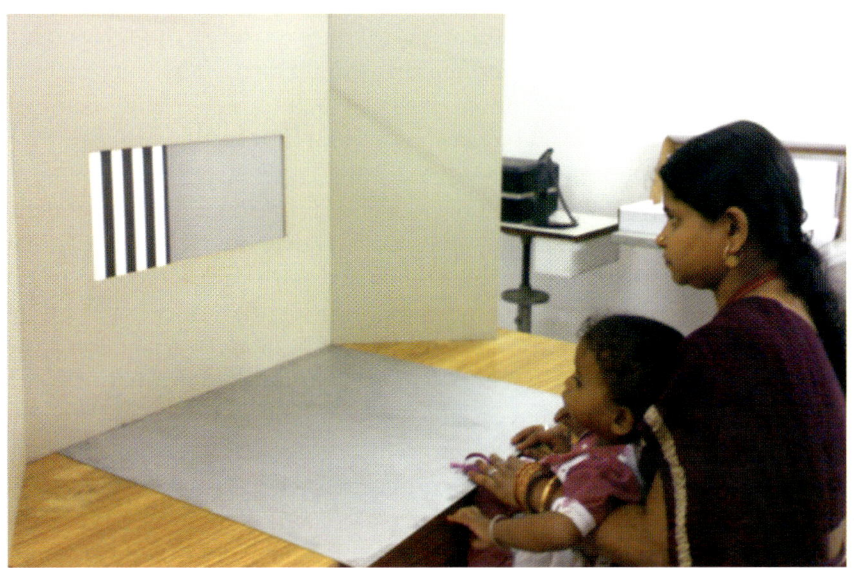

Fig. 3C: Teller's acuity cards

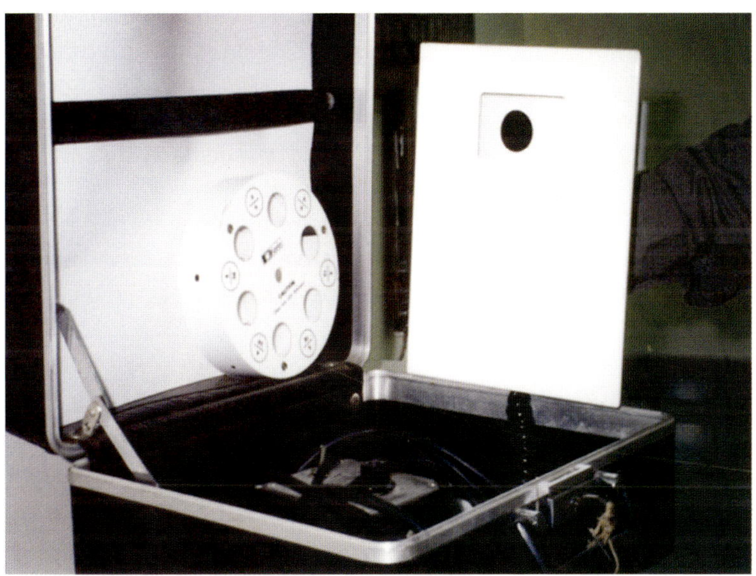

Fig. 4A: Catford drum

A lateral canthotomy is helpful in improving exposure in infants and may reduce posterior pressure. A Flieringa ring should be used in every pediatric penetrating keratoplasty. It should be fastened to the episclera with six to eight sutures. Four sutures should be left long so that they can be fastened to the drapes to gently support the eye.

Mannitol reduces vitreous volume as well as intraocular pressure and thus reduces posterior pressure. Because it causes systemic fluid shifts that can lead to hemodynamic instability, it should be used with care. The dose of 20% mannitol is 0.5 to 1.5 kg by slow intravenous infusion. To reduce the possibility of hemodynamic instability, each 0.5 g/kg should be given over a period no less than 20-30 minutes. The peak action is about 45 minutes after administration.

The scrub nurse should have a lens loop available so that an assistant can quickly use it to gently place pressure on the iris and lens if loss of lens seems imminent. The nurse should also have an "emergency suture (8-0 nylon/silk on a cutting needle) loaded and immediately available if the posterior pressure is so great that 10-0 nylon would break during placement of the cardinal sutures.

Preoperative miotic or mydriatic drops can be used depending on the procedure. If the lens is known to be clear, miotics still help protect the lens, especially in the setting of posterior pressure. If the eye has a visually significant cataract and the surgeon plans an "open sky" lensectomy, mydriatic can be used preoperatively.

A preoperative examination by a portable slit lamp and possibly pachymetry will help the surgeon avoid trephining through particularly thin areas, which would make secure wound closure more difficult.

Preoperative topical antibiotics appear to reduce the risk of postoperative endophthalmitis. If combined with preoperative irrigation of the ocular surface with dilute povidone-iodine, it reduces ocular surface bacterial counts even more.

Penetrating Keratoplasty

In infants, the cornea and anterior segment are smaller, and the cornea is often thinner and more pliable, making the surgery technically more difficult. Due to the smaller corneal size in an infant and marked posterior pressure, most surgeons use a smaller graft size in infants than in adults.

Disadvantages of Smaller Graft

1. Children often have larger pupils, so a small graft may be optically less than optimal.
2. In a smaller graft, total number of endothelial cells transplanted is lower. For instance, reducing the donor diameter from 8.0 to 6.0 mm reduces the number of endothelial cells transplanted by 44%. This reduction becomes important if the recipient rim has a low density of viable endothelial cells.

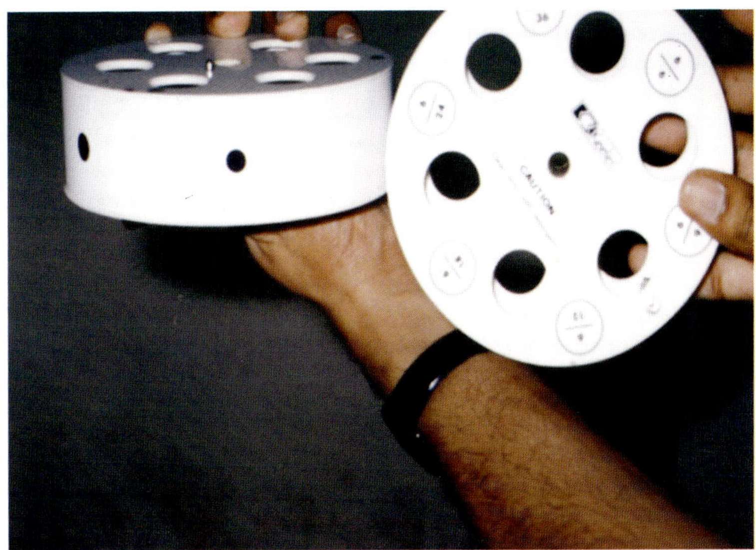

Fig. 4B: Catford drum

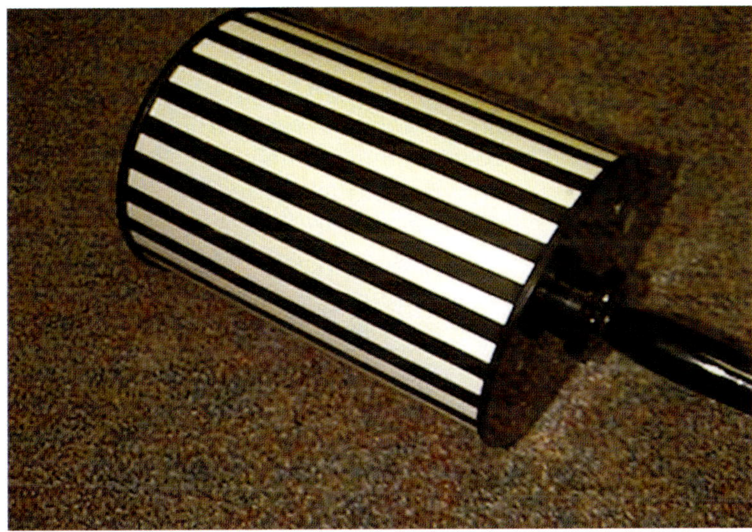

Fig. 5: OKN drum

Infants and children are more active postoperatively and probably are more likely than adults to stress the wound with crying, rubbing and injury. It is important to use a donor trephine 0.5 mm or more than the recipient trephine (0.5 mm over size) to facilitate secure closure of the eye.

Beveling in the corneal scissors after trephining two-third or three-fourth the thickness of the cornea forms the recipient bed. This technique will create a posterior lip to help form an aqueous tight wound. In a case where the entire recipient cornea is too thin and soft to hold sutures, a total corneal or corneo-scleral graft can be performed. An alternative in this situation is to perform a large lamellar keratoplasty followed by a smaller penetrating keratoplasty.

Because the graft is often needed to push the lens and iris back, copious viscoelastic agent should used liberally on the lens iris diaphragm before bringing the graft to the wound to limit endothelial trauma.

The increased fibrin production in infants and young children, combined with posterior pressure, can produce iris adhesions to the wound. These adhesions can often be avoided by placing viscoelastic in the anterior chamber as soon as the eye is opened, before the anterior chamber collapses. If adhesions form, they can be lysed by placing viscoelastic in the anterior chamber after the wound is closed, entering at a distant position from the wound with a vitreous sweep, and sweeping the adherent iris out of the wound.

Blood clot can be manually removed from the anterior chamber, and tissue plasminogen activator (25 μg) can be used to lyse a fibrin clot intraoperatively.

Wound closure is achieved with three-fourths depth 10-0 nylon sutures, as in adult penetrating keratoplasty. Because the sutures can't be removed selectively in very young patients, equal distribution of the donor tissue in the recipient bed is probably important to minimize graft astigmatism. Interrupted sutures are preferred because they reduce the chance that a broken suture will result in wound dehiscence. They also allow for staged removal if some sutures begin to erode before the wound is sufficiently healed to allow removal of all sutures.

Because of the risk of postoperative trauma, a generous number of sutures, perhaps 20 to 24 on 0.7 mm transplantation, should be placed in infants and children. All suture knots should be buried to reduce the risk of ocular surface complications.

Continuous sutures may be preferred in a symmetric vascular or avascular opacity, but never in an asymmetric vascular opacity or infected case. Contraction along the vascular, scarred area leads to early loosening of sutures there and may compromise wound healing in adjacent areas if the suture is continuous.

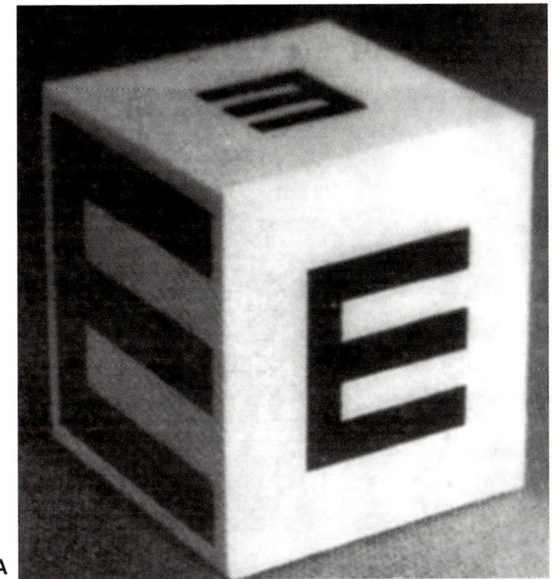

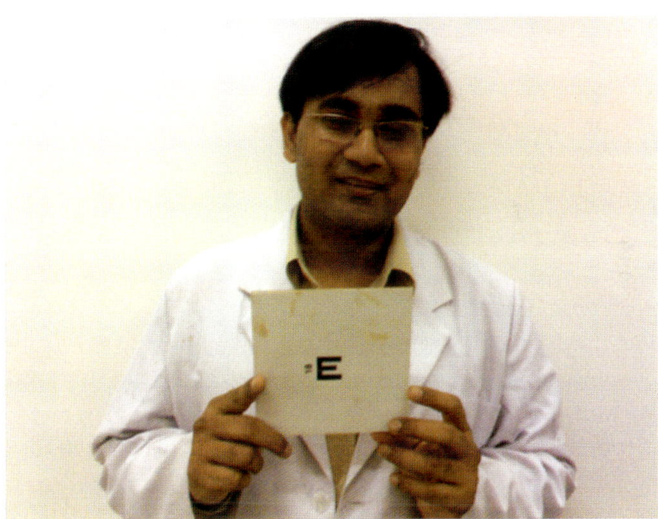

Figs 6A and B: Tumbling E

Concomitant Procedures

Iris Procedures

Peripheral Iridectomy

Indications

A. If there is posterior synechiae or persistent intraocular inflammation.
B. If associated lensectomy and vitrectomy is being performed.

Anterior Synechiolysis

If there is high positive pressure and the view is sufficient, lysis can be most easily accomplished with a vitreous sweep after making a 1 mm incision at the base of the trephine groove and injecting viscoelastic into the anterior chamber.

If the view is not sufficient, synechiolysis can only be accomplished after suturing the graft into place.

In an aphakic eye, a sector iridectomy followed by creation of a smaller pupil with 10-0 prolene suture on a noncutting needle will tighten the iris diaphgram and prevent reformation of synechiae.

Pupilloplasty

If the pupil is disfigured.

Lensectomy and Anterior Vitrectomy

Indications

i. If there is dense cataract associated with corneal pathology.
ii. In Peter's type II anomaly.

However, the decision to remove a lens with only a mild to moderate opacity during a pediatric penetrating keratoplasty should be made judiciously. Lensectomy and vitrectomy are statistically significant risk factors for graft failure and poor visual outcome. If lensectomy is performed at the time of penetrating keratoplasty, it is generally performed "open sky", as in adults.

After anterior capsulotomy and expression or aspiration of the nucleus, the cortical material is removed. Removal will be difficult in the face of vitreous upthrust. An irrigation aspiration device or anterior vitrectomy instrument with its cutting action turned off can be used for cortical aspiration.

As virtually every pediatric posterior capsule will opacify, a partial posterior capsulotomy and anterior vitrectomy should be performed in infants and perhaps children. Even though older children might cooperate for a Nd:YAG capsulotomy, in the absence of a posterior chamber lens, Nd:YAG capsulotomy usually results in vitreous prolapse into the anterior chamber. This prolapse can cause pupillary block or vitreous endothelial touch, which will threaten

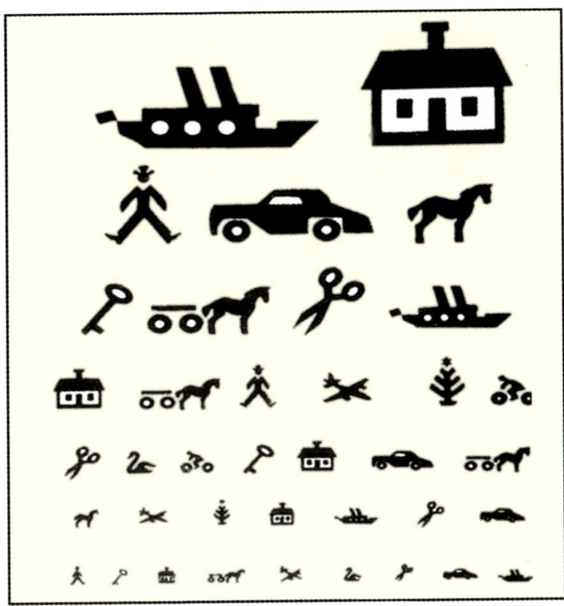

Fig. 7: Allen's picture cards

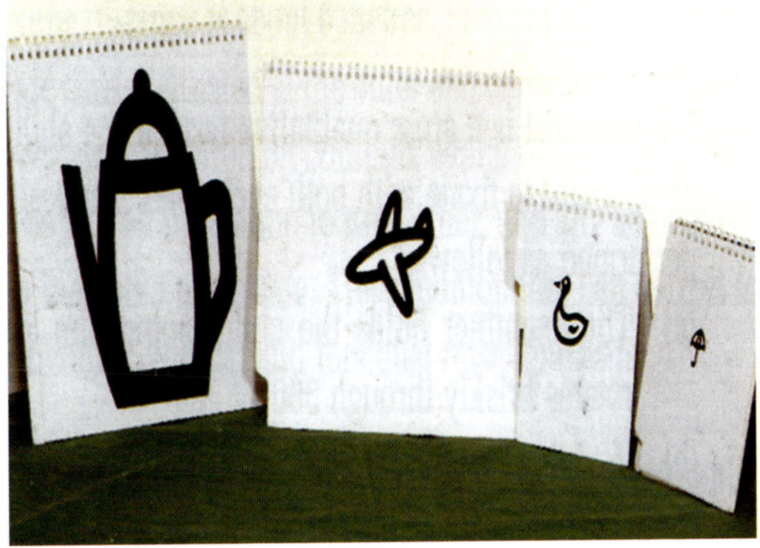

Fig. 8: Kay's picture cards

the graft. The posterior capsulotomy and anterior vitrectomy are performed with an automated vitrector with a cut rate of about 300 to 400 cycles/minute and maximum suction setting of about 80 mm Hg. The vitrector should be used to create a circular hole of about 7 mm diameter in the posterior capsule. The capsulotomy should be this large, as the capsular remnants can contract and opacify postoperatively to block the visual axis, especially in infants. If the capsulotomy is circular, it will not tear and would provide support if a posterior chamber lens is implanted later. For immediate visual rehabilitation, majority is of view of using contact lens.

Concomitant Retinal Surgery

If the eye requires pars plana vitrectomy for retinal detachment, use of an intraoperative keratoprosthesis for the retinal surgery affords the retinal surgeon a better view than through a new transplant. After the retinal surgeon completes the retinal reattachment, the keratoprosthesis is replaced with transplantation tissue.

After the transplantation is completed, subconjunctival injections of antibiotics and steroids are generally given.

It may be useful to perform a postoperative examination while the child is still under anesthesia. A portable slit lamp is useful to confirm that there is no iris adherent to the wound and can be used to provide a cobalt blue filter to perform a Siedel test of the wound.

The new transplantation may afford the surgeon the first view of the retina with an indirect ophthalmoscope. An axial eye length can be determined to help in later estimating an aphakic eye's refractive error.

Before applying a pressure patch and metal shield, a single drop of 0.5% atropine in healthy full-term infants or 1% atropine ointment in children should be applied. When seeing the family after surgery it is wise to remind them of the guarded prognosis for vision and that the transplantation is only the first step in the visual rehabilitation of the eye.

Postoperative Care

Immediate Postoperative Period

Premature infants and infants and children with systemic diseases should be monitored carefully and the recommendations of the patient's pediatrician and anesthesiologists should be sought. The child should be discharged on the first or second postoperative day if vital signs and oral intake are normal, and the eye is epithelialized.

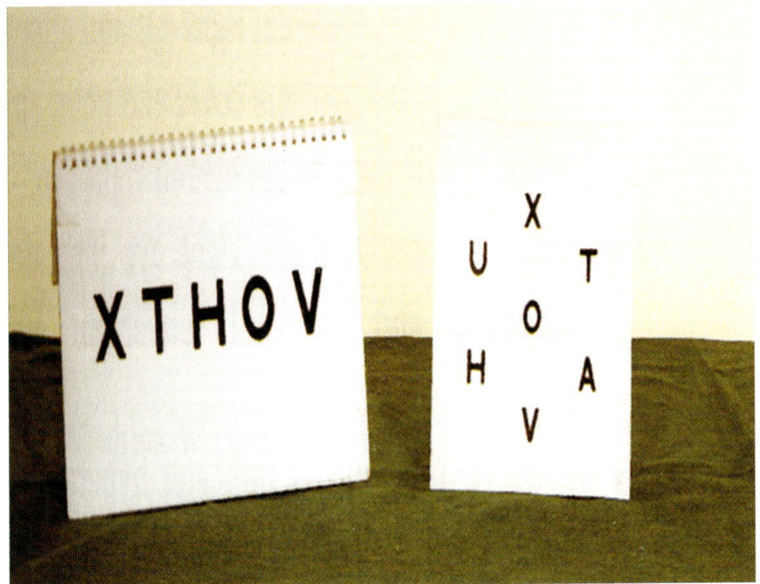

Fig. 9: HOTV chart

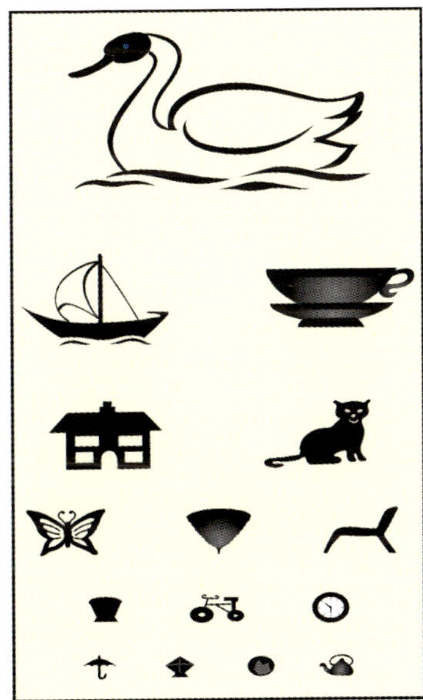

Fig. 10: Snellen's picture chart

Early Postoperative Care

The goals of the examination and interventions in the first few weeks after surgery are to make certain that the wound is secure and watertight, monitor and promote the decline in postoperative inflammation, monitor and control intraocular pressure. It is necessary to detect other postoperative complications and also begin amblyopia therapy.

The first postoperative examination should be within 24 hours after surgery. A reasonable schedule of routine postoperative examinations includes examinations on the first, second, fourth, seventh, tenth and fourteenth postoperative days.

Postoperative complications are usually the same as in adults, but infants and young children are unable to communicate effectively that they have pain, visual loss or other symptoms and hence they require frequent early postoperative examinations.

Postoperative Medications

Because infants and children can have an exaggerated inflammatory response postoperatively, it seems reasonable to use more topical steroids than in adult keratoplasty patients.

A long acting topical cycloplegic, generally atropine should also be given during first two postoperative weeks to prevent formation of synechiae.

Rest of the medications is the same as in adults.

Suture Removal

Typically all sutures can be removed safely according to the following schedule. During the first year of life, sutures are removed at 5 weeks after surgery; in one year olds at 6 to 7 postoperative weeks; in 2 and 3 years olds at 8 to 10 postoperative weeks, in 4 to year old at 3 months and in 7 to 10 years olds at 5 to 6 months postoperatively. Patients 10 to 20 years of age often require removal of all sutures because of rapid erosion by the sixth to eighth postoperative months.

Optical Correction and Amblyopia Therapy

Without effective optical correction and amblyopia therapy, a pediatric penetrating keratoplasty may be useless. The younger the patient, the deeper the amblyopia will be if the eye has a structural or refractive abnormality that limits vision. However, amblyopia is more easily reversed in a younger patient if it is treated promptly and appropriately.

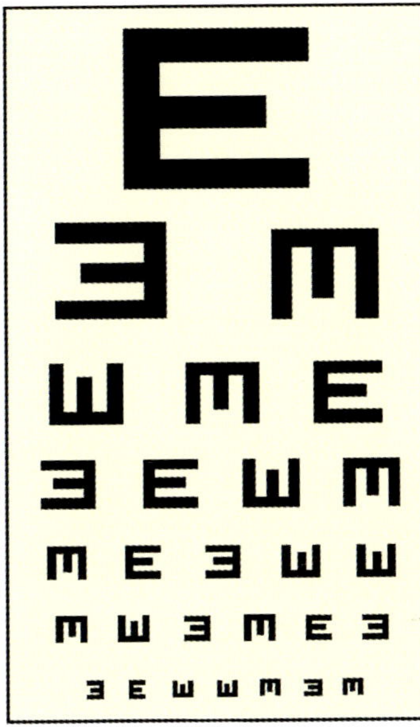

Fig. 11: Snellen's E chart

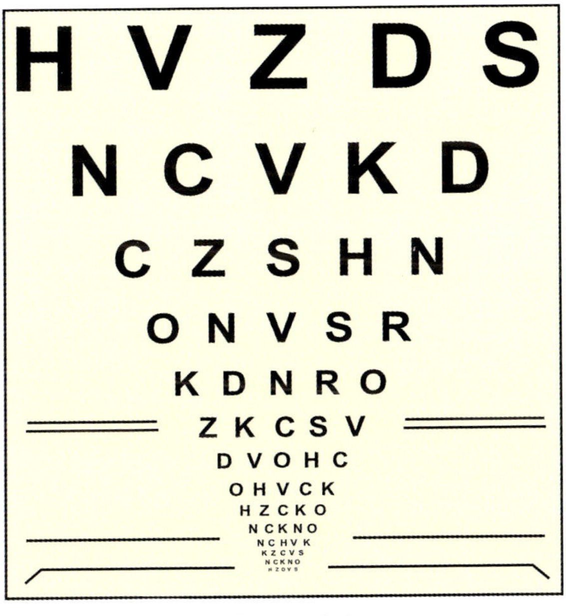

Fig. 12: ETDRS chart

Correction of refractive error is a vital part of amblyopia therapy. At about 2 postoperative weeks, the epithelium has generally healed and the graft has cleared sufficiently to perform cycloplegic retinoscopy. Retinoscopy may be difficult, and the refraction will change as the wound heals and sutures are removed; but a correction of any moderate or large refractive error should be prescribed at this time, even if it is not exact. The refraction should be repeated every 3 to 6 weeks until the sutures have been out till the age of one year. Thereafter, the refraction should be repeated at least four times a year till the age of 5 years.

Refraction of an aphakic eye may be confirmed if the axial length is known. The following formula is an approximation in an aphakic eye with a keratometry measurement of 45 diopters and a vertex distance of 10 mm

Distance spectacle power = 63.7 – (2.28 × axial eye length in mm)

The results from this formula can be modified by keratometry measurements. For an aphakic eye, an infant is generally prescribed a near correction, that is +1.00 to 2.00 sphere over the distance correction. At 1 to 3 years of age, the aphakic child should be prescribed bifocal lenses with the top of the segment at the inferior border of the pupil.

Contact lens is useful in the visual rehabilitation of pediatric keratoplasty patients. Monocular aphakic silicone lenses offer the highest oxygen permeability of all lenses and are often well tolerated by aphakic patients with normal corneas.

If the contralateral eye is normal in an infant or a young child, occlusion therapy should be started as soon as the graft has partially cleared, and refractive correction is being used. Optimally this should be no later than 2 postoperative weeks. Occlusion during the first 6 months of life is usually limited to one-fourth to three-fourths of the infant's waking hours. If the child is older than 6 months, then vision in both eyes is monitored carefully to check for improvement of the amblyopic eye or worsening of the normal eye.

If the patient has undergone bilateral penetrating keratoplasties, he or she may still have amblyopia. If amblyopia is suspected, it should be treated as outlined previously after doing everything reasonable to correct the structural and refractive abnormalities.

In all this, the role of parents cannot be overemphasized. They have to be appropriately counseled preoperatively of the child's condition and given a realistic view of the prognosis. Their participation and dedication to the whole procedure is what pays off in the long-term. Postoperatively they have to be trained to watch out for complications, as a child's ability to communicate is limited. They have to be told to recognize loose sutures and imminent graft rejection by redness in the eye, accumulations of mucus and loss of graft clarity. They may be trained in penlight examination.

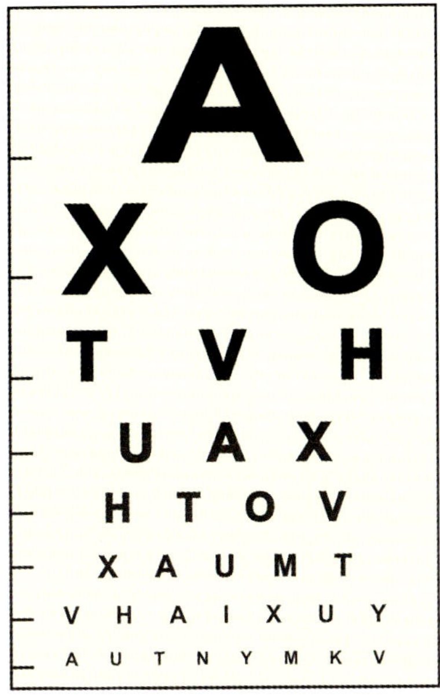

Fig. 13: Snellen's letter chart

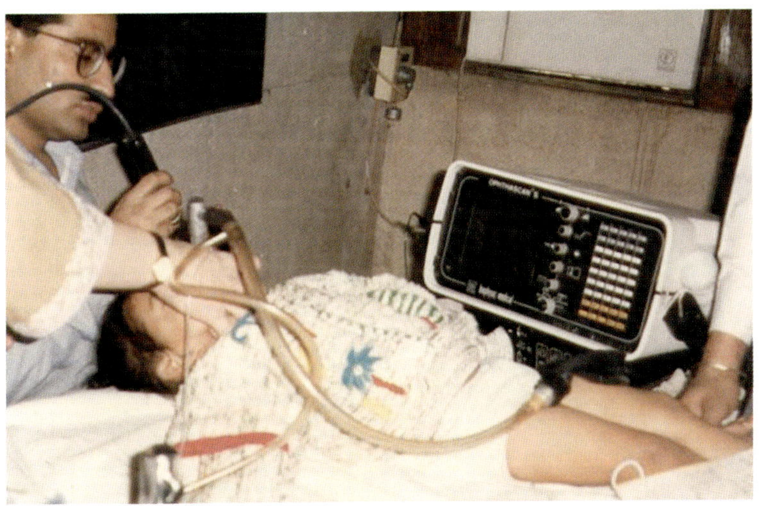

Fig. 14A: Biometry under general anesthesia

Conclusion

Because of advances in surgical techniques and postoperative care, a clear corneal graft in an infant or a child has become commonplace over the last 20 years. Although the visual results are currently disappointing, it appears that meticulous attention to the health of the graft and the eye, correction of refractive error and adequate amblyopia therapy will yield improved visual results for eyes that are otherwise normal.

Although pediatric penetrating keratoplasty patients are among the most challenging the corneal surgeon will encounter, they can also be among the most rewarding. With a great deal of effort the vision of an infant or a child, otherwise condemned to lifelong blindness, can be restored.

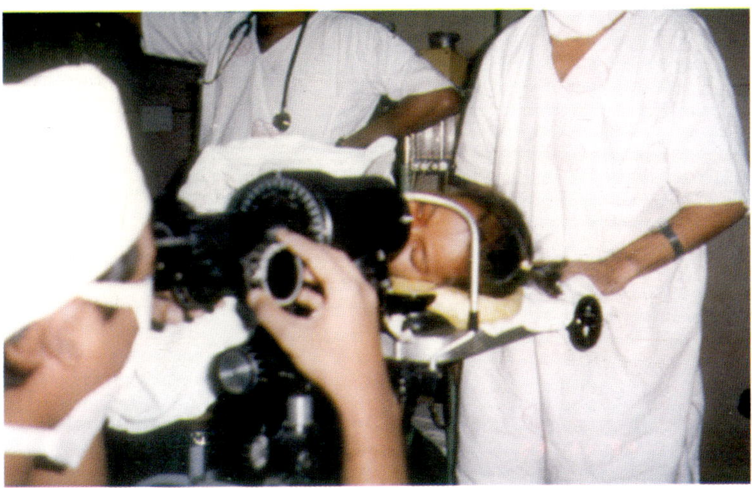

Fig. 14B: Keratometry under general anesthesia

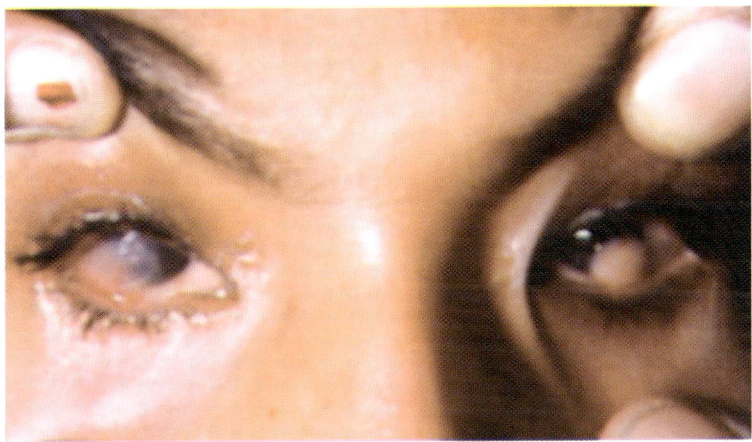

Fig. 15: Bilateral dermoid

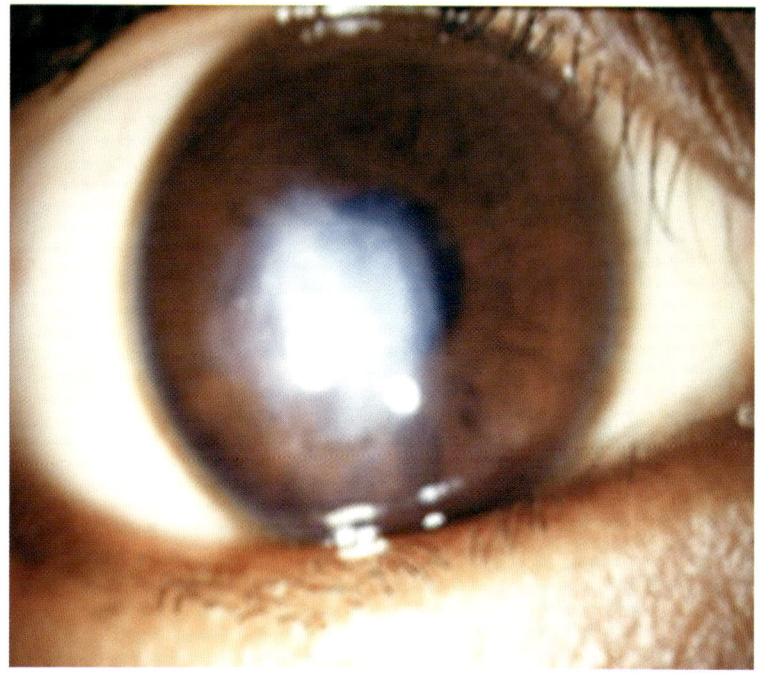

Fig. 16: CHED

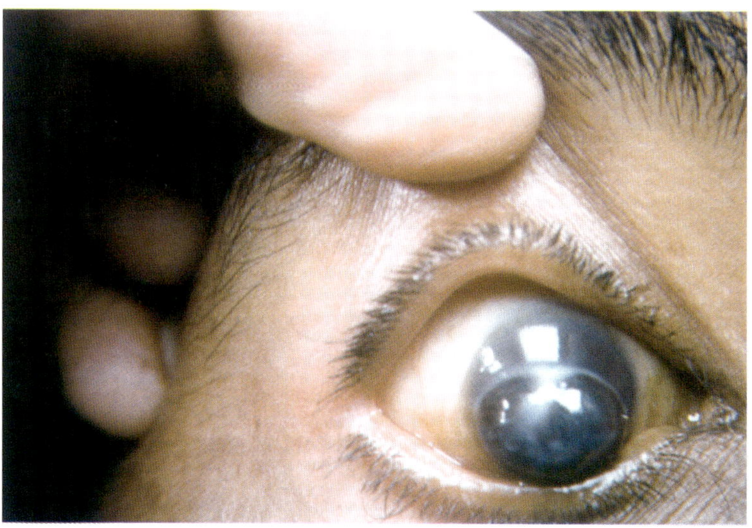

Fig. 17A: Post-traumatic corneal opacity

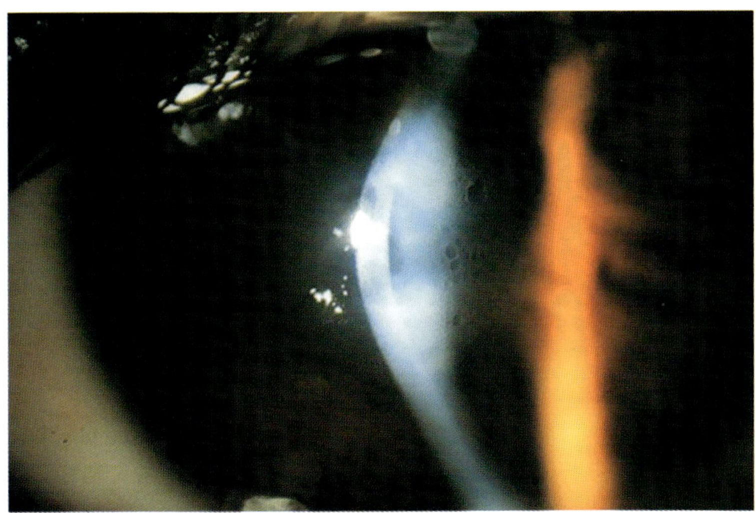

Fig. 17B: Keratoconus with healed hydrops

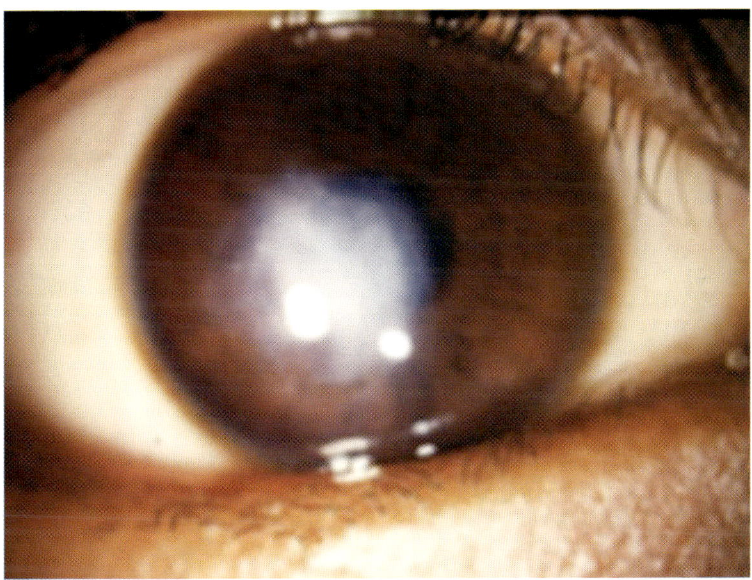

Fig. 18: Healing keratitis with partial anterior staphyloma

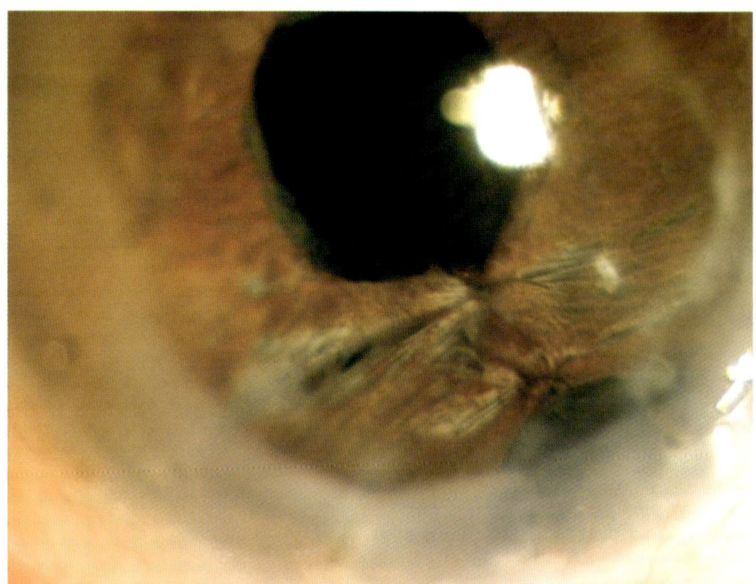

Fig. 19: Postoperative therapeutic keratoplasty

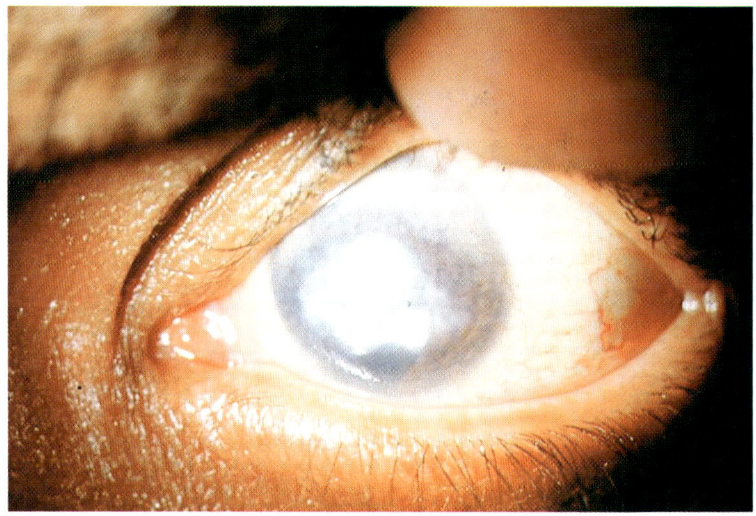

Fig. 20: Corneal opacity with cataract

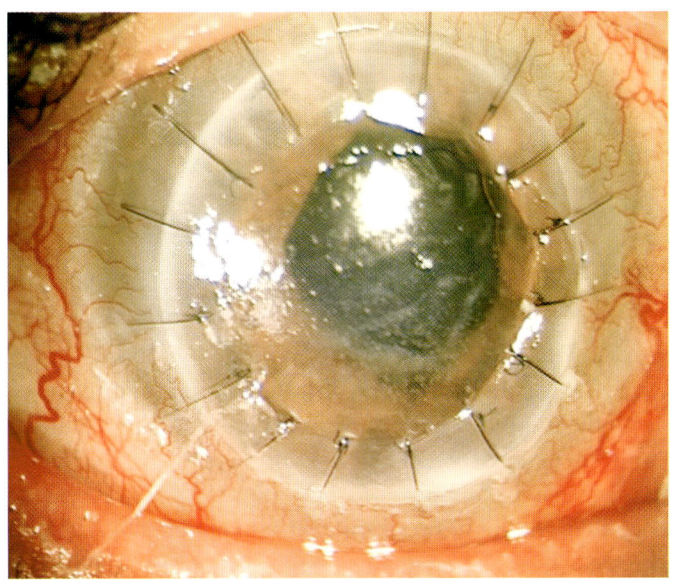

Fig. 21: Pupilloplasty in penetrating keratoplasty

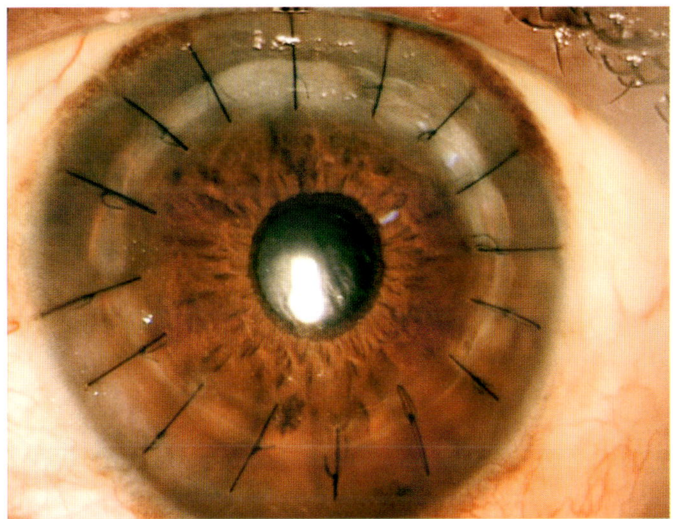

Fig. 22: Clear graft following successful optical penetrating keratoplasty

Evolution of Keratoplasty through Centuries

Anita Panda, Sandeep Kumar, Shibal Bhartiya , Abhiyan Kumar (India)

Introduction

The heritage of keratoplasty goes back to dawn of 1813. Today keratoplasty has the distinction of being the most successful of transplant surgeries, world wide. The history of the evolution of keratoplasty into a distinct clinical entity is, however, replete with bizarre and ingenious remedies, follies of misconception, and brilliant discoveries that are the basis of contemporary success. This review of milestones and challenges in keratoplasty describes the effort made by dedicated corneal surgeons who were acknowledged as the pioneers in this field for conceiving the notion of keratoplasty, stumbled along with countless failures, and laid the groundwork for what has become a twentieth century success story. It is their dynamic, incessant toil and vivid imagination that has been translated into the reality of a standard procedure in the surgical repertoire of modern ophthalmology.

Review

Franz Reisinger, coined the term "keratoplasty" and suggested the use of animal tissue to replace the scarred human cornea. His work was confined to rabbits and chickens, with most his experimental works failing because of either clouding of the graft or panophthalmitis.

The history of today´s corneal grafting dates back to the nineteenth century when K Himly of Germany suggested replacing an opaque cornea of one animal with a clear cornea of another animal (1813).

In 1837, Dr SIL Bigger reported his successful attempts at keratoplasty While traveling, Bigger was taken captive by Sahara Bedouins near Cairo in 1835. During his captivity he performed a corneal homograft on a blinded pet gazelle using the tissue of another gazelle, successfully.

Among those inspired by Dr Bigger's report was Dr Richard Sharp Kissam in New York who attempted keratoplasty in the only functional eye of an Irishman in 1838. He removed the opaque cornea with a Beer cataract knife and then with only two sutures at 3 and 9 o'clock positions, secured the donated tissue from a 6-month-old pig, into position. These sutures were removed after 36 hours, at which time the porcine graft appeared to have been united with the

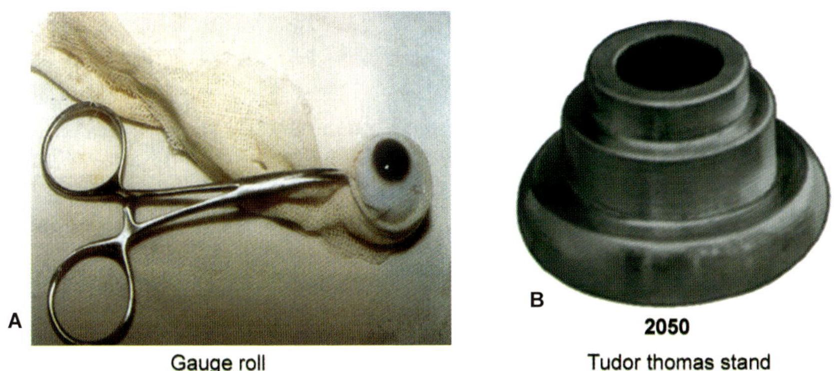

Figs 1A and B: Donor eye ball

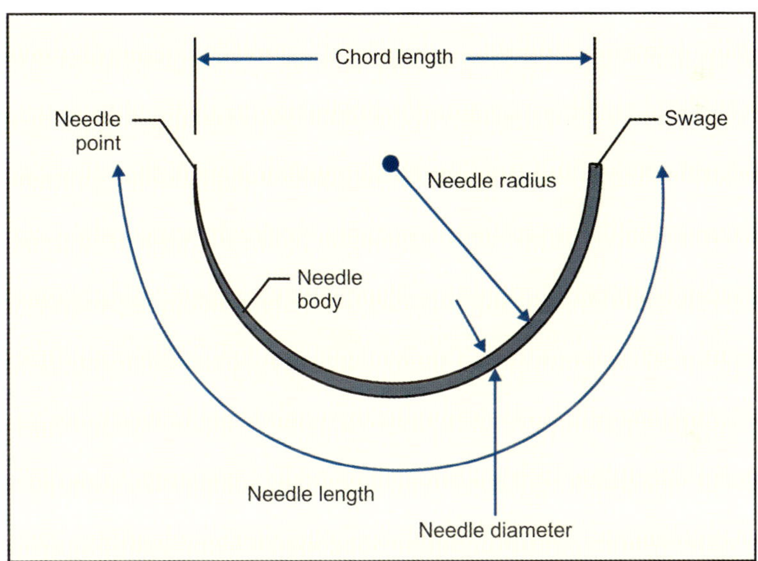

Fig. 2: Sharp cutting edge. Atraumatic long and strong needles

host tissue. Like all other surgical procedures at that time, this operation was also performed without any anesthesia. After the " severe chemosis" had subsided, the patient's vision was "improved", but the cornea opacified and absorbed over a two-week period. He postulated had the eye been normal internally. His operation might have been more successful visually.

The lack of anesthesia was only one of several conditions contributing to an unfavorable prognosis for grafts in this period. Ether was not introduced until 1846, chloroform in 1847. Cocaine came a decade later in 1858, and infiltration anesthesia was introduced in 1889. Lister's principles of antiseptic surgery were postulated in 1867, almost 30 years after Kissam's attempt at corneal transplant. The second half of nineteenth century, thus, brought increasing awareness of the importance of asepsis, careful handling and placement of graft, and the use of homografts.

In 1886, Arthur von Hippel transplanted a full thickness rabbit cornea on to the lamellar bed of a young girl's cornea, reporting an improvement in vision from finger counting to 6/60. This was the first successful corneal transplant on a human being. von Hippel used cocaine anesthesia and iodoform as an antiseptic. He focused on lamellar keratoplasty reiterating that the main determinants of corneal transparency were the integrity of corneal endothelium and Descemet's membrane. His most significant contribution was the circular trephine which is the mainstay of surgical instrumentation in keratoplasty His pioneering work initiated a new era in keratoplasty characterized by advances in surgical technique with better understanding of corneal physiology.

In 1906, Eduard Konard Zirm performed the first full thickness graft that remained clear in a 45-year-old laborer named Alois Gloat, who suffered lime burn in his both eyes while cleaning chicken coop and was left with a vision of counting fingers in both eyes. Zirm used cornea from the blind traumatized eye of an eleven-year-old boy, which he enucleated just prior to transplantation. He trephined two 5 mm buttons from the donor cornea under strict asepsis using the von Hippel trephine. He scrupulously avoided touching the tissue while performing the bilateral penetrating grafts under general anesthesia (chloroform). The left eye graft remained clear with a vision of 6/36.

Zirm elaborated the basic principles for successful keratoplasty, which with minor technical modifications, hold true even today. He recommended the exclusive use of cornea from young , healthy human donors, use of trephine, adequate anesthesia, strict asepsis, protection of the graft in a gauze moistened with physiologic saline, use of overlay sutures and careful selection of cases.

In 1908, Plange performed the first auto-keratoplasty, replacing the scarred cornea of a blind eye with a lamellar graft from the patient´s other blind eye with a normal cornea.

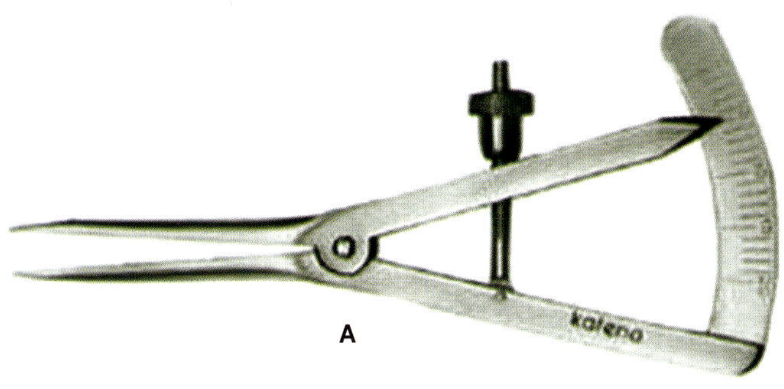

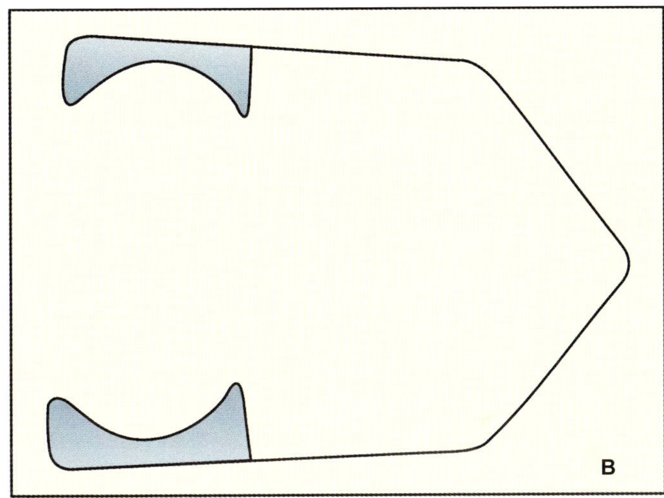

Figs 3A and B: (A) Castroveizo calipers, (B) Wire speculum

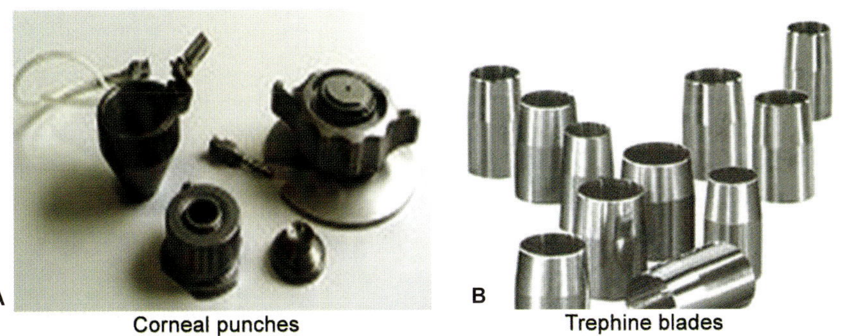

Figs 4A and B

The list of significant twentieth century contributors to the evolution of keratoplasty is long and illustrious including Arthur Elschnig , Vladimir Filatov, RT Paton, Arruga, Ramon Castroviejo, Barraquer, Paufique, Sourdille and Franceschetti, Forstot and Kaufman have all made significant technical and biological advances in the evolution of the art and science of keratoplasty.

VP Filatov is considered as the father of modern eye banking. He used an egg membrane to fixate the graft. His work also involved the usage of cadaver cornea stored in moist chamber as the donor material and he highlighted the importance of protecting the intraocular tissues while trephining the host tissue and advocated direct suturing.

In 1940s, corneal transplant surgery evolved dramatically with the availability of antibiotics and introduction of the use of steroids in corneal surgery.

In late 1950s small fine needles were used for first time for suturing. At the same time, Paufique and Charleux popularized lamellar corneal grafting, and introduced limbal and eccentric grafts.

Although, most of the corneal transplant surgery has evolved in the first half of the 20th century, the greatest advances in corneal grafting have taken place in the last 30 years. The understanding of corneal anatomy and physiology especially with regard to the corneal endothelium, introduction of microsurgical techniques, advances in corneal preservation, the elucidation of corneal immunology and the development of usage of antiinflammatory and immunosuppressive agents have resulted in a high success rate of corneal grafting.

Corneal graft rejection is the greatest limiting factor in graft survival and Edward Maumenee was the one to recognize this clinical entity. The classic scientific experimental models were elegantly designed by Khodadoust.

Ramon Castroviejo performed the world´s first successful human corneal transplant and devised numerous instruments including the castroviejo calipers, forceps, corneal scissors, corneal punch, cyclodialysis spatula, needle holder, tying forceps, suturing forceps, etc. His original suturing technique used a continuous silk suture coursing across the external surface of a square graft , with many of his square grafts providing good visual acuity for many years.

Richard Troutman designed a microscope and numerous microsurgical instruments. He was the pioneer in the field of astigmatism control, he invented surgical keratometer and technique of wedge resection.

Townly Paton was the first to set up an eye bank in New York in 1959, and the Eye Bank Association of America was founded in 1961. This organization laid down the standards for obtaining, preservation, storage and usage of donor tissue.

The specular microscope developed by Maurice provided the means of studying donor and transplanted endothelium, proving that a healthy functioning endothelium is the key to success of a corneal graft.

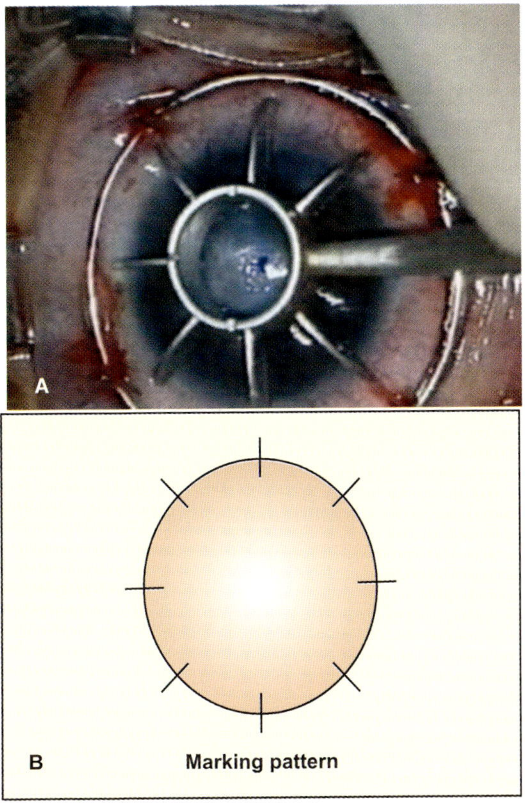

Figs 5A and B: RK marker

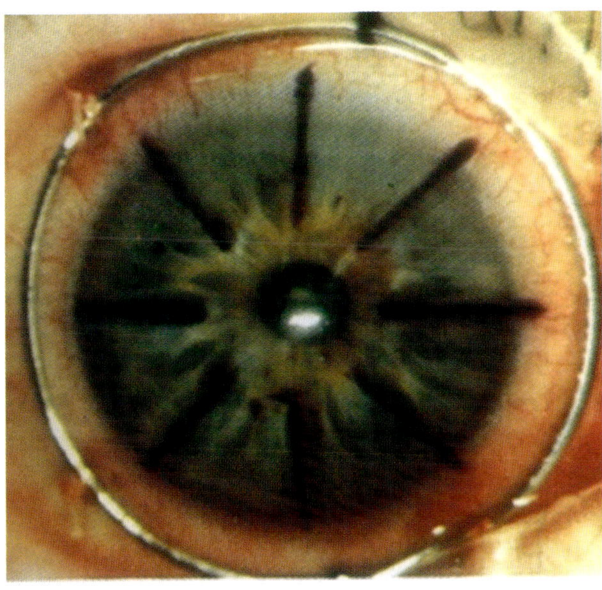

Fig. 6: Fliringa ring

Eye Banking and Corneal Storage

.The preservation of donor cornea influences the outcome of surgery to a great extent. A preservation procedure besides ensuring the endothelium viability also enables safe transportation of material and increases the duration of storage, so that an efficient use of donor cornea can be made.

First successful transplantation using a cryopreserved human donor tissue was reported by East Cott in 1954. Capella and Kaufman developed the basic method of cryopreservation in 1965.

Introduction of the MK medium by McCarey and Kaufman in 1974 was a significant development, heralding a revolution in corneal preservation. This medium proved to be reliable for storage of donor cornea for at least 3-4 days, allowing the elective planning for surgery.

Anterior segment and corneal surgery have undergone significant change and greater emphasis is now placed on quality of visual rehabilitation. Increasing interest has developed in alterations of the cornea to effect refractive change. There are bound to have successes and failures. One only hopes that attempts to make present day corneal surgery more useful are guided by the same care and determination that led to keratoplasty, as we know it.

Lamellar Keratoplasty

Though penetrating keratoplasty is considered to be the standard procedure, it was gradually realized that all 3 layers of the cornea may not be needed in eyes where the disease is limited to certain layers. Thus, the different lamellar procedures are popularized.

Recent advancements in lamellar keratoplasty have two aspects: the refinement in surgical technique, which has improved postoperative visual outcomes and the transplantation of specific tissues of the donor cornea, such as limbal stem cells. Stem cell transplantation has expanded dramatically as a method of ocular surface reconstruction. Long-term prognosis for limbal allograft transplantation has recently been reported, and postoperative treatments including epithelial management and immunosuppression are now major topics to be studied.

The increased precision in deep stromal dissection, the refined automation and sophisticated processing available for the donor tissue has lead to extension of application of anterior lamellar keratoplasty (ALK) for optical purposes. Revolution in the investigative procedures, surgical instruments, equipments, orbscan, confocal and techniques more refined suture materials, and better postoperative care have made the procedure more advanced and popular.

Deep anterior lamellar keratoplasty (DALK) was first described by Archila in 1985. The procedure consisted of a full thickness donor corneal button placement over a near total dissected recipient bed. However, the outcomes of

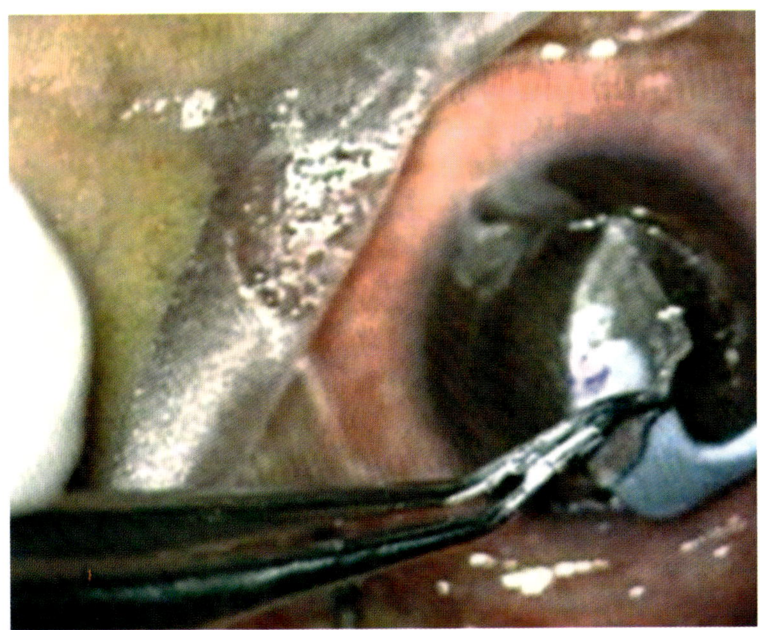

Fig. 7: Lamellar dissection

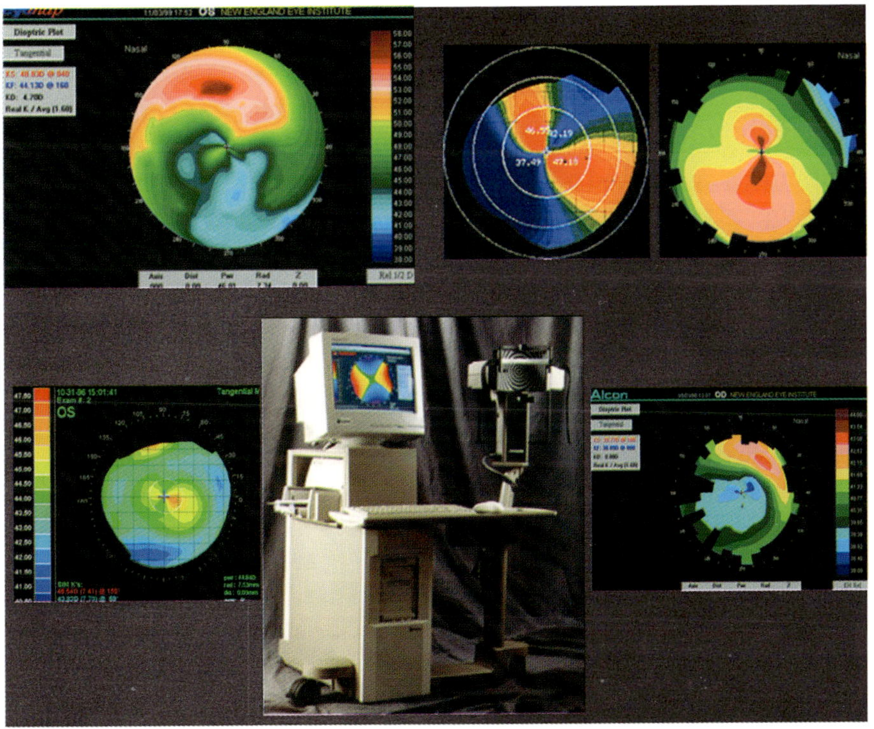

Fig 8: Corneal topography

these grafts were suboptimal in terms of subsequent loss of graft clarity. This could be attributed to the donor endothelium, which was having a constant insult from the recipient corneal tissue over which it was placed. Price in 1989 modified the procedure by structural matching of the donor and recipient tissue, by dissecting the donor tissue right up to the endothelium.

Limbal Stem Cell Transplantation

After the establishment of lamellar keratoplasty, limbal epithelial cells were the next targets for corneal surgery. To replace the damaged epithelial cells either autologous/homologous/allogenic limbal stem cell transplants are performed. However, this was associated with 50% failure, for which the cultivated epithelial transplantation has been developed.

Corneal Collagen Cross Linking

A number of surgical modalities such as PK, LK and DLK have been advocated for advanced keratoconus depending upon the extent of the opacity. Epikeratophakia has been introduced by Kaufman and Werblin in early cases of keratoconus to arrest progress. Intrastromal corneal ring segments have also been used to get the ecstatic cornea to its more natural curvature. Recently, it has been observed that the riboflavin when activated by UV-A light, augments the collagen cross links in the stroma, thus increasing the strength of the cornea by 328.9%.

New Technology

Blades are being replaced by microtome and then high speed lasers in order to make surgical incisions more precise. These improved incisions allow the cornea to heal more quickly and may not require more sutures and also the sutures can be removed sooner. The healing is much more stronger than that of standard blade operations. Also it provides quicker rehabilitation.

Cano et al in 1995 and Buarratto et al in 1998 added a new dimension towards further refinement of the technique by using the Excimer laser to prepare the recipient bed and then to shape fresh donor tissue to appropriate thickness and refractive power with the microkeratome.

Till late eighties, there was no procedure, which could overcome the existing problems of PKP and get an equivalent optical outcome. Ko et al have been credited for initiating a technique of posterior lamellar keratoplasty (PLK) in 1993 in experimental animals (rabbit) wherein the donor button was inserted in place to the recipient bed through a limbal incision without applying any sutures, thus preserving the preoperative corneal topography. Thereafter, Melles et al in 1998 described and applied this technique in clinical situations such as corneal lesions involving the endothelium and posterior stroma . The quest for

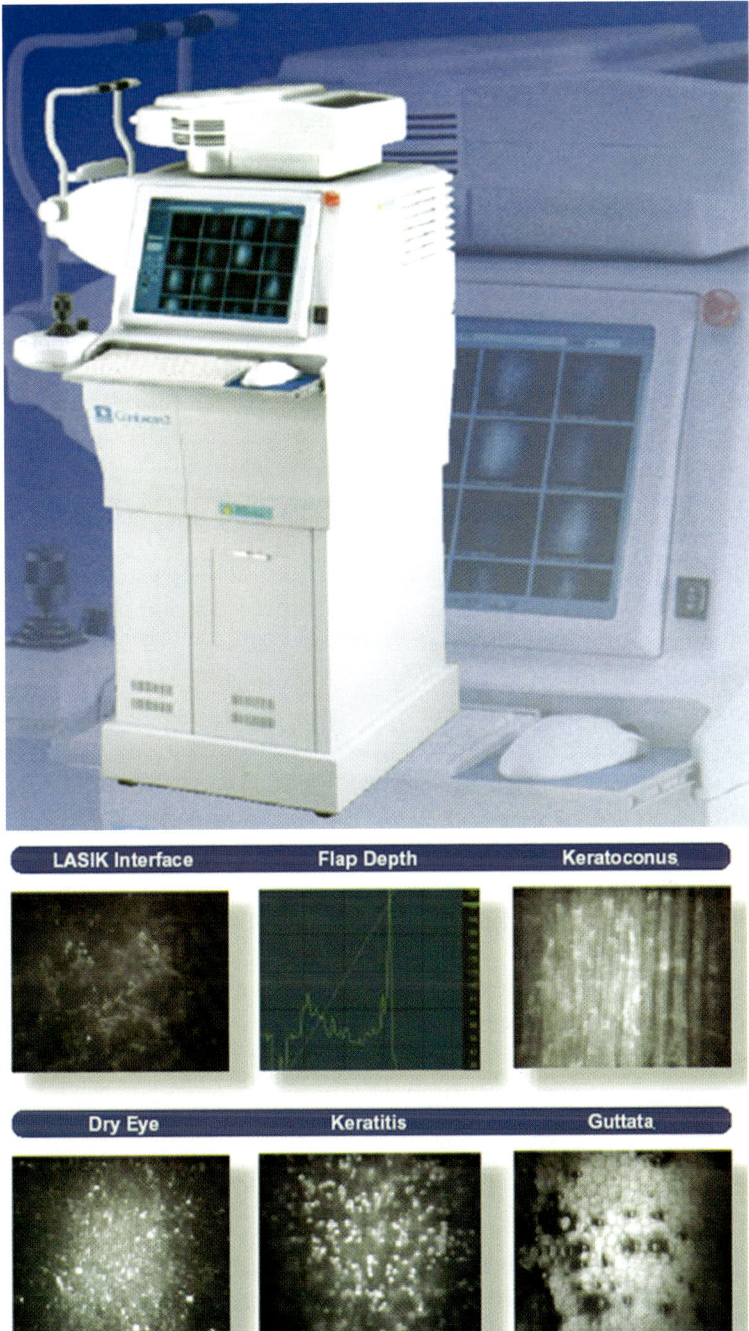

Fig. 9: Confocal microscope (Invented Marvin Minsky—1957)

a lamellar surgical technique for Endothelial transplantation has evolved in two directions: the corneal flap technique and the corneal lamellar dissection technique

Jone's and Culbertson in 1998 and Busin et al in 2000 described the flap technique wherein they used a microkeratome to create a 480 μ thick-hinged flap. This was followed by stromal trephination after retracting the flap. A slightly larger diameter posterior corneal donor button was then placed over the stroma and the flap was reposited in place and sutured with a resultant smooth interface.

Jones et al used a microkeratome to create an anterior cornea flap that was retracted to gain access to the mid and posterior stroma. The posterior diseased cornea was trephined and removed, the donor cornea was secured in place with one or more sutures and the anterior corneal flap was sutured back in position. This technique was termed endothelial lamellar keratoplasty (ELK) by Jones et al (1998), endokeratoplasty by Busin et al (2000) and microkeratome-assisted posterior keratoplasty by Azar et al (2000, 2001). Although this procedure had the advantages of a microkeratome assisted smooth dissection and easy 'open-sky' access for other intraocular procedures, it suffered from the same inherent problems as PK in terms of surface corneal incisions and sutures.

The pocket technique involved creating a corneal stromal lamellar pocket through a limbal or scleral incision. The posterior stromal disc along with the diseased endothelium is excised using an intrastromal circular trephine and healthy donor posterior stroma and endothelium is placed endothelial side down on a viscoelastic covered spatula for insertion into the recipient eye through a 9 mm limbal/scleral incision. A large air bubble placed in the anterior chamber intraoperatively pushes the donor 'disc' towards the recipient stroma, to which the donor disc adheres through the endothelial pump mechanism, thereby eliminating the need for any corneal sutures, requiring only scleral sutures to close the scleral/limbal wound. This technique was first described by Gerrit Melles in a laboratory study in 1998 and he coined the term posterior lamellar keratoplasty (PLK). The preliminary clinical results of PLK were promising with respect to postoperative astigmatism as well as endothelial cell viability.

As a modification of this technique, Melles described the sutureless PLK in which a 5 mm superior scleral tunnel incision was fashioned through which custom-made corneal stromal microscissors were used to excise the recipient posterior lamellar disc. In a whole donor globe a deep corneal pocket was dissected at 80-90% stromal depth using custom-made blades (DORC International, Zuidland, Netherlands). The corneoscleral rim was excised and an 8.5 mm trephine was used to punch the cornea from the endothelial side. The donor endothelium was protected with a viscoelastic and the disc was folded and inserted into the AC through a 5 mm scleral wound. The disc was unfolded within the AC and was positioned against the recipient stroma, a large air bubble helping the donor disc to adhere. During this time Mark Terry

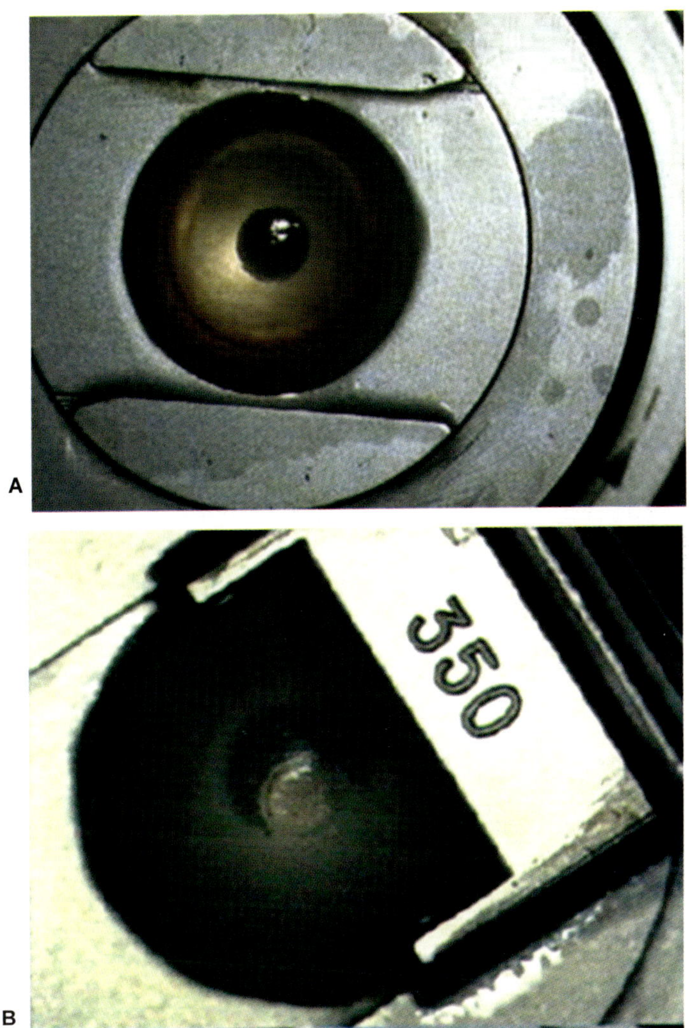

Figs 10A and B: Microkeratome

from Portland, Oregon, USA, using Melles principle, modified the instrumentation and surgical technique and popularized this technique in the USA as deep lamellar endothelial keratoplasty (DLEK).

He later described the technique of small-incision DLEK in 2005. Both short-term (up to 6 months) and medium-term (up to 3 years) studies have shown that both PLK and DLEK offer early and rapid visual rehabilitation, with minimal induced astigmatism and ECDs comparable to that obtained with traditional PK's.

Frank Price from Indianapolis, USA was the first surgeon to publish clinical results of this descemetorhexis technique, renaming it Descemet's stripping endothelial keratoplasty (DSEK).

DSEK has now evolved into DSAEK (Descemet's stripping automated endothelial keratoplasty) in which a motorized microkeratome is used to harvest the donor posterior lamella and endothelium. This technique has rapidly gained in popularity among corneal surgeons as it is technically easier to perform in comparison to PLK/DLEK since these involve a difficult lamellar stromal dissection and excision of the posterior lamellar disc using either an intrastromal trephine and/or scissors.

Descemet's stripping with endothelial keratoplasty (DSEK) has several advantages over PLK and DLEK procedures as it is a technically easier procedure to perform and is less traumatic to the cornea and to the anterior segment .It maintains the structural integrity of the corneal stroma and leads to a smoother interface, as the stromal lamella is not dissected. With the recent introduction of an artificial AC and an automated motorized microkeratome the need for manually dissecting the donor cornea is also avoided (DSAEK). The automated microkeratome not only reduces the intraoperative time required to prepare the donor disc but also provides a smoother interface which may also improve visual acuity.

In 2006, Melles described a new technique of pure Descemet's membrane transplantation through a small incision—termed Descemet's membrane endothelial keratoplasty (DMEK). It is hoped that with further developments in eye banking, provision of endothelial discs using either an automated microkeratome or femtosecond laser will make the surgical technique much easier and more reproducible. Clearly, further advances are on the way and are only limited by the imaginations of the practitioners of ophthalmology!

Evolution of New Nomenclature in Corneal Transplant Surgery

- ELK (endothelial lamellar keratoplasty) (Jones and Culbertson 1998)
- PLK (Posterior lamellar keratoplasty) (Gerrit Melles 1998)

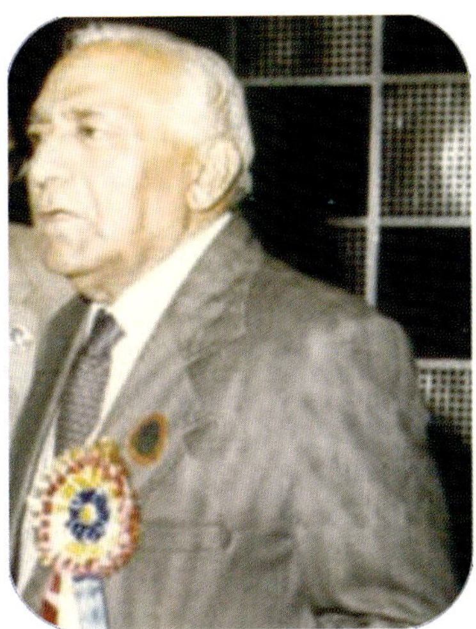

Fig. 11: Dr RP Dhanda

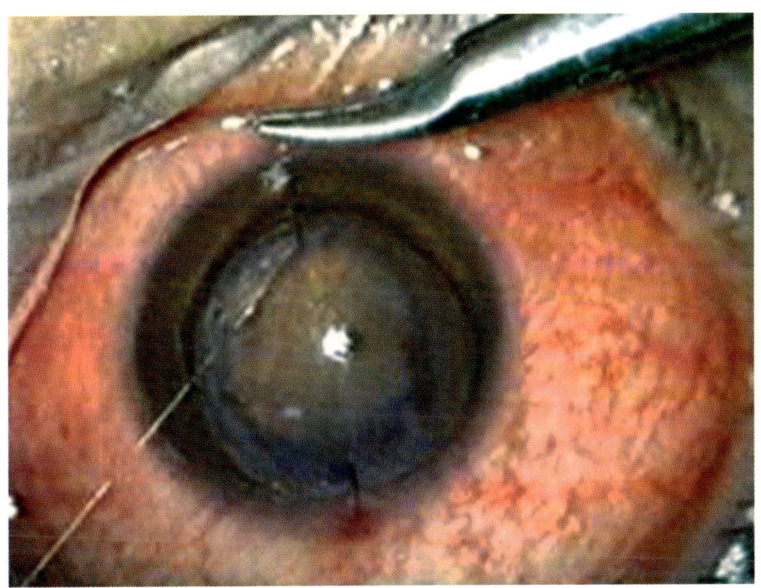

Fig. 12A: PK

- Large incision PLK (Gerrit Melles 1999)
- Sutureless PLK (Gerrit Melles 2002)
- Sclerokeratoplasty (Anita Panda 1999)
- DLEK (Deep lamellar endothelial keratoplasty) Mark Terry 2001
- Large incision DLEK (Mark Terry 2001)
- Small incision DLEK (Mark Terry 2004)
- Descemetorhexis (Gerrit Melles 2004)
- DSEK Descemet's stripping endothelial keratoplasty (Francis Price 2005)
- DSAEK (Descemet's stripping and (automated) endothelial keratoplasty) (Goroyov 2006)
- DMEK (Descemet's membrane endothelial keratoplasty) (Gerrit Melles 2006).

Evolution of Keratoplasty: Indian Scenario

RP Dhanda has been honoured with the epithet "father of keratoplasty in India" as he was the pioneer in this field, introducing corneal transplantation in the early sixties. He also introduced anterior lamellar keratoplasty in association with, Kalevar. Under his dynamic leadership, eye banking and corneal surgery got an increasing impetus.

The work of Madan Mohan from Dr RP Centre, New Delhi in the field of eye banking and keratoplasty in early seventies is remarkable. In 1976, he introduced keyhole pattern LK in recurrent pterygium and also further popularized the technique of anterior lamellar keratoplasty using a microkeratome. In 1980, cresentic graft was also introduced by him.

The first annular keratoplasty was performed by Panda et al in 1982 in a case of ring dermoid. In the same year, Panda et al introduced the use of MK medium for corneal storage and specular microscopy evaluation for assessment of endothelial function.

The author is also credited for pioneering work in the field of epikeratoplasty in 1988, using a manually prepared donor lenticule in keratoconus and made the procedure of anterior lamellar keratoplasty more popular. Advancement in eye banking and establishment of Eye Bank Association of India in 1989 improved the eye donation movement and tissue collection. Considering the untoward effect of suture induced strengthened by the effort astigmatism on suturing sutureless sclerokeratoplasty was advocated for total corneal lesions such as anterior staphyloma and total corneal ulcer in 1992, which are not amenable to simple keratoplasty, with great success. In the early nineties limbal stem cell transplantation, deep lamellar keratoplasty in addition to ALK and frozen section guided excision and anterior lamellar keratoplasty for recurrent ocular surface squamous neoplasia were initiated.

In the subsequent years, stem cell culture for sheet transplantation was initiated by the two dynamic institutions in southern India; namely, Sankara Nethralaya and LV Prasad Eye Institute.

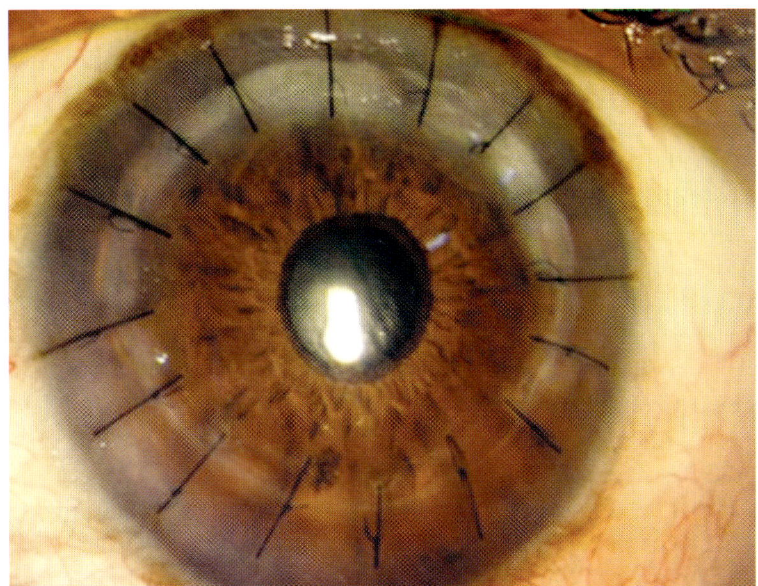

Fig. 12B: PK

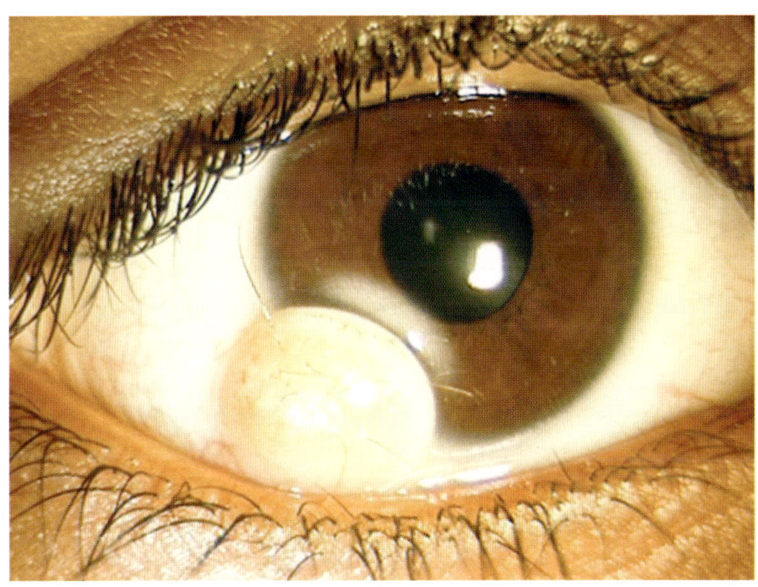

Fig. 13A: Limbal dermoid (Pre- and post ALK)

In 2000, while initiating PLK using flap technique Panda et al announced their pathbreaking technique of multiple recipients benefiting from one donor eye. They harvested two limbal lenticules , one anterior and one posterior lamella from the same donor eye, revolutionizing modern day eye banking practices. The PLK technique, however, was slowly but surely displaced by the growing popularity of DSAEK.

R Fogla and S Basak popularized DSAEK and are eminent proponents of innovations in this field.

In 2002, Panda et al introduced the concept of simultaneous lamellar keratoplasty and phacoemulsification, resulting in prompt visual rehabilitation of patients with coexistent corneal opacity and cataract. Another major step in this direction was the introduction of the modified PK-Phaco: in this a lamellar dissection is first performed to improve anterior chamber visualization followed by closed chamber phacoemulsification and foldable IOL insertion.

In 2003, Fugo blade was introduced for corneal surgery, the aim being two folds: (i) To cut and (ii) to prevent bleeding. They carried out histopathological study and declared that the blade does not produce any deleterious effect on cornea.

Thereafter, the diseased endothelium is removed and replaced by a fullthickness donor corneal button. As is evident from the glorious history of corneal transplantation all over the world, the history is one of extreme grit, single minded devotion and scientific imagination.

To quote Dr Dhanda, a teacher and corneal surgeon par excellence "curiosity is stronger than passion and passion overtakes interest. Keratoplasty is not a toy of curiosity for an occasional surgeon to play with. It will be pertinent to say that acquired dexterity in cataract surgery and a training in corneal carpentry with a sense to face disappointments inspite of a job well done, are prerequisites for practising routine corneal grafting."

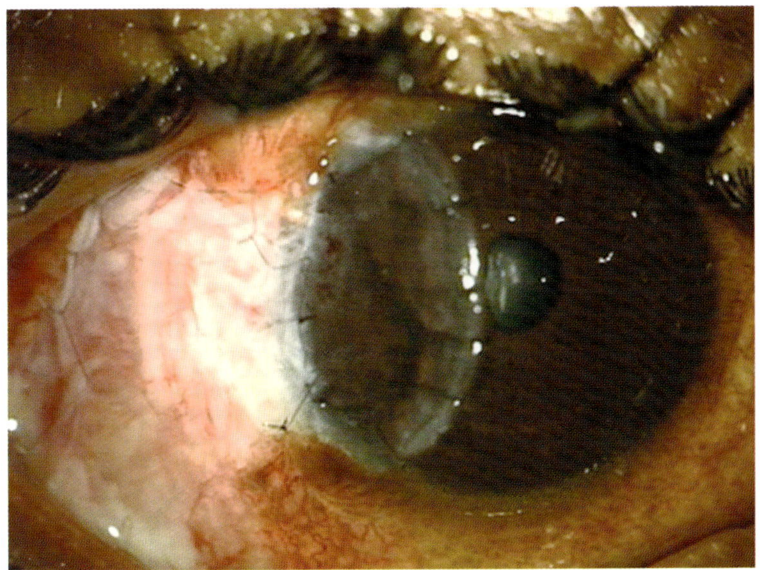

Fig. 13B: Limbal dermoid (Pre and post ALK)

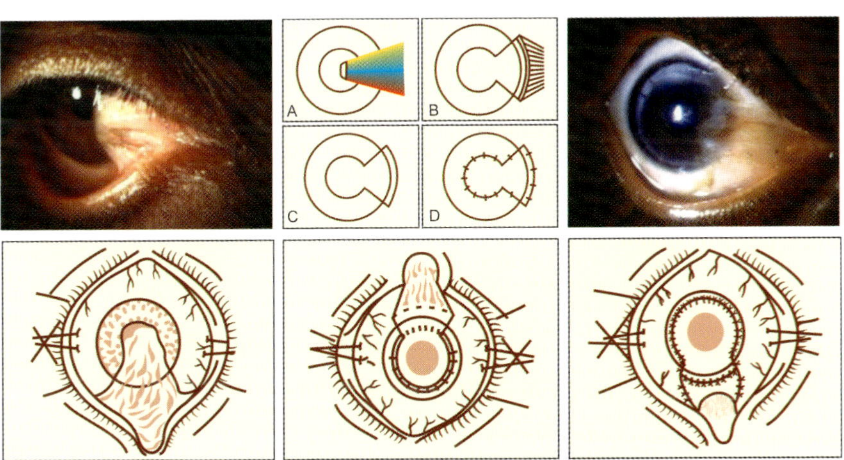

Fig.14: Key hole keratoplasty for pterygium

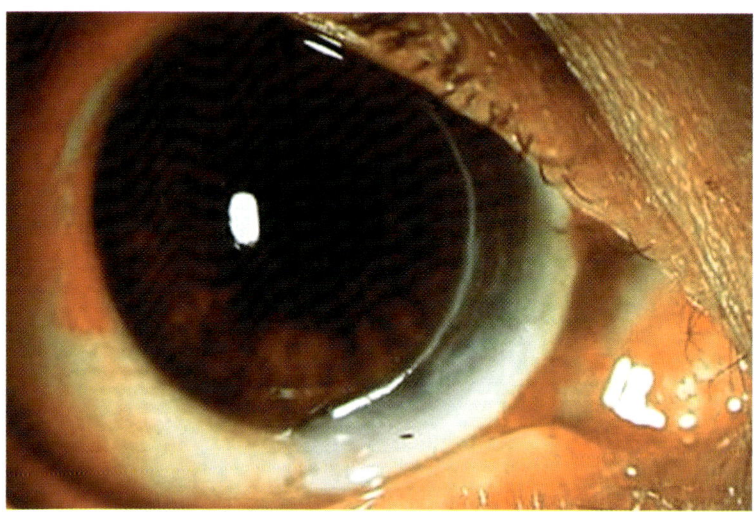

Fig. 15: Crescentic graft

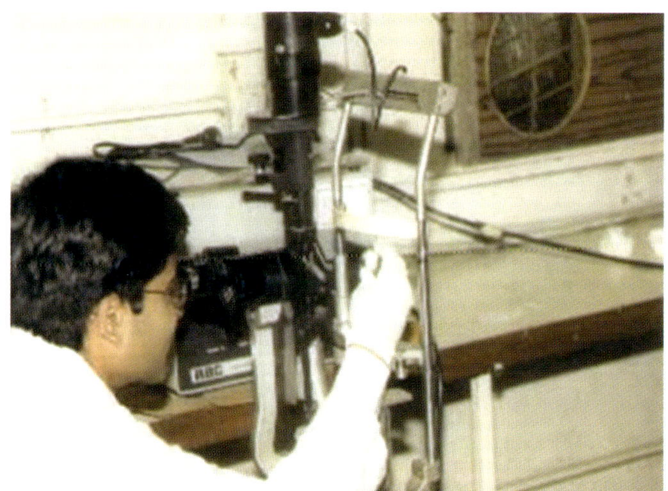

Fig. 16: Eye ball evaluation

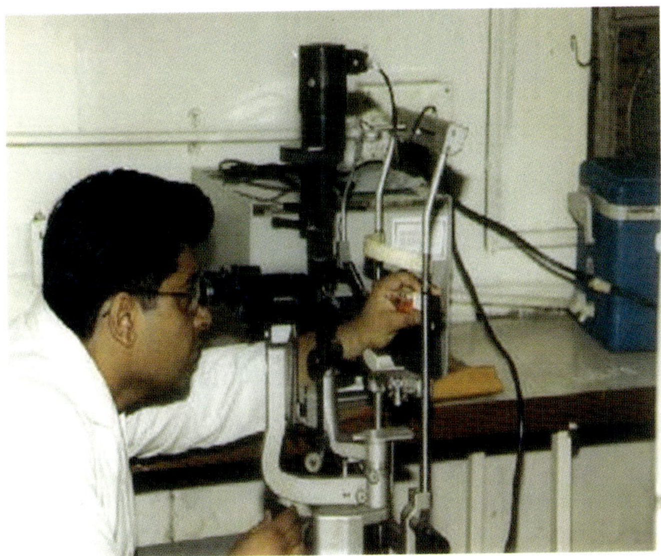

Fig. 17: MK medium stored corneal tissue evaluation

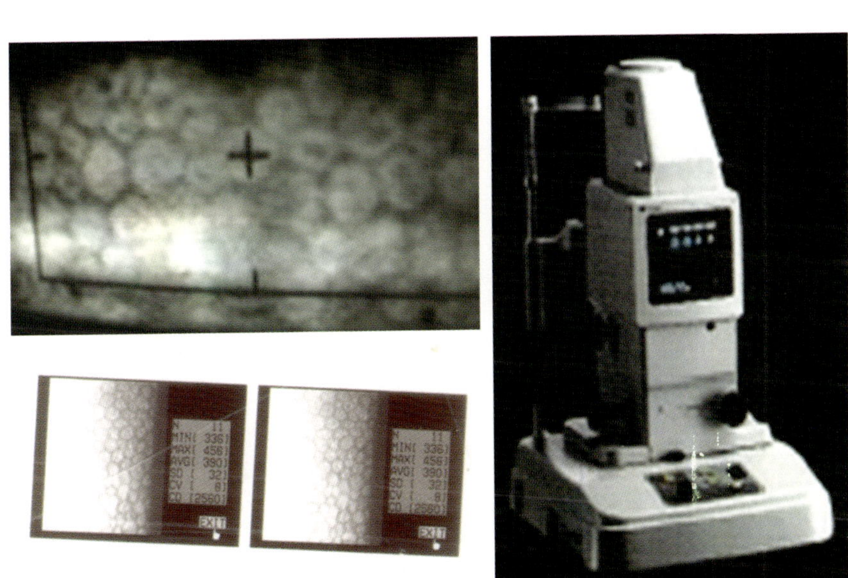

Fig. 18: Specular microscope

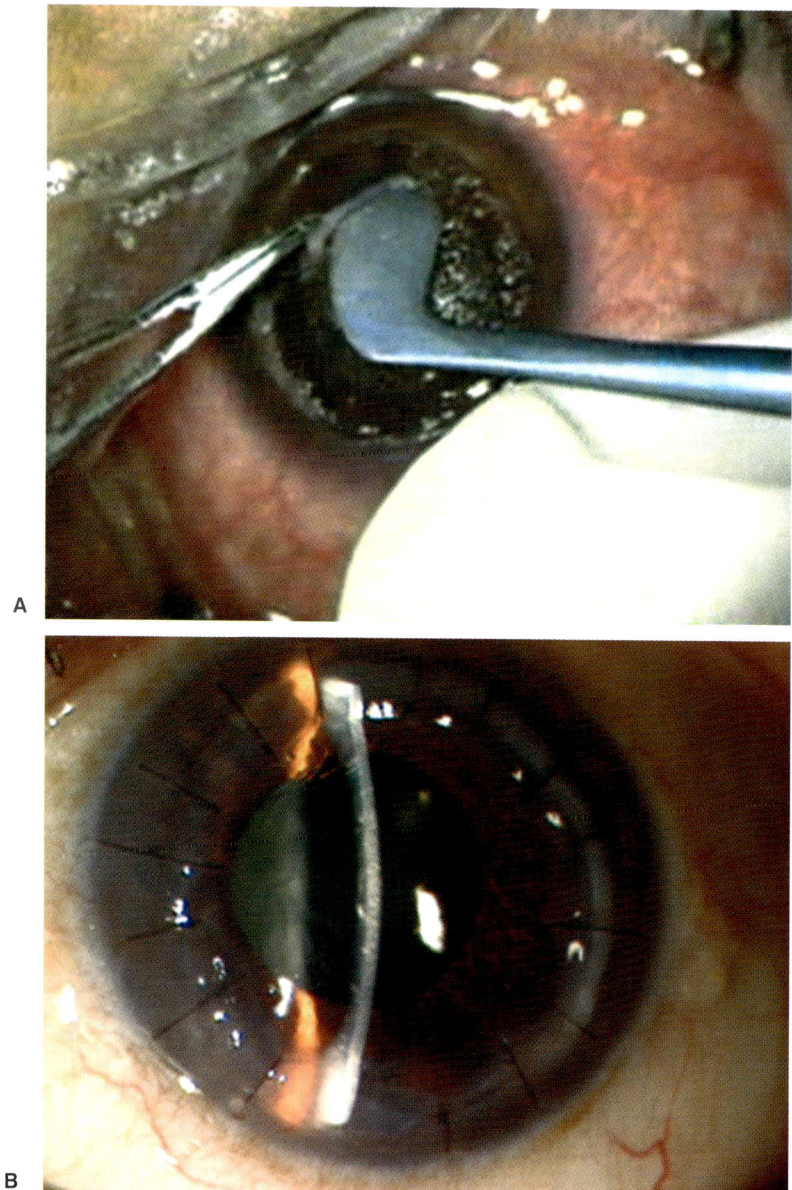

Figs 19A and B: ALK

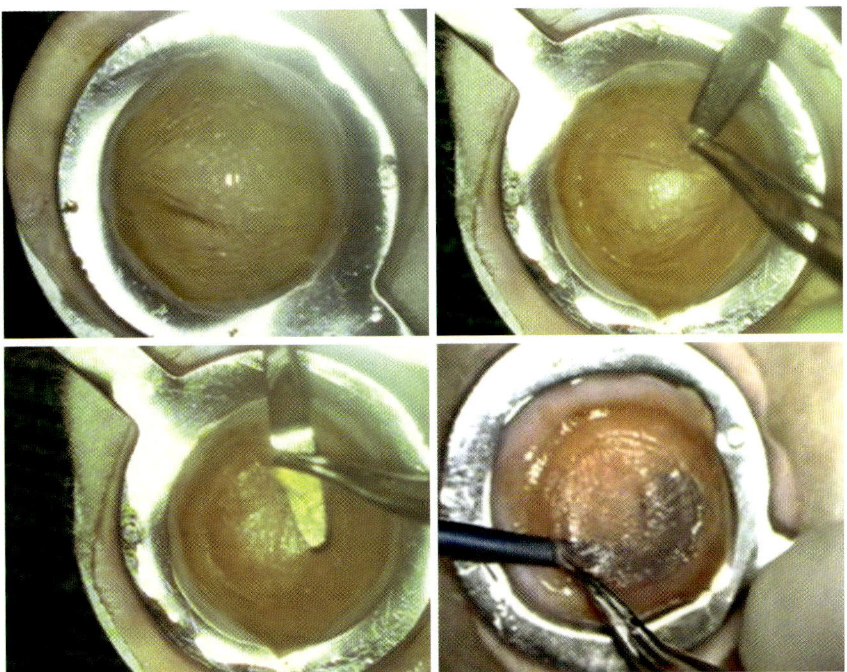

Fig. 20: Donor button preparation for ALK

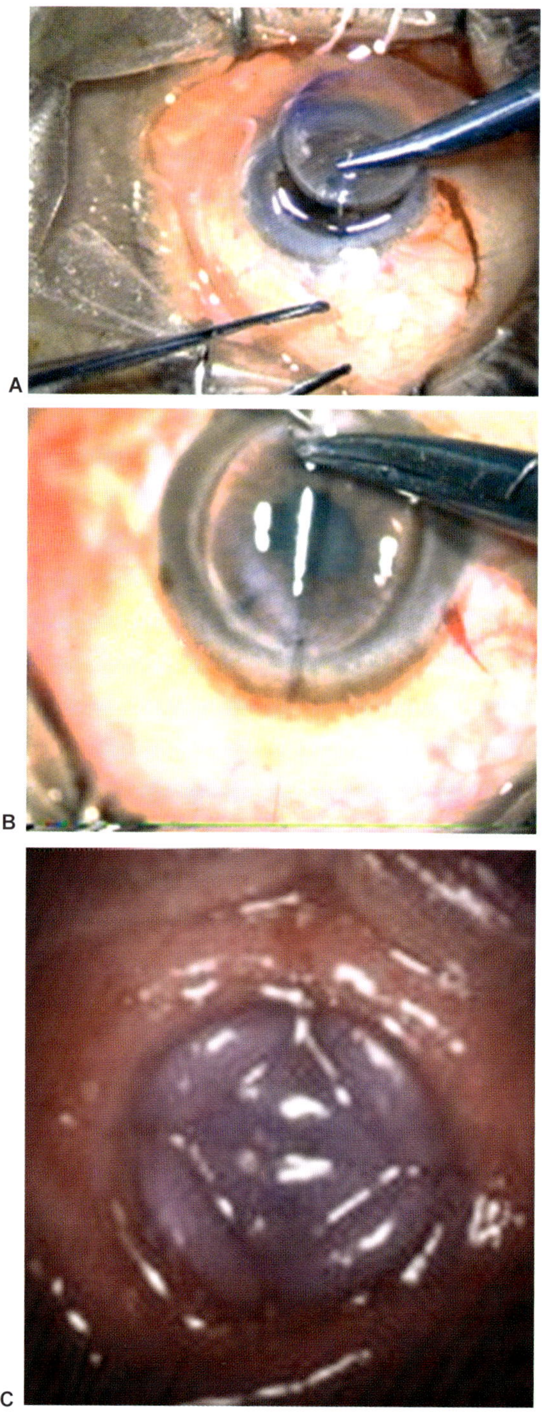

Figs 21A to C: Cardinal sutures in PK

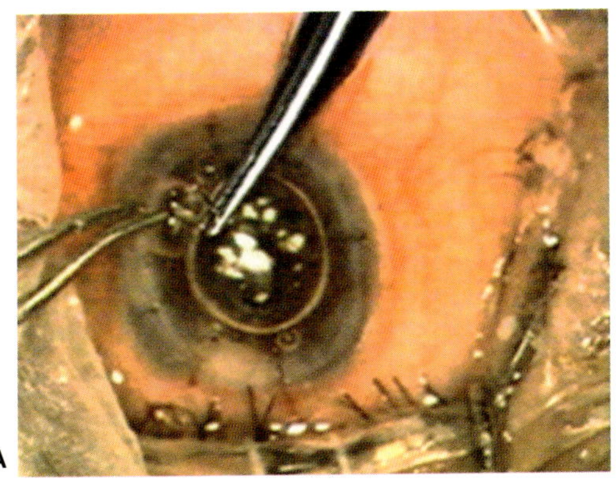

A

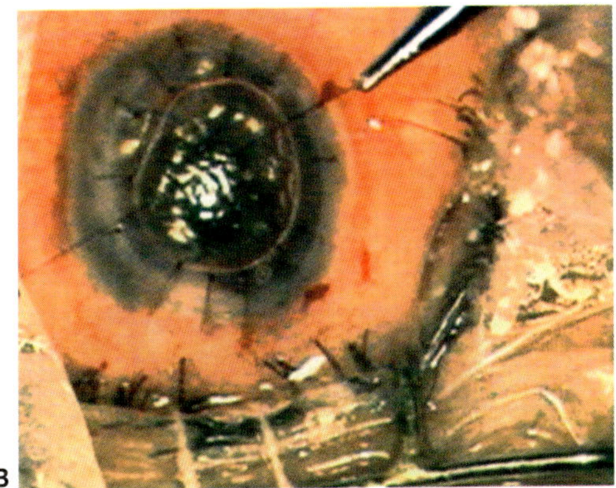

B

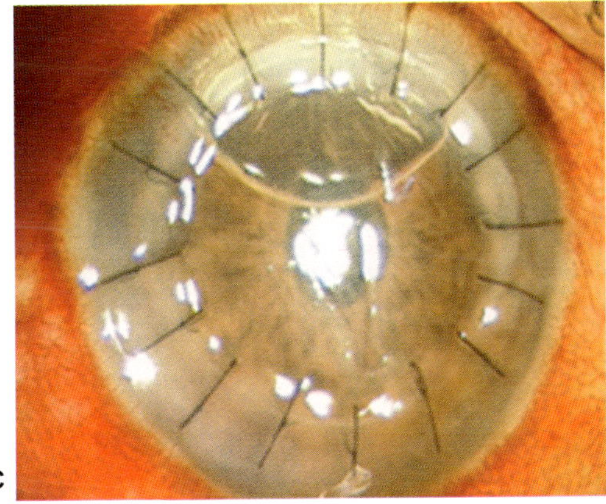

C

Figs 22A to C: Suturing in PK

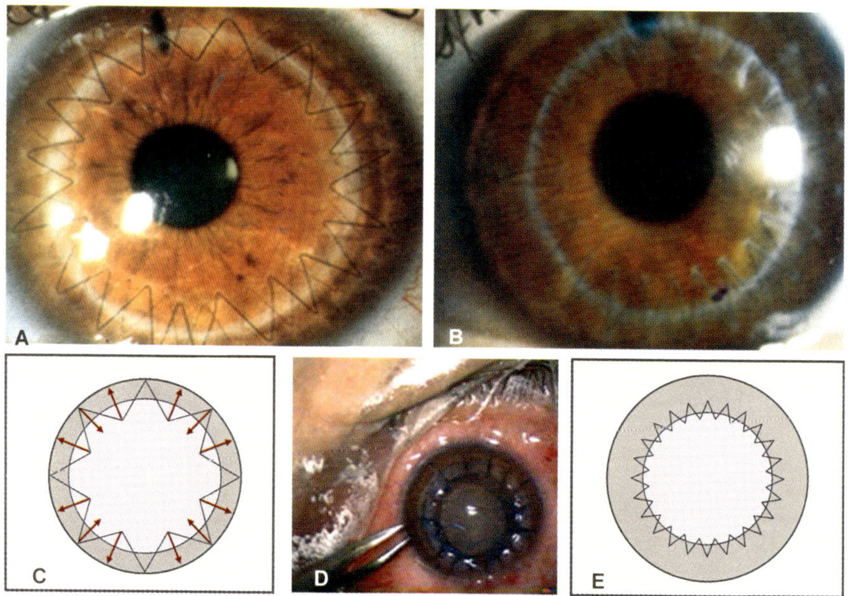

Figs 23A to E: Suturing in PK

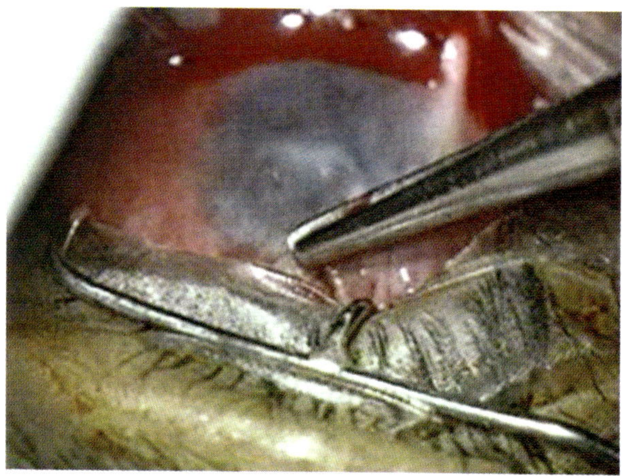

Fig. 24: Recipient

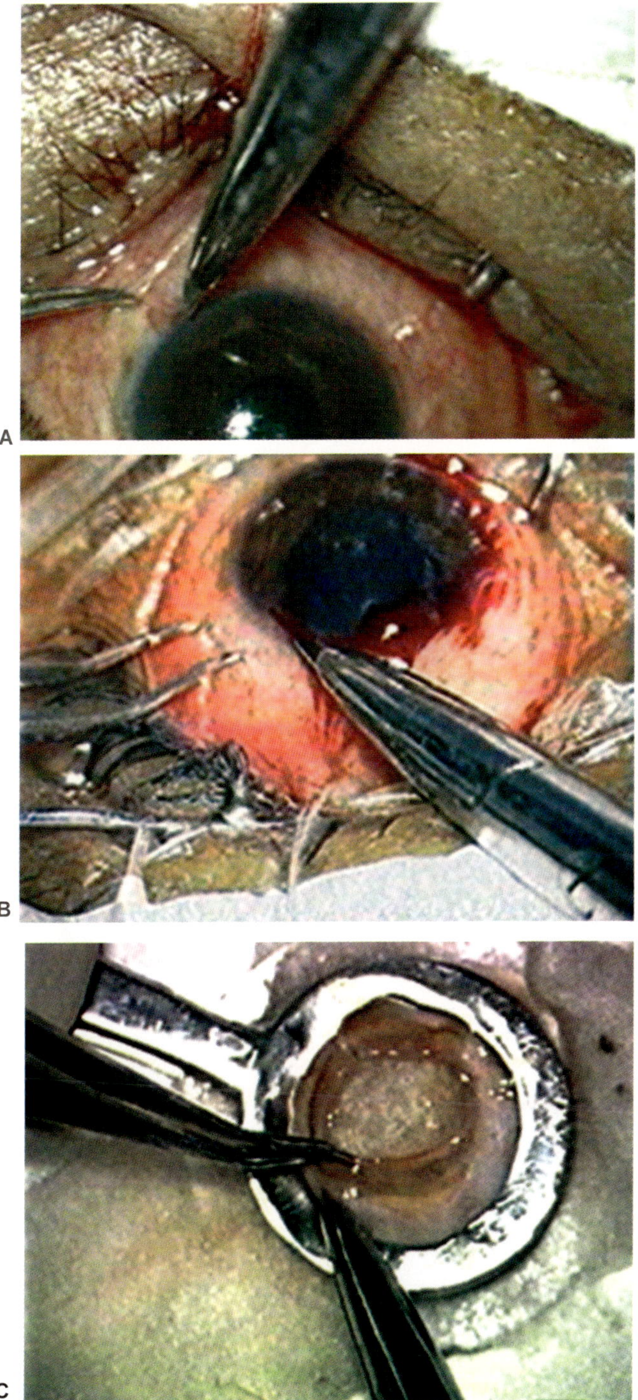

Figs 25A to C: Donor lenticule harvesting
(Fellow eye, blood related donor and used corneoscleral rim)

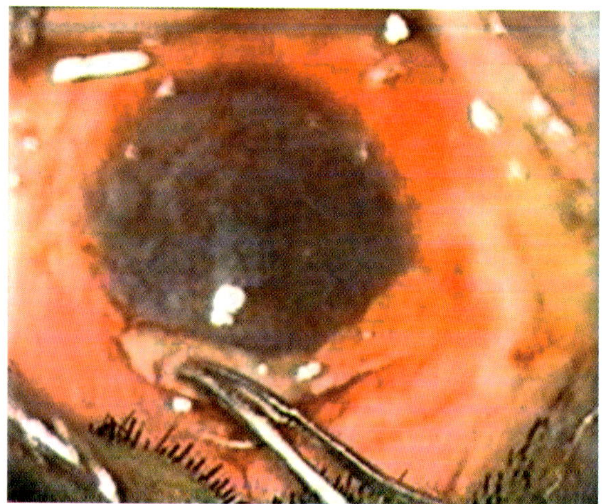

Fig. 26: Recipient with LCT

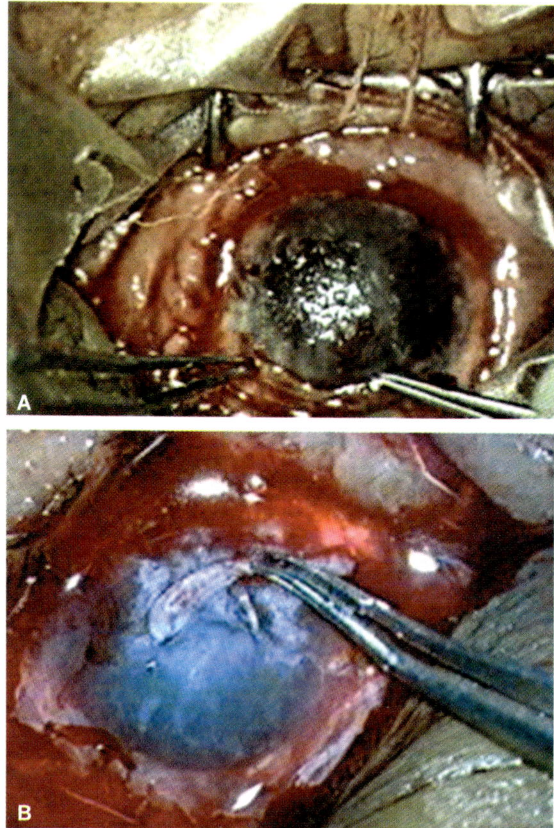

Figs 27A and B: Recipient with LCT(Inlay/onlay AMT)

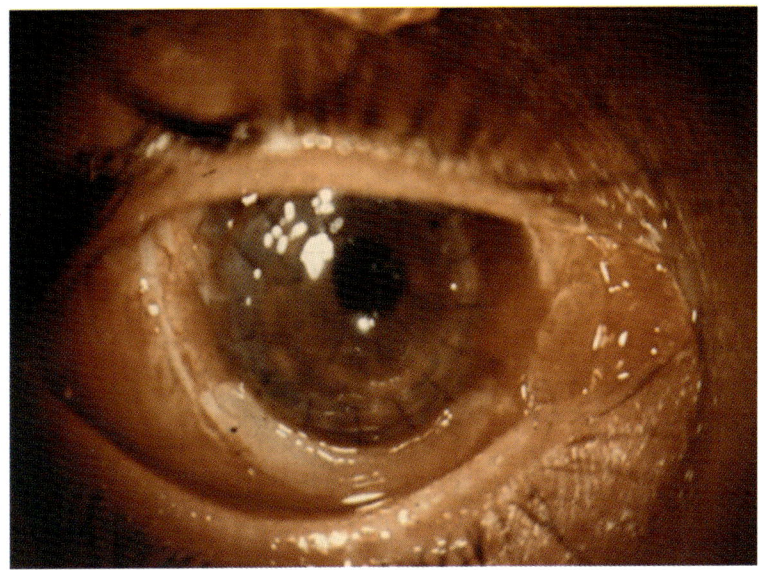

Fig. 28: Recipient, LK with LCT

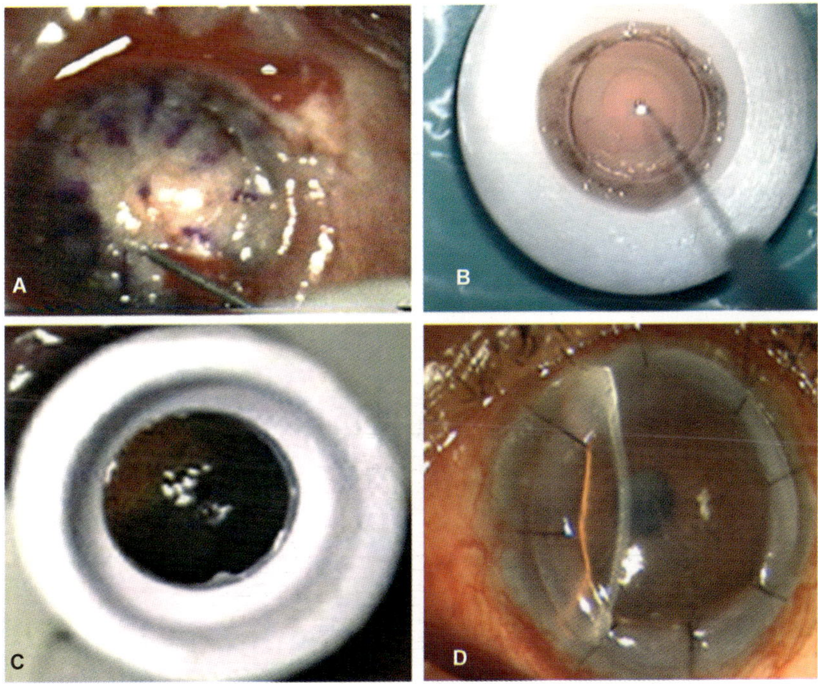

Figs 29A to D: DLK

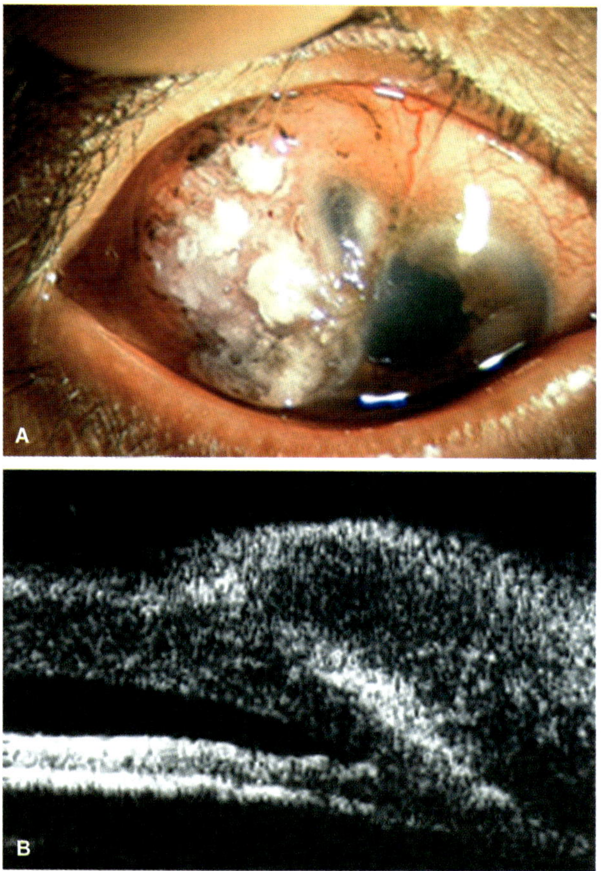

Figs 30A and B: OSSN. UBM to confirm the extension to ocular structures

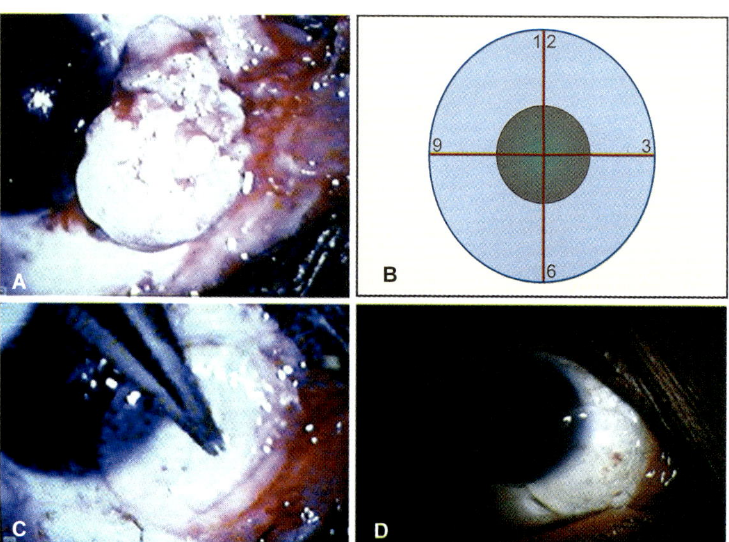

Figs 31A and B: OSSN FSGE

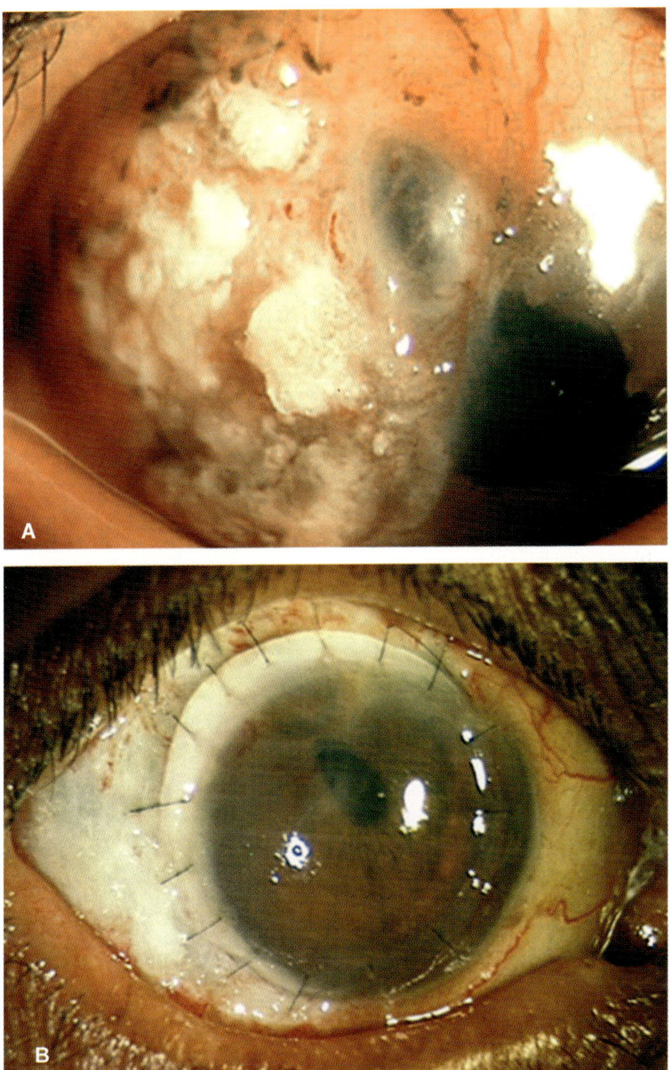

Figs 32A and B: OSSN (A) Preoperative, (B) Postoperative

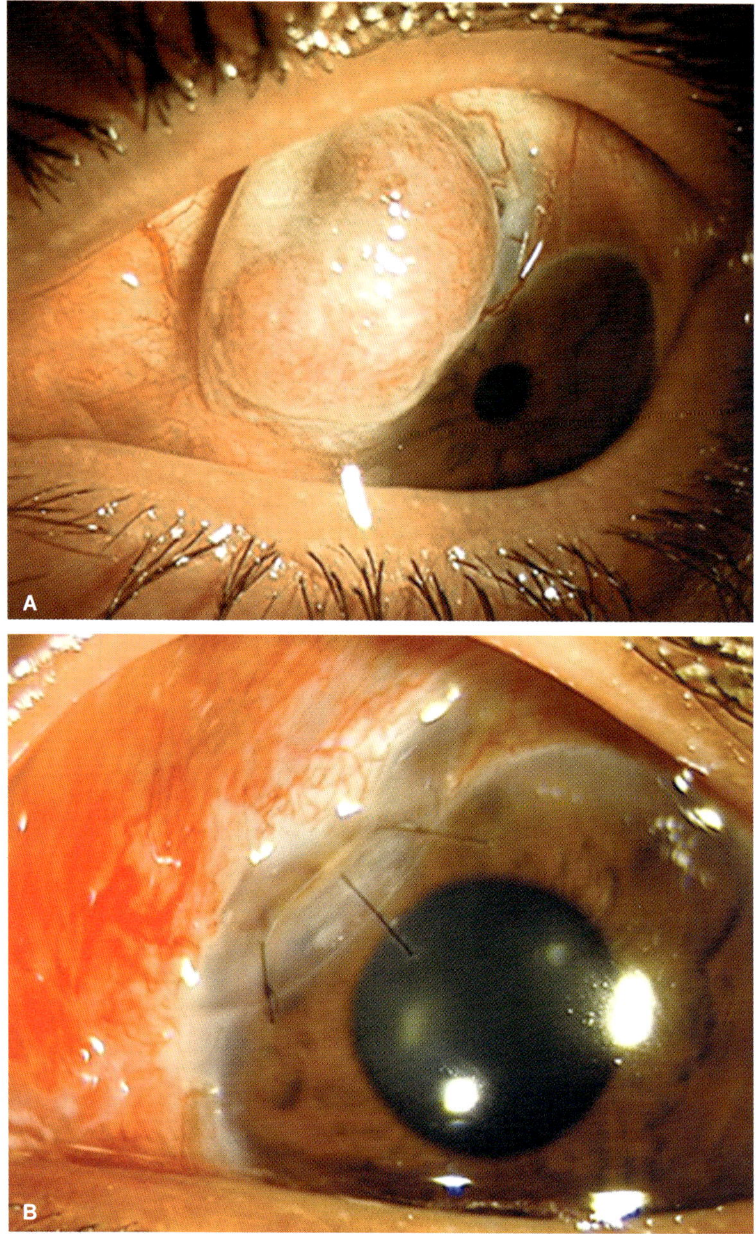

Figs 33A and B: OSSN (A) Preoperative, (B) Postoperative

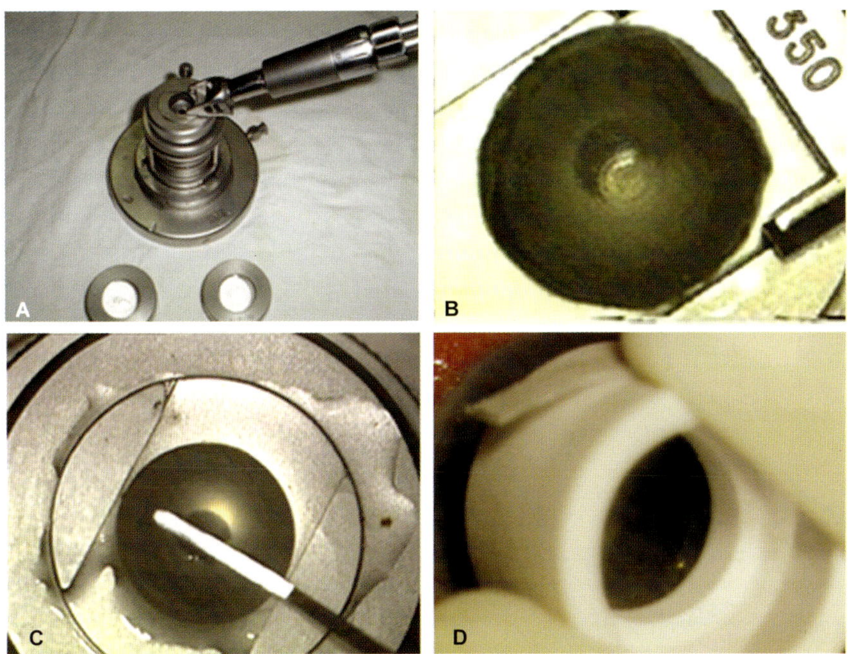

Figs 34A to D: PLK (Flap technique)

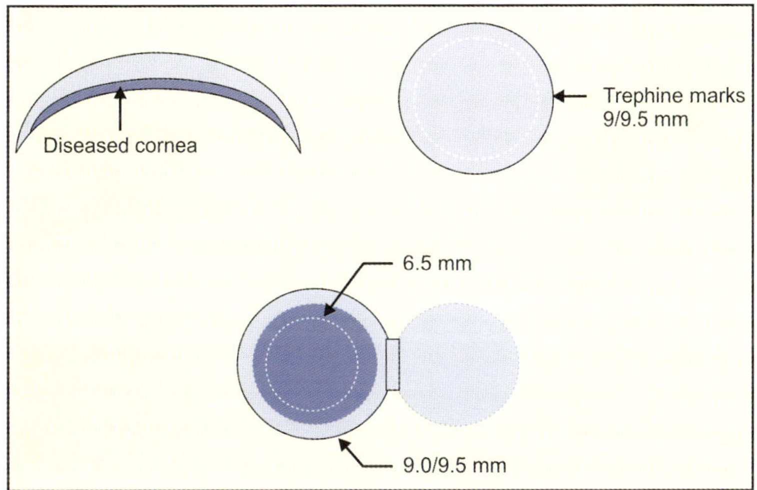

Fig. 35: PLK (Flap technique) (Host)

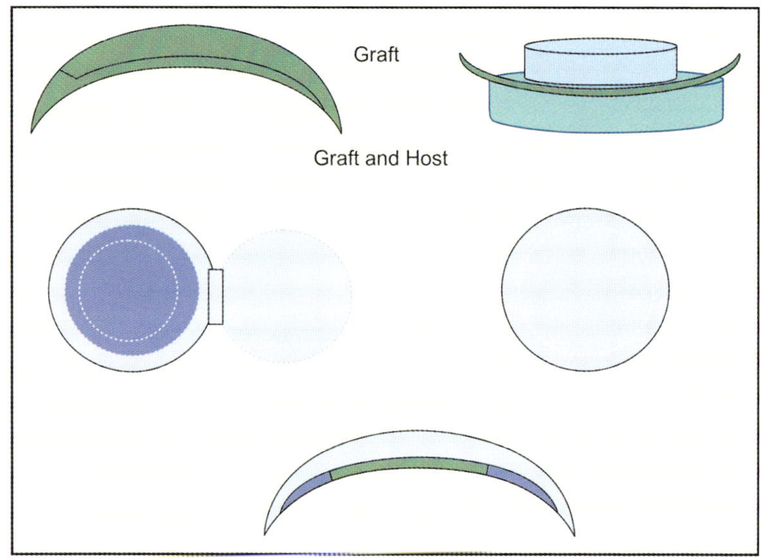

Fig. 36: PLK (Flap technique)

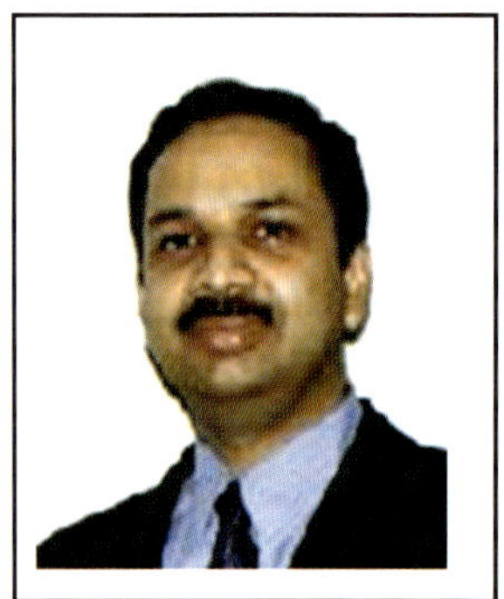

Fig. 37: Dr Rajesh Fogla

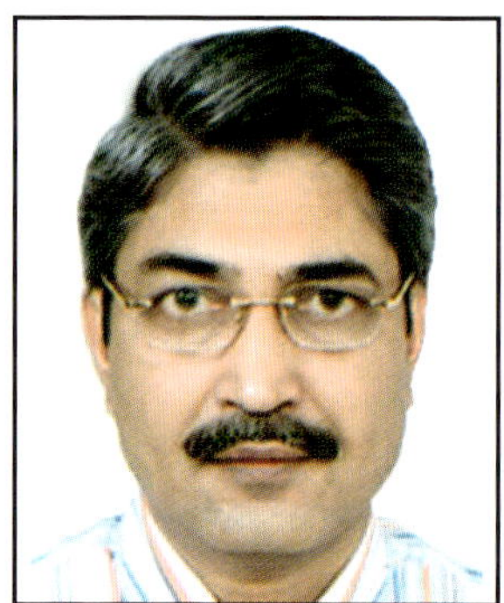

Fig. 38: Dr Samar Basak

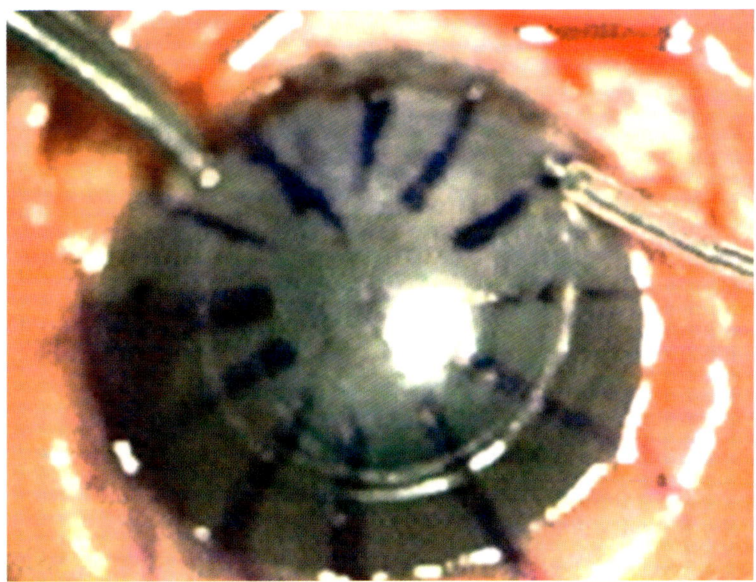

Fig. 39: FUGO blade in corneal surgery

Current Concepts in Pediatric Corneal Transplant Surgery

Ashok Sharma (India)

Introduction

Visual rehabilitation of pediatric corneal blinds is a major challenge to corneal transplant surgeons. Penetrating keratoplasty is the only way to restore vision and prevent irreversible blindness due to amblyopia in children. Performing penetrating corneal grafts in children poses difficulty in evaluation, technical difficulties during surgery and problems during follow-up. Younger children do not cooperate for proper examination at slit-lamp and need to be examined under general anesthesia. In addition, the complications encountered during adult corneal transplant surgery, including allograft rejection, post penetrating keratoplasty astigmatism and post penetrating keratoplasty glaucoma are more frequent. In case the graft is successful the child will require rigorous treatment for amblyopia. Parents need to be counseled before surgery and possible visual outcome and chances of obtaining clear graft should be discussed.

Indications of Penetrating Keratoplasty

Indications of penetrating keratoplasty may be grouped into congenital corneal opacities and acquired corneal opacities. Among the congenital causes Peter's anomaly, congenital hereditary endothelial dystrophy (CHED), posterior polymorphous dystrophy, sclerocornea, dermoid and mucopolysaccharidosis are common indications for performing surgery. Of the acquired causes traumatic corneal opacities, infectious keratitis, keratoconus, post cataract surgery corneal edema, non-penetrating corneal edema, are the main indications. Corneal edema due to endothelial cell decompensation in patients with buphthalmos has been successfully treated by penetrating keratoplasty. In the acquired group it can be traumatic in nature. In case of traumatic corneal scars the visual outcome depends upon the extent of injury to the posterior segment. The occurrence of indirect optic nerve injury, choroidal rupture and retinal detachment may limit the visual prognosis after penetrating keratoplasty. In developing countries corneal opacities resulting from healed infective keratitis (bacterial, viral and fungal) constitute a major group of indications among the acquired causes. Corneal opacities following keratomalacia is

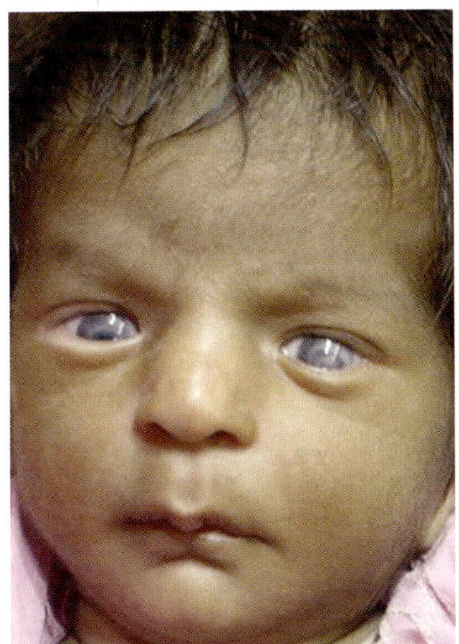

Fig. 1: Bilateral congenital corneal opacity

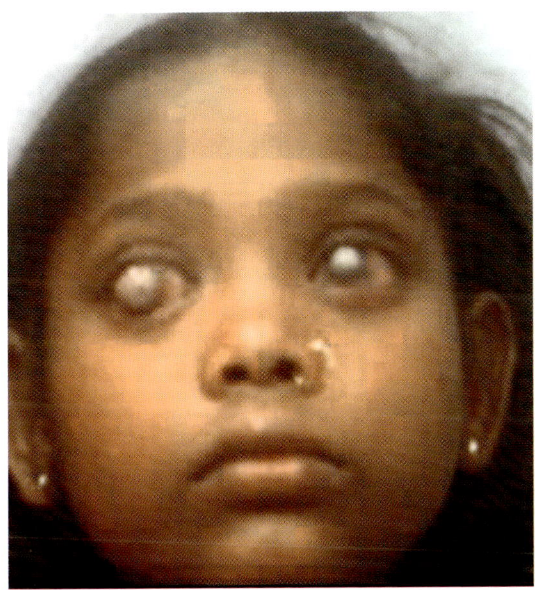

Fig. 2: Bilateral acquired corneal opacities

another frequent indication in developing countries. Congenital corneal opacities are usually bilateral, where as acquired corneal opacities are mostly unilateral.

Age at the time of Penetrating Keratoplasty

Recent studies have shown that penetrating keratoplasty in children should be performed at the earliest to prevent irreversible amblyopia In neonates with congenital corneal opacities, penetrating keratoplasty is advocated as soon as the child is fit for general anesthesia. In case of acquired corneal opacities the waiting period for penetrating keratoplasty should be minimized. In case the waiting list for penetrating keratoplasty is long, the child is given priority over the adults. Penetrating keratoplasty in neonates and very young children is technically difficult and the risk of graft failure is high. In a study children having undergone unilateral cataract surgery before the age of four months had better visual outcome as compared to those after four months. The study indicates that penetrating keratoplasty in children should be performed early to have better visual outcome. The youngest neonate reported to have undergone successful penetrating keratoplasty for large corneal perforation is, a 34 week post conception infant weighing 1 lb.

Neonates due to immunological immaturity are less predisposed to graft rejection. The immune system in neonates develops very early in gestation and is fully developed by birth. Neonatal immune system has characteristically dominance of T suppressor cells and qualitatively less functional B cells. It has been well documented that the anterior chamber is a privileged site for transplantation. This is mainly due to the absence of blood supply and access to lymphatic system. This makes antigen presentation, which is the part of the afferent limb of rejection, ineffective. Immunization schedules for neonates also avoid the first 4 weeks of life to avoid tolerance to the subsequent dose of antigen leading to less than optimal antibody response in future. Clinical studies have also shown that in neonates with isolated corneal opacities, corneal transplantation in the neonatal period resulted in better prognosis in terms of both graft clarity and vision improvement. The success of these grafts has been attributed both neonatal immune tolerance and clear visual axis during the most initial period of visual development.

Evaluation of Infants or Neonates with Congenital Corneal Opacities

Detailed examination of infants and neonates with congenital corneal opacities is essential to plan treatment. The visual acuity must be

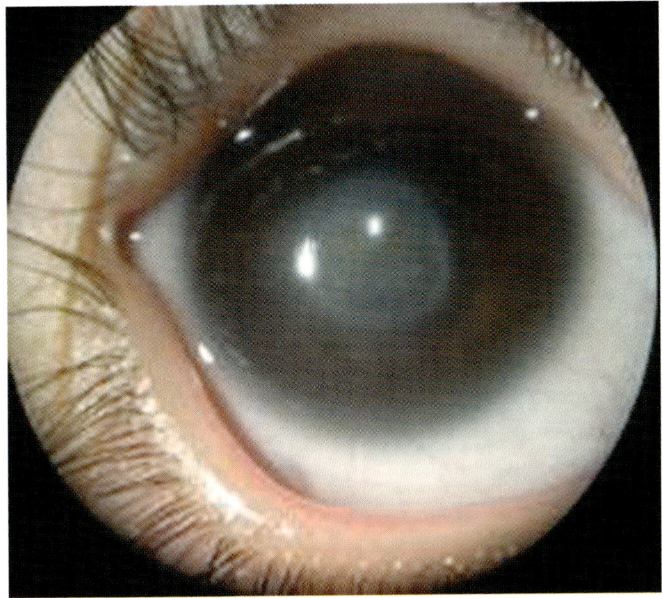

Fig. 3: Unilateral acquired corneal opacity

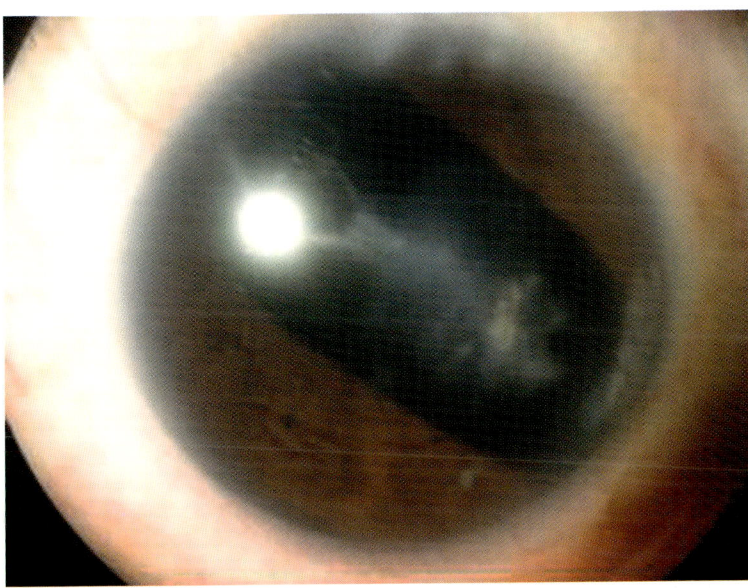

Fig. 4: Healed corneal laceration for RG P contact lens fitting

ascertained. Response to light stimulus, fixation at light source and following of the movement of illuminated object or light source are helpful. Responses are to be observed carefully and even parents should be demonstrated these tests. Detailed personal history, obstetric history and family history in a child with congenital corneal opacity is recorded. Detailed ocular examination may not be possible in the consultation chamber as the neonates and infants will never be steady and fixate to allow detailed slit lamp biomicroscopy. This part of the examination is better performed under general anesthesia. These days risk of general anesthesia in case of the newborns or infants is minimal. The amount of information on detailed examination we get out weigh the risk of general anesthesia. Under general anesthesia, detailed anterior segment examination, measurements of corneal diameters (both horizontal and vertical) and recording of intraocular pressure evaluation are recorded. Details of corneal opacity, whether central or peripheral, localized or diffuse, are recorded. Peripheral corneal opacities occur in partial sclerocornea and peripheral corneal ulcers. Central corneal scars may occur in Peter's anomaly. Perforated corneal ulcer may require therapeutic penetrating graft. Direct and indirect ophthalmoscopy to visualize retina is performed details of retina, macula and disc are recorded.

Investigations

Ultrasonography, A scan and B scan are performed to evaluate vitreous and retina status. In case eye is microphthalmic there is always possibility of associated ocular anomalies. The ultrasound biomicroscopy (UBM) give more details of intraocular pathologies. UBM is of special importance in patients with corneal opacity and associated glaucoma. Configuration of anterior chamber angle, details of angle structure and ciliary body are better delineated by UBM. In patients with anterior staphyloma, UBM may provide correct position of the iris and details of iris incarceration or iris adhesions. UBM has been of immense values on studying the structural alterations in pathological conditions including Peter's anomaly, aniridia and ocular trauma. The status of lens and the integrity of the posterior capsule should be evaluated. In case the cataract is present, an additional procedure of cataract extraction and post chamber IOL implantation along with penetrating keratoplasty should be performed.

Pediatric Keratoplasty Constraints

Pediatric penetrating keratoplasty is a challenge to corneal surgeons. The major constraints to perform corneal transplants in neonates include technical difficulties due to small eyes and positive posterior pressure. Low scleral rigidity cause extreme positive posterior pressure, resulting a forward bulge of iris lens diaphragm and make the surgery difficult. At times the positive pressure is extremely high and causes extrusion of lens, lose

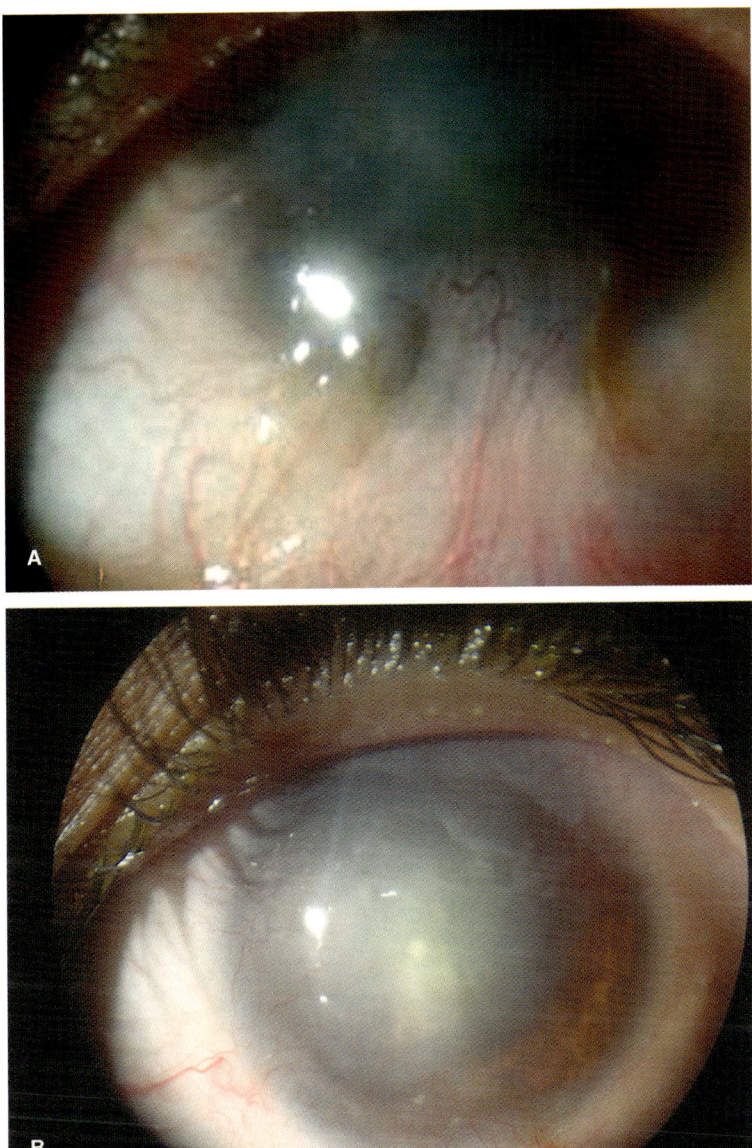

Figs 5A and B: Chemical eye injury: (A) Before amniotic membrane transplant, (B) After amniotic membrane transplant

of vitreous. Associated ocular abnormalities, i.e. cataract, glaucoma and microphthalmia make the surgical procedure complicated and increase the operating time significantly. In the immediate post operative period severe inflammatory response is encountered. In case surgery is delayed, immaturity of the visual system leads to amblyopia.

Preparation before Corneal Transplant Surgery

The aim of the corneal surgeons is to attain clear visual axis and prevent amblyopia by performing corneal transplant at an early age. Corneal transplants have been recommended as soon as the child is fit for general anesthesia. Corneal opacification should not be considered in isolations. There is always a possibility of associated eyelid and adnexal abnormalities. These abnormalities should be first corrected so that the graft surface following surgery is well protected and the integrity is not affected. Intraocular pressure, in case it is high is controlled and brought to normal range either with medical treatment or surgical (glaucoma filtering surgery) intervention. Associated posterior segment anomalies, including retinal detachment or vitreous hemorrhage should be evaluated and treated. Child should be examined by a pediatrician before surgery and cleared for surgery under general anesthesia. Most of the children with congenital corneal opacities may be having associated cardiac abnormalities.

Donor Tissue

Exact age matching between the donor and the recipient may not be possible, however excellent grades of tissue from younger donor should be used. Donor's age between 4 to 30 years is best suited for children. Donor corneas from young than 4 years are relatively difficult to handle during surgery and subsequently. Donor cornea from infants and very young children have steeper cornea and may result increase corneal curvature of the graft. In routine, oversized graft (0.5 mm) is used. Unusually high myopia (6.0 D) has been reported from steeper donor cornea from young donors. This makes amblyopia treatment difficult. The donor cornea for corneal transplants in children has endothelia cell count close to 3000. In published data donor age, donor cell count and death storage time did not affect grafts surgery. However, decreased death to corneal transplant surgery has been associated with better graft.

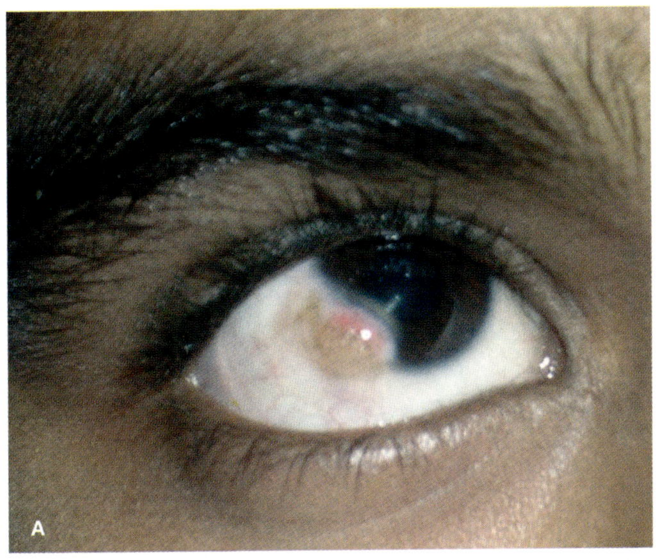

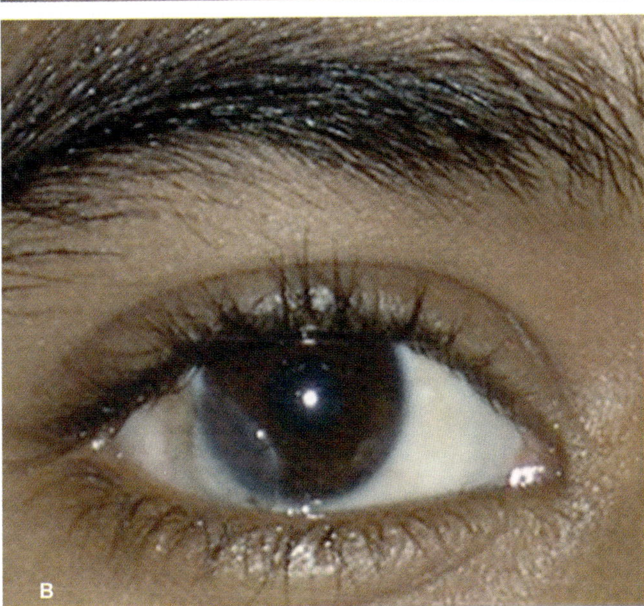

Figs 6A and B: (A) Limbal dermoid preoperative, (B) Limbal dermoid postsurgery, DALK

Surgery

Extremely high positive posterior pressure is a major intraoperative problem encountered during corneal transplant surgery infants and neonates. Although it is impossible to eliminate the positive posterior pressure, however every effort should be make to keep it minimum. In case of smaller palpebral aperture lateral canthotomy reduce posterior pressure. Use of preoperative mitotic drops or intra cameral miotic may be useful to keep iris lens diaphragm behind. An experienced anesthetist may be asked to keep the neonate at deeper plan of anesthesia. A sudden increase in intraocular pressure have posterior pressure and may even suddenly loss the lens. A non depolarizing muscle relaxant eliminates the risk of movements and contraction of extraocular muscle. Keeping head at a higher level than feet may be helpful. Anesthetist may be asked to hyperventilate child in case posterior pressure is extreme. Hyperventilation decreases posterior pressure and vitreous pressure.

Digital pressure or application of Honan's balloon is another good option to keep posterior pressure down. External pressure on the globe due to speculum should be avoided. Flieringa's ring should be applied in every case. Pre placed mattress suture is helpful in securing the graft immediately and pushing the iris lens diaphragm behind by injecting viscoelastic substance. One may use one mattress suture or two mattress sutures depending upon the requirement. These sutures if needed can also be applied after trephination of host cornea. Use of 8 '0' silk or monofilament to place cardinal sutures in case of extreme positive pressure is a good option. It secures the graft and one can inject viscoelastic substance to push iris lens diaphragm back. A cohesive viscoelastic suture, i.e. healon GV or healon 5 may be used to keep positive posterior pressure down and allows suturing.

Surgical procedure should be completed in a shortest possible time. After punching the donor tissue all the instruments required for recipient trephination and donor button suturing should be kept ready. Neonates or infants may be given intravenous mannitol 20% (0.5 to 1.5 gm / KBW) to reduce the vitreous volume and thus decreasing the positive posterior pressure. At times the positive posterior pressure is extremely high and it may not be possible to suture the graft unless we reduce it. Some of the surgeons have advocated placement of flat instrument (lens spatula) over the iris to prevent lens extrusion and vitreous loss. We routinely leave the recipient corneal button attached at 3 'o' clock position and do not excise it completely. We place donor button in the recipient opening and start suturing. After securing donor corneal button with 4 cardinal sutures we excise the host corneal button and continue suturing. This intact recipient bed in situation of extreme positive posterior pressure is put back on the recipient open. Few more cardinal sutures are applied and posterior pressure

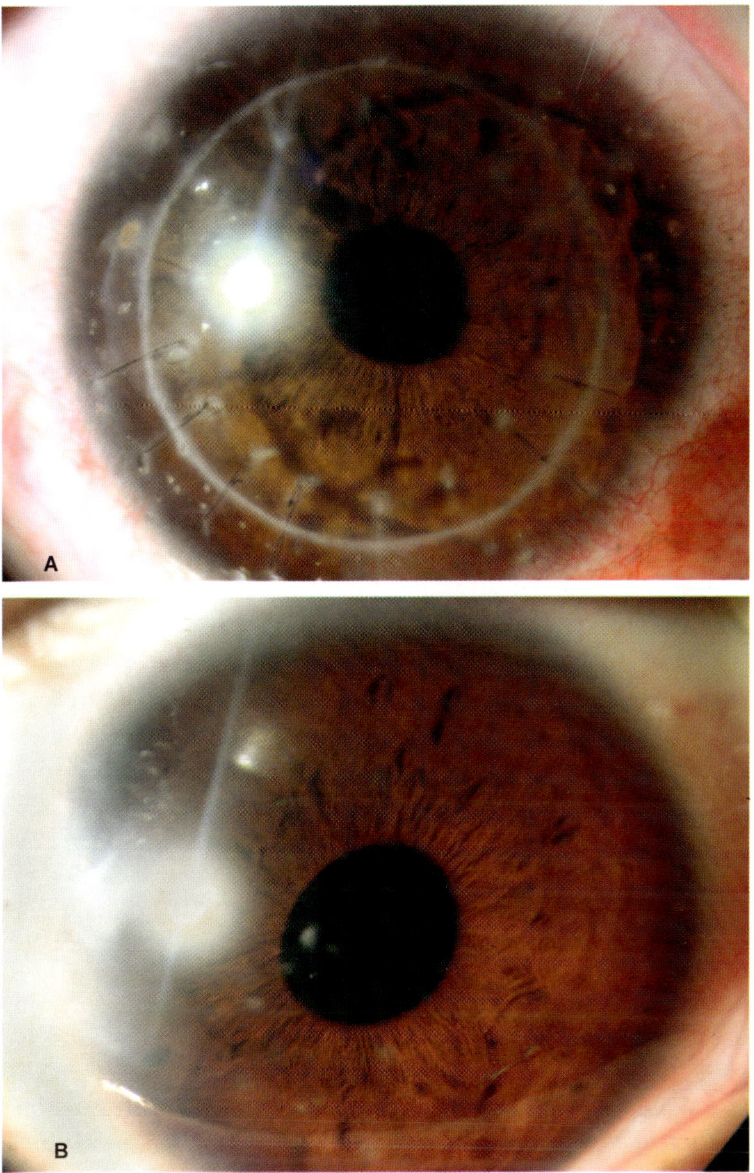

Figs 7A and B: (A) (RE) DALK for multiple stromal foreign bodies, (B) (LE) Few corneal foreign bodies

is reduced. Then the donor button is sutured. We have found this simple method extremely useful in combating high posterior pressure (Nirankari and Sharma, unpublished data). In case positive pressure is extreme and passing of 10 '0' nylon is difficult and it is not holding, it is wise to use 8 '0' nylon / silk suture and replace these sutures after the suturing in complete. Pars plana vitrectomy before trephination has been advocated to prevent posterior pressure for patients who are at higher risk for developing extreme positive posterior pressure during penetrating keratoplasty.

Size of the Graft

In a large multicentric study, this average graft size was 7.1 mm diameter. Graft size may be determined according to the diameter of the cornea. For a normal sized cornea (10.5 mm) 7.5 mm diameter graft should suffice. However in case of microophthalmia/microcornea graft size may be decreased according to the diameter of the cornea. Small grafts are required in the small diameter corneas because placing a normal sized graft (7.5 mm) in a small diameter cornea brings host graft junction very close to the limbus. This may predispose the graft to allograft rejection and its failure. Use of small diameter grafts in otherwise normal cornea may have several disadvantages. This may result in higher astigmatism. With the use of small grafts the number of viable endothelial cells decreases significantly. In case the graft size is reduced from the size 8 mm to 6 mm diameter the number of viable endothelial cells on the graft decreases by 44%. Thus smaller grafts will be predisposed to graft failure as the redistribution of endothelial cells will result a final cell count of the graft well below 1000 per mm. It is advisable to use over sized donor corneal button (0.5 mm) routinely. In a study, 1 mm over sizing for pediatric case has been advocated to decrease incidence of peripheral anterior synechia. This option should be used with extreme caution as this may cause difficulty in suturing of the donor button. In patient with anterior staphyloma the recipient cornea is under stretch due to raised IOP. On trephination the recipient opening decreases as the tissue is relaxed and IOP is low. In such a situation 1 mm oversizing further increases and may result in malposition of the host graft junction and difficulty in suturing. In addition if the donor happens to be young less than 2 years of age, the donor cornea is steeper and 1 mm oversizing will result in high myopia, and amblyopia therapy may be difficult.

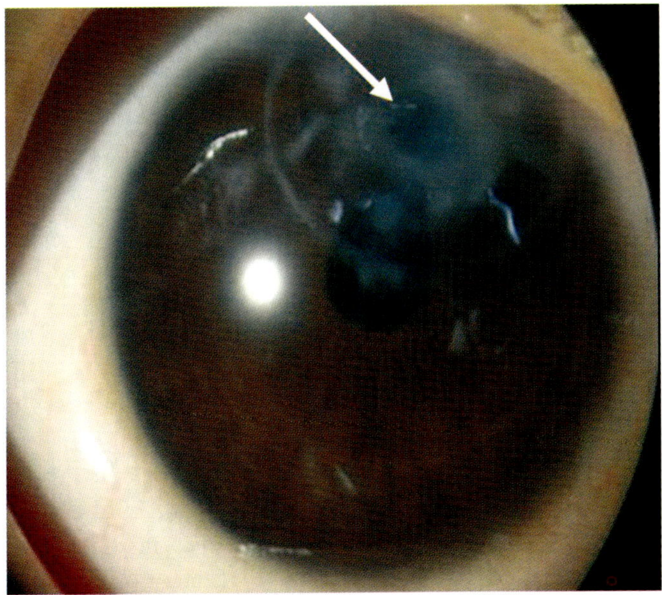

Fig. 8: DALK for chronic corneal perforation with anterior staphyloma (Arrow corneal perforation)

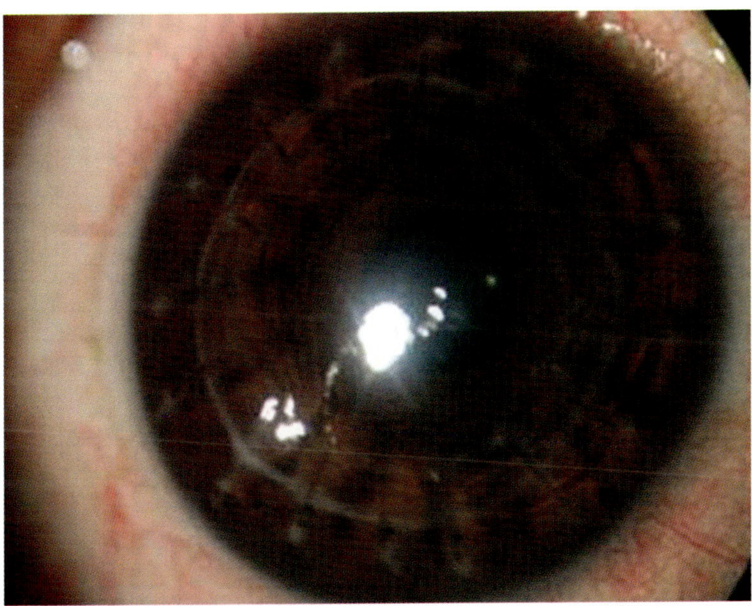

Fig. 9: Penetrating keratoplasty for keratoconus

Alternatives to Penetrating Keratoplasty

Corneal opacities partially obscuring the visual axis, gas permeable contact lens may be tried. Majority of the patients suffering from opacities resulting from traumatic corneal lacerations can be managed by fitting rigid gas permeable contact lenses. Most of the children are cooperative for fitting and monitoring the follow-up. Patients are usually apprehensive of gas permeable contact lenses. Majority of children learn quickly how to insert or take out rigid gas permeable contact lenses. They take care of contact lenses as per directions.

In case opacification is central and peripheral cornea is clearer one can evaluate the child for autorotational keratoplasty. The significant advantage is that the risk of allograft rejection is eliminated and chance of graft success is enhanced. However, postkeratoplasty astigmatism and other problem of operating up on neonates/infant remains unchased. Risk of high astigmatism is more as the disparity or defect occurs in both host cornea as well as donor cornea. In case of oval due to oblique placement of corneal trephine both host corneal bed and the donor button are oval. Placement of oval donor cornea button in an oval recipient opening with long axis at different angles result in high astigmatism.

In case corneal opacity is central and larger part of the inferior cornea is clearer, one can consider optical iridectomy. Optical iridectomy performed on the superior half of the iris do not serve any purpose as large part of it will be covered by the eyelids. Optical iridectomy is best performed in the lower nasal quadrant however one can opt for lower temporal in case opacity is extending into the lower nasal quadrant. In our experience patients are not happy with an optical iridectomy. Most of the times it does not provide an adequate vision to prevent amblyopia. Large optical iridectomies iridoplasty and pupilloplasty difficult during penetrating keratoplasty.

Infants and children with superficial corneal disease may be evaluated for superficial keratectomy. Most of the children suffering from pannus or conjunctivilization due to partial limbal stem cell deficiency can be treated with superficial keratectomy. Once a dissection plane is reached, it is extremely easy to remove the superficial corneal tissue. Children suffering from vernal ulcer and plaque formation need epithelial debridement and plaque removal in addition to medical treatment. The objective should be to achieve smooth and transparent corneal surface. To promote epithelialization, bandage contact lens may be applied. Children suffering from chemical eye injury and having conjunctivalization due to partial limbal stem cell deficiency need superficial keratectomy with amniotic membrane transplant.

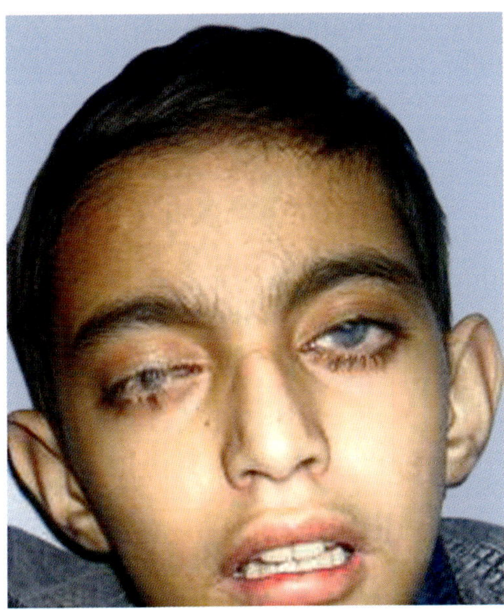

Fig. 10: Regraft in a child with bilateral Peter's anomaly (LE)

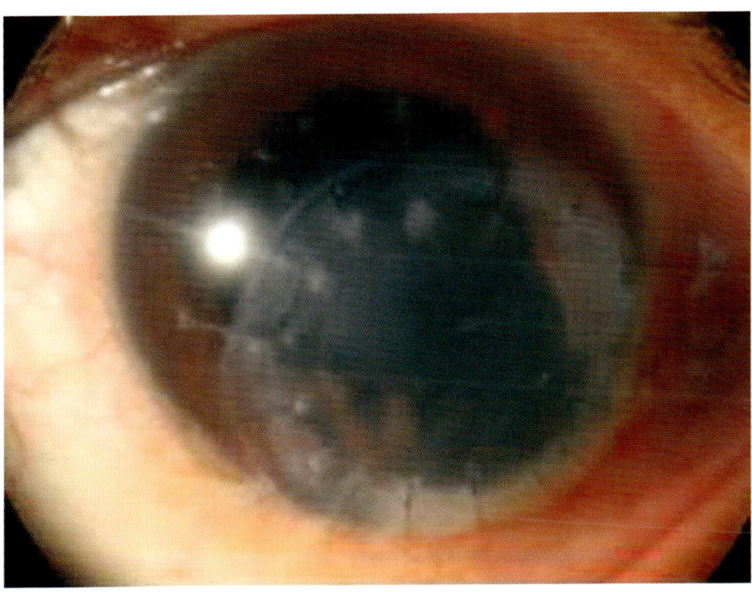

Fig. 11A: Regraft for opaque therapeutic graft: before regraft

In case of partial thickness corneal opacities or in condition where endothelium is healthy, lamellar corneal surgery, lamellar keratoplasty or deep anterior lamellar keratoplasty may be advised. In case of superficial corneal opacities due to healed bacterial or fungal corneal ulcers one should consider lamellar keratoplasty. Corneal endothelium is healthy in these cases. Depending upon the depth of involvement of cornea one may chose to perform either lamellar keratoplasty or deep anterior lamellar keratoplasty. Advantage of DALK/LK are that all the intraoperative problems (extreme positive posterior pressure, danger of extrusion of extrusion of lens and difficulties of suturing peripheral anterior synechia) may be avoided. In addition, risk of allograft rejection in DALK / LK is significantly less as compared to penetrating keratoplasty. In addition post-PK astigmatism is lower and visual rehabilitation is faster. These procedures may not be suitable for children with corneal opacities and deep corneal vascularization. Patient developing corneal opacities following recurrent herpes simplex keratitis are also a not suitable candidate either LK or DALK, as they may develop recurrence of HSK infection from residual corneal tissue. Cornea has been documented as site of viral latency and recurrence may occur from corneal tissue alone. Limbal dermoids are best treated with LK / DALK depending upon the level of involvement. We have treated a child suffering from corneal scarring due to multiple intrastromal foreign bodies in the right eye following cracker injury by performing DALK. We have also treated corneal perforation with anterior staphyloma by performing DALK.

High Risk Penetrating Keratoplasty

Presence of deep corneal vascularization in two quadrants or more predisposes the corneal grafts to higher risk of allograft rejection. Children having undergone penetrating keratoplasty for herpes simplex keratitis are at higher risk of graft rejection, recurrence of disease and failure. Children should be put on oral acyclovir prophylaxis. Children undergone regraft are at higher risk of allograft rejection due to prior sensitization. Patients having corneal opacities in association with limbal stem cell deficiency and ocular surface disease are also at higher risk of developing graft failure due to allograft rejection. Children suffering from corneal opacification and associated ocular surface disease should undergo limbal stem cell transplant and amniotic membrane transplant prior to penetrating keratoplasty. Patients with severe ocular surface disease due to chemical eye injury, Steven's Johnson syndrome may undergo deep lamellar keratoplasty. Deep lamellar keratoplasty has lower risk of allograft rejection.

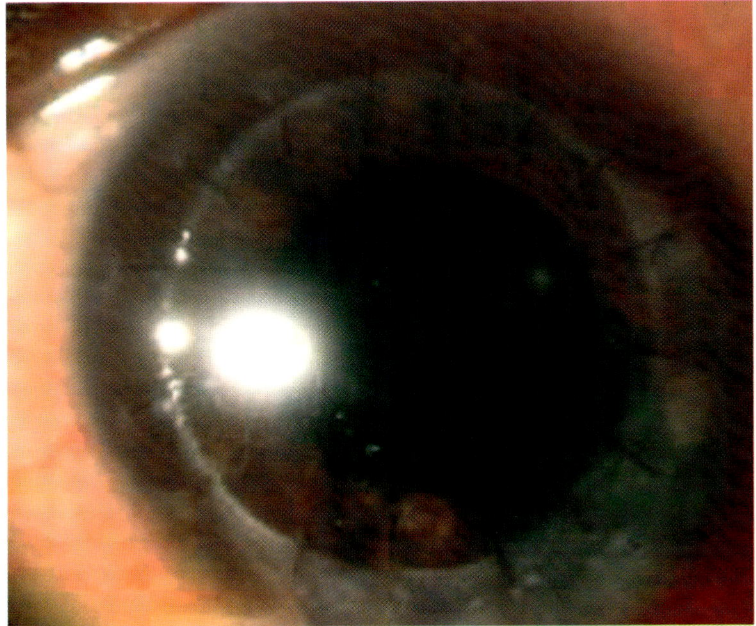

Fig. 11B: Regraft for opaque therapeutic graft: after regraft

Perioperative Care

Success of corneal transplant surgery is determined by meticulous perioperative care. Thorough examination of child including slitlamp biomicroscopy should be performed. During the follow-up visits parents should be explained danger signs and should be asked to report immediately as soon as the danger signs appear. The younger children and infants do not communicate their symptoms. However in case the child is irritable or crying without any obvious reason, he should be brought for eye checkup. The first examination is usually at 24 hours intervals. Status of the graft clarity, wound integrity, epithelial healing, intraocular inflammation and intraocular pressure every visit. Infants or children should be examined daily for one week and an alternate day for two weeks. After that every week examination is carried out. In case child develops any problem child may be examined early to the start treatment.

Complications

Early

Delayed epithelization, disruption of host graft junction, fibrinous reaction, high intraocular pressure are the common problems encountered in the first few days. Infective keratitis although rare (5%) may occur and need intensive topical antibacterial treatment. Fibrinous exudative reaction should be treated with topical and systemic steroids. Delay in epithelization may be secondary to severe uveitis or high intraocular pressure. In these cases severe uveitis is treated with topical or systemic steroids. Once uveitis or high intraocular pressure is controlled epithelial defect heals completely. Rarely endophthalmitis following penetrating keratoplasty in children may occur.

Intermediate

Neonates and infants need to be examined under general anesthesia at around 3 weeks even if they have no visible problem. Wound healing in neonates and infants is past and sutures become lose. At 3 to 4 weeks lose suture should be removed. At 6-8 week complete healing occurs and sutures may be removed at 6-8 week period. In older children 2 to 4 years may be observed for lose suture and may be removed little later. Children above 6 years behave more or less similar to adults and selection suture removal may be performed.

Late

Allograft rejection, suture related infections, recurrence of disease (HSK, keratoconus) post keratoplasty astigmatism and postkeratoplasty glaucoma may occur. Suture related complications can be prevented by immediate removal of lose sutures. Lose suture may cause an epithelial defect, secondary inflammation and trigger allograft rejection due to inflammation and graft vascularization. Postkeratoplasty astigmatism is higher with PKP as compare to lamellar procedure (LK/DALK). Selective suture removal can be done to reduce astigmatism in children aged 6 years or more.

Allograft Rejection

Parents should be explained that allograft rejection might occur any time after surgery. Studies have shown that 30 to 70% pediatric grafts fail within first six months and 65 to 85% within first year. Neonates and infants should be closely maintained for development of allograft rejection in the first year of life. Children are unable to complain about the symptoms and usually present late for treatment. Parents should be educated to bring the child for examination on observing any redness, discomfort, and opaqueness in the graft or decrease in vision. On every visit child should be examined at slit lamp to detect early signs of allograft rejection. Infant and children may not present with characteristic signs of allograft rejection. Graft edema even in the absence of keratic precipitates should also be treated as allograft rejection. Intraocular pressure should be monitored in these cases, they may have associated secondary glaucoma. Once allograft rejection is diagnosed, the child is put on prednisolone acetate (0.1%) eye drop every one hour and atropine ointment twice daily. In addition oral prednisolone (1 mg/kbw) should also be started. In recent studies topical cyclosporine A (2%) has been found successful in treating graft reaction. Topical cyclosporine A has also been used to prevent graft rejection in high risk cases. Cyclosporine A being lipid soluble, topical cyclosporine A (2%) need to be prepared in castor oil in the hospital pharmacy. At times young children may not tolerate it, as it causes significant ocular irritation. It has also been reported to cause persistent epithelial defects and delayed epithelial healing. Recent studies have shown that topical cyclosporine A prepared in the aqueous solution is also effective and can be prepared in preservative free artificial tear solution. Topical cyclosporine A has been reported to be equally effective in concentrations ranging from 0.05% to 1%. Topical cyclosporine A 0.05% (Restasis, Allergan) has been found effective in treatment and prevention of graft rejection in high risk cases. The formulation of the drug is such that it releases large number of microdroplets in the tear film..

Glaucoma

Treatment of glaucoma prior to penetrating keratoplasty or after it includes medical treatment, trabeculectomy with adjuvants and/or trabeculotomy. Treatment of refractory glaucoma is a real challenge as it will not only damage the optic nerve but also corneal graft resulting graft failure. Glaucoma drainage implant procedures have shown encouraging results in the treatment of refractory postpenetrating keratoplasty glaucoma. Several authors have reported favorable results of pediatric penetrating keratoplasty following control of IOP using glaucoma drainage implant procedures. Although conventionally glaucoma is first controlled and then only penetrating keratoplasty is performed. At times due to the risk of development irreversible amblyopia glaucoma implant surgery may be combined with penetrating keratoplasty to provide early visual rehabilitation and preventing the development of amblyopia.

Treatment of Amblyopia

Amblyopia treatment should be started as early as possible following surgery. Cycloplegic refraction should be done and glasses should be prescribed. Parents should be explained that the normal eye of the child need to be patched so that he uses the operated eye. The schedule for patching may be the same as used for standard amblyopia treatment. In children upto 2 years (2 : 1), 2 to 3 years (3 : 1), 3 to 4 years (4 : 1), 4 to 5 years (5 : 1) and 6 years or above (6 : 1) should be used.

Outcome

Anatomical success rate following penetrating keratoplasty in childhood including infants and neonates has increased significantly. The incidence of vision restoration in children following penetrating keratoplasty is still low. Visual prognosis has been reported better in younger children and is likely determined by the incidence and severity of amblyopia. In recent study of 65 grafts on 58 eyes of 52 children (mean age 10.6 years SD 4.3 years) 38% achieved BCVA 6/9 or better and 60% had BCVA 6/18 or better. Visual acuity has been reported significantly better for the acquired as compared to congenital indications. Significant numbers of patients in this study had keratoconus as an indication for penetrating keratoplasty. Results from developing countries are less favorable. In a study from India nearly 1/3rd patients achieved > or = 20/400 vision and nearly 50% of these achieved > or = 20/50. Allograft rejection, infective keratitis and glaucoma were major causes of graft failure. The overall long term (10 years) probability of maintaining clear graft after initial penetrating keratoplasty for Peter's anomaly is 35% +/– 0.6%. Eyes with severe disease, larger donor cornea, co-existing central nervous system abnormalities and anterior synechia were reported to have significantly poorer outcome than eyes without these factors. Children with severe form of Peter's anomaly may required multiple grafts to have functional vision. One of our patient with severe Peter's anomaly had undergone four corneal transplants during 14 years and enjoyed good vision. He finally died recently due to severe CNS disease.

Repeat Corneal Graft

In case the child develops graft failure a repeat graft should be considered. Parents need to be explained that subsequent corneal grafts have less chances of success. In one of the studies, of 27 repeat grafts undergoing second graft 19% were successful and of six graft undergoing third graft none succeeded. Repeat graft may be indicated to prevent dense and irreversible amblyopia. However in case child is having unilateral corneal capacity, parents should be explained that even if the graft may becomes opaque, later on chances of improvement of vision by performing repeat graft will be there. In adults if the grafts is fail due to the graft rejection, it is advisable to wait for 6 months before a repeat graft is performed. It is aimed to bring down the inflammation in the graft to minimum and to decrease the incidence of allograft rejection. At times it may be difficult to ascertain whether the graft failed due to allograft rejection or due to some other cause. It is better to treat it as allograft rejection. In younger children it may not be possible to wait for 6 months due to danger of development of amblyopia. In these cases the repeat graft may be performed at 3 months after the initial graft has failed. One can wait a little longer in case the child is six years old or more. Children suffering from perforated corneal ulcers need therapeutic penetrating keratoplasty and these grafts usually become opaque due to chronic inflammation. However, successful regraft can be performed for these patients at later date and both vision improvement and graft clarity can be obtained.

Keratoprosthesis

Infants and children who are at high risk of graft rejection and subsequent graft failure may be benefited with keratoprosthesis or artificial corneal transplantation. Keratoprosthesis transplantation means placing an optical device in the host cornea. It is immunologically inert and has the advantage that graft rejection does not occur. Recently, a custom made Boston type 1 keratoprosthesis is available and can be designed to correct refractive errors including aphakia. AlphaCor, a synthetic cornea made up of hydrophilic polymer poly (2-hydroxyethyl methacrylate) is another keratoprosthesis used in high risk cases for corneal transplant surgery. The AlphaCor is implanted in a corneal stromal lamellar pocket in a two stage procedure. In the first stage 360° peritomy and debridement of corneal epithelium is done. A superior 180° limbal incision at 50% of depth is extended into the corneal stroma forming an intralamellar pocket is made. A central 3.5 mm posterior corneal trephination is performed. The device is placed with in the corneal pocket and paralimbal incision is closed. After 8 to 12 weeks anterior trephination (3 mm) is done to expose the optic of the device. Keratoprosthesis helps the corneal surgeon to rehabilitate those corneal blinds having visual potential, but are unlikely to be benefited by performing penetrating keratoplasty using human donor cornea.

Pediatric corneal transplant surgery is a team effort it involves combined effort of corneal surgeon assisted by glaucoma specialist pediatrician, anesthetis, counselors and rehabilitation team.

Rehabilitation of Blinds due to Corneal Disease

Children with bilateral corneal opacities either congenital, chemical burns, Stevens Johnson syndrome may not be successfully visually rehabilitated even after performing repeated corneal grafts. The parents of these children should be counseled to get their children admitted to blind schools to provide educational and vocational training to these children. These children can lead independent life and contribute to the development of the society if proper facilities and opportunities are provided.

Summary and Conclusions

Advancement in microsurgical techniques, quality eye banking and better anesthesia facilities have made possible to undertake corneal transplant in a neonate as soon as the diagnosis is made and corneal transplant surgery is advised. Although surgery is technically demanding but it is possible to provide clear visual axis during critical period of visual development. Treatment and prevention of development of amblyopia in neonates is extremely important even after successful penetrating keratoplasty.

Index

A

B

C